Edited by Patrick Callaghan, John Playle, Linda Cooper

Mental Health Nursing Skills

OXFORD
UNIVERSITY PRESS

Great Clarendon Street, Oxford OX2 6DP

Oxford University Press is a department of the University of Oxford.
It furthers the University's objective of excellence in research, scholarship,
and education by publishing worldwide in

Oxford New York

Auckland Cape Town Dar es Salaam Hong Kong Karachi
Kuala Lumpur Madrid Melbourne Mexico City Nairobi
New Delhi Shanghai Taipei Toronto

With offices in

Argentina Austria Brazil Chile Czech Republic France Greece
Guatemala Hungary Italy Japan Poland Portugal Singapore
South Korea Switzerland Thailand Turkey Ukraine Vietnam

Oxford is a registered trade mark of Oxford University Press
in the UK and in certain other countries

Published in the United States
by Oxford University Press Inc., New York

© Oxford University Press 2009

British Library Cataloguing in Publication Data
Data available

Library of Congress Cataloging in Publication Data
Data available

Typeset by SPI Publisher Services
Printed in Great Britain
on acid-free paper by
L.E.G.O. S.p.A. –Lavis TN

ISBN 978-0-19-953444-9

1 3 5 7 9 10 8 6 4 2

Foreword

I am delighted that *Mental Health Nursing Skills* provides pre-registration students of mental health nursing and nurses with such an excellent resource to complement and enhance their educational experience. The book sets out how students can acquire, develop, and demonstrate the best practice competencies and capabilities identified as part of *From Values to Action: the CNO Review of Mental Health Nursing in England*. It provides a strong foundation for their future career, ensuring that mental health nurses are well equipped to deliver high quality health care to people with mental health problems.

The way in which we are prepared for practice underpins our ability to deliver quality. We know there are inconsistencies in care, for example in the experience of service users across acute inpatient units, and getting the quality of care consistently high for all service users of the NHS is important for us all. Mental health nurses in particular, deliver a great deal of the care that the NHS provides to people with mental health problems and therefore have a great influence over the quality of healthcare.

Marking the 60th year of the NHS, '*High Quality Care for All*', the final report of Lord Darzi's NHS Next Stage Review set out how the NHS can become fairer, more personalised, effective and safe for its patients and users. Much progress has been made on this already but there is still much to be achieved. The Review places nursing right at the forefront in driving up standards of care and improving the patient experience. Mental health nurses working at the frontline across the NHS are ideally placed to drive improvements in quality. It is true to say that service user and carer experience is often determined by the quality of nursing, and good nursing care plays a key role in health, in healing, and in recovery from illness, so we have to get it right.

What patients want most of all is to be kept safe, cared for, respected, and involved. These are the constants of nursing for today and for the future. In focusing specifically on the attitudes, values and behaviours, competencies and capabilities needed at the point of registration, this volume helps to reaffirm these essential attributes and characteristics, ensuring today's mental health nursing students are well prepared to provide high quality care now and well into the future.

I have no doubt that this volume will go a long way to making a positive impact on the implementation recommendations of *Form Values to Action: the CNO Review of Mental health nursing*.

Chief Nursing Officer Dame Christine Beasley

How to use this book

Mental Health Nursing Skills explores and demonstrates the skills required of mental health nurses through the use of specific features and learning tools. This brief tour shows you how to get the most out of this textbook package.

Clearly mapped against professional benchmarks

Table 1.1 in Chapter 1 maps the best practice competencies and capabilities of mental health nurses against each chapter in the book. Learning outcomes at the start of each chapter highlight the specific knowledge and skills set that readers will acquire by reading on.

Learning outcomes

By the end of this chapter you should be better able to:

1 Consider the concept of caring in terms of the language of caring and its ethical underpinnings

2 Demonstrate an awareness of the relevance of caring to contemporary mental health nursing practice when working with people towards their recovery from mental health problems

3 Display the interpersonal and intrapersonal skills required to adopt a caring approach to practice

4 Transfer these skills into your mental health nursing

Theory and practice balanced

Clear sections on theory, step-by-step guidance, and practice are provided in each chapter so readers can see what to do and why. The policy and evidence base for each skill is explored to promote rigorous practice before the authors outline a step-by-step description of that skill and then demonstrate how to apply it in practice.

The evidence base

The person-centred approach

The central premise of the person-centred approach is that the therapeutic relationship is sufficient in itself for change to take place. Rogers (1957) proposed that the use of warmth, **empathy**, **unconditional positive regard** and **genuineness**, in the immediate therapeutic encounter, are necessary and sufficient conditions for therapeutic gain. He argued that, for constructive psychological change to occur, certain core conditions should be in existence: the client's state of incongruence and the helper's congruence and experience of unconditional positive regard for the client. The helper should demonstrate

Health and Clinical Excellence 2004). However, the recency of these new evidence reviews (Cuijpers et al. 2007, Ekers et al. 2007) means that BA is certainly being included as a treatment option in revisions of these guidelines, and is likely to be recommended in future editions. Our new understanding of the evidence base strongly suggests that BA should be offered to patients as a routine choice in care.

Step-by-step description

The following protocol for BA is drawn from a clinical trial of depression management in the UK (Richards et al. 2008). It was developed from the clinical methods described by Martell et al. (2001) and Hopko et al. (2003a).

Skills are applied to practice

'Practice Examples and Tips' boxes clearly demonstrate how to develop and use the skills in nursing practice through the use of realistic scenarios, suggested activities, and sample material. Dark blue in colour, these are easy to find for a quick reminder.

✖ Practice Example and Tips

Case

A young man, John, has been admitted to the ward where you work. He has never been in hospital before or had contact with mental health services. Recently he has had troubling experiences of voices, which prompted him to harm himself in the hope that this would help stop them. John is fearful and suspicious of help, and you, as his primary nurse, must reassure him and begin to engage him. Based on this chapter what would you do? Once you have finished this chapter, you can go online at

- Engage meaningfully in order to facilitate later and ongoing work.
- Spend time getting to know the person as a whole person and not simply as a service user.
- Offer opportunities to talk and listen.
- Do not automatically expect trust—nurses must work to achieve it.

Sustaining therapeutic relationships

1 Carry out a focused assessment to identify the service user's priorities for recovery.

2 If applicable, facilitate opportunities for the service

Online support

Where you see the icon and web address in the text, the authors have devised a specific online resource to help readers practise and develop their skills.

---

ent-centred approach is often useful in engendering hope and realistic optimism.

A fictitious case example is included in the web-based material accompanying this book www.oxfordtextbooks.co.uk/orc/callaghan. We would encourage you to examine the findings of assessment and answer the short answer questions based on what has been learnt from this chapter.

Assignments and developing your knowledge further

Each chapter finishes with directions to our online resource centre where scenarios, quizzes, and other activities can help you develop your skills further. Directions to useful websites and further reading are given in addition to the references employed by the authors.

Website

You may find it helpful to work through our short online quiz and scenario intended to help you to develop and apply the skills in this chapter

www.oxfordtextbooks.co.uk/orc/callaghan

Further reading

Khan, K., ter Riet, G., Galanville, J., Sowden, A., and Kleijnen, J. (2002). **Undertaking Systematic Reviews of Research on Effectiveness CRD's Guidance for Those Carrying Out or Commissioning Reviews. Report 4,**

Mowrer, O. H. (1950). *Learning Theory and Personality Dynamics.* New York: Arnold.

Skinner, B. F. (1953). *Science and Human Behaviour.* New York: Macmillan.

✚ References

American Psychiatric Association (1994). *Diagnostic and Statistical Manual of Mental Disorders,* 4th edn (DSM-IV). Washington, DC: APA.

Beck, A. T., Rush, A. J., Shaw, B. J., and Emery, G.

Ekers, D., Richards, D., and Gilbody, S. (2007). **A meta-analysis of randomized trials of behavioural treatment of depression.** *Psychological Medicine* 35(5), 611–23.

Hopko, D. R., Lejuez, C. W., Ruggiero, K. J., and Eifert,

Glossary terms

Technical terms particular to mental health nursing are highlighted in colour in the text and explained in the glossary at the start of the text.

---

brief contact between mental health workers and patients, as well as being used as a more traditional **high-intensity psychological treatment**, in which therapists and patients work together for longer and more numerous sessions. It has shown to be as equally effective as both **cognitive therapy** and **antidepressants** (Dimidjian et al. 2006). Competence in applying BA will equip any nurse with a highly effective and acceptable psychological technique to assist people with depression.

This chapter outlines the theory, history, and evidence base for BA and describes a seven-step BA protocol (Richards et al. 2008) illustrated by practice examples. Details of how BA can be used in **relapse prevention strategies** is also described, followed by key references and further reading.

How to use the online resource centre

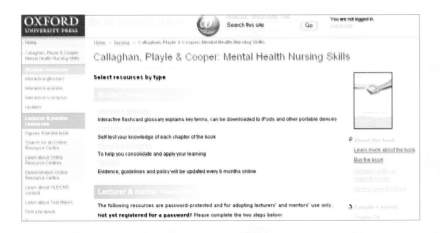

This textbook is accompanied by a free online resource centre (website) that provides students and lecturers with interactive resources to develop and practise mental health nursing skills. You can access the online resource centre from any computer with internet access. You will find it helpful to save the web address in to your 'favourites' at the earliest opportunity:

www.oxfordtextbooks.co.uk/orc/callaghan

Scenarios

Interactive scenarios give students the chance to try out their skills in a safe environment prior to placements. A short description of a service user or a challenge in practice is outline before a set of questions prompt the student to consider how they would employ their mental health nursing skills. There is an opportunity to note these down and compare them to the author's suggested answer.

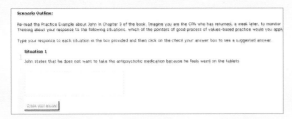

Quizzes

To register as a nurse, students need to demonstrate their knowledge and understanding of nursing practice. To help you, the authors have written short online quizzes for each chapter to reinforce your learning. Feedback is provided for each question and page references signpost where to find the topic in the book for further investigation.

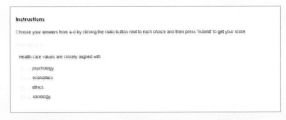

Updates

Major developments in evidence, policy, and guidelines in the field of mental health skills will be posted to the online resource centre on a regular basis. Sign up to be alerted to the updates by clicking on the link 'Keep me updated about this site' (on the main home page of the online resource centre www.oxford-textbooks.co.uk/orc/callaghan) and send us an email as instructed there.

Interactive glossary

Technical terms from the book are presented in an interactive 'flashcard' format to help students learn and revise terms and concepts.

Preface

This book emerged following the publication of the Reviews of Mental Health Nursing in England and Scotland in 2006, and discussions with colleagues about mental health nursing in Wales and Northern Ireland. The purpose of writing the book was to unpack for mental health nursing students how they might **demonstrate**, in their day-to-day practice, the capabilities and competencies they are expected to have acquired at the point of registration.

There are many mental health nursing textbooks out there for students, but *Mental Health Nursing Skills* differs from the others in several respects. The book was written specifically for mental health nursing students, has an evidence-based focus, maps the content to national benchmarks of essential skills and capabilities, shows how mental health nursing students can demonstrate the best practice competencies and capabilities required to practise effectively, and has an interactive companion website that students can use alongside the text. We have attempted in this book to discuss skills that mental health nurses will need, irrespective of where they practise. In our experience of working in mental health, it strikes us that the core skills required of mental health nurses are similar; with this in mind we have written a text that we believe will be of use to all students of mental health nursing. We also recognize, however, that mental health nursing students are being educated in different health and social care contexts and in different parts of the world. Although this text should stand alone as essential to all mental health nursing students, in some countries it will be read alongside complementary country specific texts.

Mental Health Nursing Skills is written by expert and experienced mental health nurses and others working in the mental health field. We selected each contributor on the basis of their expertise in the topic, in addition to their skills in applying the knowledge in practice. Each contributor is involved regularly in the education of student nurses and other mental health students, and they are experienced teachers. Each contributor's regular contact with students has informed the content of their chapter. Many of the contributors have regular contact with mental health service users and carers, as well as other mental health stakeholders; some have used services themselves. These contacts have also influenced the content and style evident in each chapter.

Alexander Graham Bell, the inventor of the telephone, once remarked that it takes the cooperation of many minds to realize good things. We think that this book is a good thing and we wish to acknowledge our gratitude to the people who helped us to realize it: our fellow contributors for meeting the ever-imposing deadlines with good grace; the reviewers of each chapter for their critical and helpful comments; colleagues and students at the Universities of Nottingham, Manchester, and Cardiff, for their sharp insights; Oxford University Press for stamping its distinguished imprimatur on our thoughts; our editor at OUP, Geraldine Jeffers, for her kind support and timely reminders. We wish to acknowledge the contribution of Mental Health Nurse Academics UK (MHNAC/UK) from where the original idea for the book originated. Many of the contributors are members of MHNAC/UK; Patrick Callaghan was previously Chair of the group; John Playle and Linda Cooper are the current Chair and Vice Chair respectively. Lastly we acknowledge the unstinting support and love of our family, friends, and loved ones, who tolerated with patience the occasional distractions that editing this book entailed.

Patrick Callaghan
John Playle
Linda Cooper

Contents

Part 1 – Putting values into practice

Part 2 – Improving outcomes for service users

Part 3 – A positive, modern profession

Detailed contents

Part 3 – A positive, modern profession

Contributors

Martin Anderson is Associate Professor in Mental Health and Deputy Director of Research within the School of Nursing, University of Nottingham, UK. He is a Senior Fellow of the Institute of Mental Health. Over the past four years he has been directly involved in the implementation of the UK national suicide prevention strategy at a regional and national level. An experienced researcher in the field of mental health and suicidal behaviour, he has 12 years of experience in the education of mental health professionals.

Penny Bee is a Research Fellow at the University of Manchester, UK and has been involved in a wide range of research studies. She has published a number of papers from her research and is currently leading a research trial into telephone treatment for mental health problems.

Geoff Brennan is Nurse Consultant in Psychosocial Interventions (PSI) for Berkshire Healthcare NHS Foundation Trust. Geoff has practised and supervised PSI for more than 20 years and is closely involved with acute inpatient care, including recent involvement in the City Nurse Project in East London.

Dan Bressington is a Senior Lecturer in Mental Health Nursing at Canterbury Christ Church University, UK. Prior to this current academic role Dan worked as a Research Nurse and Tutor at the Institute of Psychiatry, London. Dan's teaching interests relate to medication management and psychosocial interventions for adults with serious mental illness. He has completed the THORN course and his clinical experience includes working as a psychosocial therapist in the community and as Senior Clinical Charge Nurse on inpatient units. He has published work around medication management and psychopharmacology.

Neil Brimblecombe is a mental health nurse who chaired the Chief Nursing Officer's Review of Mental Health Nursing (2006). He is currently Director of Nursing for two mental health foundation Trusts: South Staffordshire and Shropshire Healthcare and the Tavistock and Portman.

Patrick Callaghan is a mental health nurse and Chartered Health Psychologist. He is Professor of Mental Health Nursing at the University of Nottingham, UK, and Nottinghamshire NHS Healthcare Trust where he heads a research programme designed to enable people to recover from mental distress, leading on service evaluation, testing the effect of psychosocial interventions on health and well-being, and investigating links between mental health nursing and service user outcomes.

Michael Coffey is a Lecturer in Community Mental Health Nursing, Department of Public Health and Primary Care, School of Health Science, Swansea University, Wales. His current research is exploring re-integration and identity work in the talk of conditionally discharged people.

Linda Cooper is a Senior Lecturer and Professional Head of Mental Health, Learning Disabilities and Psychosocial Care at the School of Nursing and Midwifery Studies, Cardiff University, Wales. She is a strong advocate for the development of psychological mental health nursing skills and is published in the area of clinical supervision research. She is a member of the All Wales Senior Nurse Advisory Group for Mental Health and is Vice Chair of the national group: Mental Health Nurse Academics (UK).

Paul Crawford is Associate Professor of Health, Language and Communication at the School of Nursing, University of Nottingham, UK, where he directs interdisciplinary research on mental health language and literature. He is also a novelist and literary critic.

Sarah Eales is a Lecturer in Mental Health in the Department of Mental Health and Learning Disability at City University, London, UK. She has a clinical and research interest in mental health care in non-mental health settings and Liaison Mental Health Care.

Clare Fox is a research assistant at the University of Lincoln, UK. Her interests lie in child and adolescent mental health and in criminal justice and mental health.

Judith Gellatly is a Research Fellow at the University of Manchester, UK. Her research interests include developing accessible and effective psychological interventions for common mental health problems. Her current research is examining decision-making in mental health, focusing on the health professional's perspective as well as that of the service user.

Richard Griffith is a Lecturer in Health Law at Swansea University, Wales. Richard has a particular research interest in mental health and mental capacity law, and has written extensively on these subjects. He is currently examining the implications of the deprivation of liberty safeguards for nursing and social work practice.

Dr Ben Hannigan is a Senior Lecturer in the Mental Health and Learning Disabilities Team, School of Nursing and Midwifery

Studies, Cardiff University, Wales. He has published widely in the fields of mental health policy and practice.

Jeanette Hewitt is a Lecturer in the Centre for Philosophy, Humanities and Law in Health Care, School of Health Science, Swansea University, Wales. Her current research is exploring moral perspectives on suicide.

Julia Jones is Senior Research Fellow in the Department of Mental Health and Learning Disability at City University, London, UK. She has conducted a number of research studies in acute inpatient psychiatric settings, including a study of service users' experiences of being observed closely by nurses.

Karina Lovell is Professor of Mental Health at the University of Manchester, UK. Most of her research is centred on developing and testing accessible treatments for people with anxiety and depression. Karina is past president of the British Association for Behavioural and Cognitive Psychotherapies and patron of Anxiety UK.

Jean Morrissey is a mental health nurse and an accredited counsellor. She is a Lecturer in Mental Health Nursing, School of Nursing and Midwifery, University of Dublin – Trinity College. Her current research is exploring mental health nurses' responses to clients with suicidal behaviour.

Sara Owen is Professor of Nursing and Dean of the Faculty of Health, Life and Social Science at the University of Lincoln, UK Her research interests include women and mental health, and mental health workforce development and education.

Rachel Perkins is Director of Quality Assurance and User/Carer Experience at South West London and St George's Mental Health NHS Trust, UK. She has co-authored a number of books including: Repper, J. and Perkins, R. (2003). *Social Inclusion and Recovery: A Model for Mental Health Practice.* London: Baillière Tindall.

Peter Phillips is a Senior Lecturer in Mental Health in the Department of Mental Health and Disability, City University, London, UK. He specializes in substance misuse and has written widely on this issue in national and international publications.

John Playle is Professor of Mental Health Nursing at the University of Manchester, UK. He has published and presented widely on various aspects of mental health nursing and mental workforce issues, arguing strongly for a greater voice for service users in the design and delivery of mental health education services and care.

Julie Repper is Associate Professor and Reader in Mental Health Nursing and Social Care at the University of Nottingham, UK. She has co-authored a number of books including: Repper, J. and Perkins, R. (2003). *Social Inclusion and Recovery: A Model for Mental Health Practice.* London: Baillière Tindall.

Dave Richards is Professor of Mental Health at the University of Exeter, UK. He campaigns to improve access to mental health care and leads a multicentre research programme that investigates new methods of care delivery. He is the author of more than 100 peer-reviewed scientific publications, books, and book chapters.

David Riley is a Registered Mental Nurse who works as a Personal Safety Co-ordinator for Mersey Care NHS Trust, UK. He has delivered training in the prevention and management of challenging behaviour for the past 11 years and has collaborated on a number of research projects with the School of Health Sciences at Liverpool University.

Greg Rooney is Principal Lecturer and Professional Lead for Mental Health Nursing at the University of Hertfordshire, UK. He has a background in cognitive behavioural psychotherapy and psychosis, and his research interests include the professional education of mental health nurses.

Alan Simpson is a Postdoctoral Research Fellow and Lecturer in Mental Health Nursing at City University, London, UK. Alan has conducted extensive research in acute inpatient and community mental health services and has a special interest in developing user and carer involvement in practice, research, and education.

Gemma Stacey is Lecturer in Mental Health at the University of Nottingham, UK. She has a specialist interest in developing nursing education to equip students with the values and skills needed to support people with mental health problems towards recovery. Her research focuses on the influence of professional socialization on the development of values in mental health nurses.

Theo Stickley is Associate Professor of Mental Health at the University of Nottingham, UK. Theo has practised as a mental health nurse and counsellor for many years. The focus of his research is mainly the arts and mental health.

Helen Waldock is the Director of Nursing with the Health and Social Care Advisory Service, UK. She also works part-time as a mental health liaison nurse within a primary care practice at the University of Kent. Experience has been clinical, operational, and strategically introducing and promoting high standards of patient care in mental health and general nursing at a local and national level.

Keith Waters is a Clinical Nurse Specialist and Team Leader of a Mental Health Liaison Team working for the Derbyshire Mental Health Trust, UK, providing an assessment service predominantly to the Accident and Emergency Department of the Derbyshire Royal Infirmary. Keith has worked in the area of self-harm for more than 20 years, maintaining an active clinical role as well as pursuing research interests and service developments in the area of self-harm and suicide prevention.

Richard Whittington is Reader in Health Sciences at the University of Liverpool, UK. He is a chartered psychologist with a background in mental health nursing. He was co-editor (with D. Richter) of *Violence in Mental Health Settings* (Springer 2006), lead author on *Best Practice in Managing Risk* (Department of Health 2007), and is chairman of the European Violence in Psychiatry Research Group (www.liv.ac.uk/eviprg).

Mark Wilbourn is Principal Lecturer, Department of Mental Health and Learning Disabilities, Faculty of Health and Social care, London South Bank University, UK. His teaching interests are in pathology and psychopharmacology, and he has published in this area. Mark also has research interests in non-medical prescribing, the subject of his current PhD research and the focus of his clinical consultancy work with a local NHS Trust.

Glossary

A

acceptance · not judging a person, by treating the individual with respect, not criticizing, and seeing the person not just the behaviour

activity scheduling · a forerunner of behavioural activation consisting of increasing positive activities only and often undertaken as the first stage in cognitive or cognitive behavioural therapy

advance patient directives · plans agreed between care providers and patients/service users while they are well, specifying what should be done for the person's health in the case of relapse where he or she is no longer capable or competent to make decisions due to the effects of illness

aggression · behaviour intended to injure others physically or psychologically

akathisia · restlessness of arms and legs; this can be a side effect of antipsychotic treatment

amendment · a change to legislation

anhedonia · a reduction in or the total loss of the feeling of pleasure in acts that normally give pleasure

antidepressants · pharmacological agents (drugs) that act on neurotransmitters in the body to improve mood

approved clinician · a person approved by the Secretary of State or Welsh Ministers to act as an approved clinician for the purposes of the Mental Health Act 1983

attentive listening · thinking and acting in ways that connect you with the speaker in order to communicate an interest in what someone is saying

autonomy · the right to self-determination, to decide what should happen

axilla · hollow area under the arm where it joins the body (the armpit)

B

behavioural activation · a psychological treatment that aims to increase behaviours that were previously avoided or reduced in frequency in order to produce improvements in mood

behavioural interventions · intervention strategies that focus on and aim to enable clients to change or modify behaviours

bibliotherapy · a type of therapy achieved through the use of books or other types of literature. Self-help books are the most common form of bibliotherapy

break away · removal of yourself from an aggressor in a safe manner

brief psychotherapy · approaches that focus on developing insight and subsequent character development through interpersonal relationships with the therapist, including brief interpersonal therapy or brief psychodynamic therapy

C

care coordinator · the care coordinator or case manager coordinates and oversees the care plan, and often has the closest therapeutic relationship and most contact with the service user

case management · known in the UK as the Care Programme Approach (CPA), case management provides a framework in which the strengths and needs of users are assessed and care plans written, implemented, and reviewed in consultation with the user, family, and other carers

clinical supervision · a process that aims to bring practitioners and skilled supervisors together to reflect on practice, to identify solutions to problems, to increase understanding of professional issues, and, most importantly, to improve standards of care

cluster randomized controlled trial · participants are clustered together; there are similarities within clusters and therefore participants are less likely to be independent of one another

cognitive behavioural therapy (CBT) · the mixture of evidence-based cognitive and behavioural treatments for emotional disorder

cognitive restructuring · a way of looking at and challenging unhelpful thoughts; aims to challenge and evaluate one's irrational, counter-factual beliefs and replace them with more accurate and beneficial ones

cognitive therapy · a therapy that seeks to identify and teach patients to modify negative thinking, cognitive distortions, and underlying dysfunctional beliefs that are hypothesized as being related to the patient's current mood state. Behavioural 'experiments' may also be part of the clinical method in cognitive therapy, specifically designed to challenge thinking

compliance aids · devices to help service users remember to take medication that separate medications into daily doses (e.g. Medidos/dosette boxes)

confinement · the state of being detained

contextual · a theory that argues that the contexts in which human activity takes place—the time, the space, and the place in the sequence of events—are crucial to the nature of that activity

continuing professional development · a systematic and planned approach to the maintenance, enhancement, and development of knowledge, skills, and expertise that continues throughout a professional's career and is to the mutual benefit of the individual, the employer, and the professional body

continuity of care · defined by Freeman et al. (2001, p. 7) as 'the experience of a coordinated and smooth progression of care from the patients' point of view'

D

de-escalation · communication skills designed to prevent physical violence

deprivation of liberty · a situation in which a person is being kept in conditions where the hospital or care home has complete and effective control over the incapacitated person's residence, assessment, treatment, and movement. It is often characterized by a situation where the person is under continuous supervision and control, and is not free to leave (HL v United Kingdom [2004])

detention · being kept in official custody and not free to leave

dual diagnosis · the combination of a mental illness and substance use. As far as the literature is concerned, this means a severe and enduring mental illness (such as schizophrenia) and harmful use or dependence. Clinically, a wider range of presentations is accepted as a dual diagnosis (e.g. depression and heavy drinking after bereavement)

dyskinesia · an involuntary movement, such as irregular blinking, grimacing, tongue movements, and protrusion of the tongue, and worm-like movements of fingers and toes, sometimes caused by use of antipsychotic drugs. The effect of these drugs can be tardive, meaning the dyskinesia continues even after the drugs are no longer taken

dyslipidaemia · a disorder in which blood lipid levels are abnormal; the main cause of atherosclerosis (hardening, clogging, or narrowing of the arteries)

dystonia · prolonged muscle spasm, which can be extremely painful, affecting various parts of the body, causing unusual movements and postures. It can be a side effect of antipsychotic drugs

E

empathy · imagining yourself into the place of the client so that you become aware of their inner world and private meanings

evidence-based practice · using the best available evidence, clinical acumen, and patient preferences to make clinical decisions within available resources

exposure therapy · when we are afraid of a situation or object such as spiders, meeting new people, or going out, we often try to avoid it. Avoidance can relieve anxiety, but often for only a short time. Avoidance can often lead to long-term difficulties because a vicious circle of anxiety and avoidance builds up. Exposure therapy is useful to break this cycle. It teaches you slowly to confront the feared object or situation until anxiety falls

F

FPS (Framingham Points Score) · evidence-based coronary disease risk prediction score using age, total cholesterol, smoking status, high-density lipoprotein, and systolic blood pressure to calculate risk levels

G

genuineness · responding authentically with reference to own thoughts and feelings and without professional façade or pretence

guided self-help (GSH) · refers to self-help evidence-based interventions that require minimal therapist contact. Such interventions are based on CBT principles and are usually mediated through a health technology (e.g. bibliotherapy, computer-administered therapy), but with some facilitation/guidance by a practitioner

H

habilitation · to train to function in a role

harm reduction · a pragmatic, public health-oriented approach to the management of drug-related harms that focuses on the reduction of harms rather than drug use *per se*. The central tenet of harm reduction (used interchangeably with harm minimization) is that some ways of using substances are clearly safer than others

harmful use · drug or alcohol use that persistently causes or exacerbates harm to physical, psychological, social, and occupational health/function. An important feature of harmful use is continued use despite subjective awareness of harm

high-intensity psychological treatments · traditional psychological treatments involving a large (12 or more) number of sessions, usually face to face, between mental health workers and patients/service users

hyperglycaemia · higher than normal blood glucose level

hyperlipidaemia · high levels of one or more of the lipid substances in the blood, especially cholesterol or triglycerides

hyperprolactinaemia · excess production of the hormone prolactin in both males and females; may cause ovulation and menstrual disorders in females, and sexual dysfunction in males. There are many causes including hypothyroidism, side effects of certain drugs, and pituitary tumour

hypokinesia · reduced number of movements

I

ideology · a system of ideas and ideals

interpersonal communication · the verbal and non-verbal ways in which we interact with others

intrapersonal communication · our relationship with ourselves, the way we know ourselves, and how we process thoughts, feelings, and emotions

K

Knowledge and Skills Framework (KSF) England and Wales · a competency framework and a human resources tool that defines and describes the knowledge and skills that UK NHS staff need to apply in their work in order to deliver quality services

L

learned helplessness · a psychological condition in which someone has learned or come to believe that they have little influence or control over a situation, often resulting in them becoming passive, apathetic, or withdrawn

lifelong learning · lifelong learning is about growth and opportunity, about making sure that staff, teams, and organizations can acquire new knowledge and skills, both to realize their potential and to help shape and change things for the better

ligature · an item that can be used for tying or binding in suicide (a rope, wire, bedding, or clothing)

low-intensity psychological treatments · treatments that involve small amounts of contact between mental health workers and patients. Examples include computerized cognitive behavioural therapy, exercise, guided self-help. Low-intensity treatments are often also delivered using the telephone or by email

M

motivational interviewing (MI) · the working principle of MI is that it is the business of the individual to change their life and the business of the therapist to assist this change. Taking the position that any change can be understood as a process, MI allows both parties to understand the stages of change and to work collaboratively to support the change process

multidisciplinary team · team of workers providing care for service users and support for families and carers. Often includes psychiatrists, mental health nurses, social workers, occupational therapists, psychologists, and other support workers

N

negative obligation · an obligation under Human Rights Law not to breach an individual's fundamental rights and freedoms

negative reinforcement · the strengthening of a response as a consequence of its being followed by the cessation or avoidance of an aversive stimulus

neuropathy · a problem in peripheral nerve function (any part of the nervous system except the brain and spinal cord) that causes pain, numbness, tingling, swelling, and muscle weakness in various parts of the body; also called peripheral neuropathy

nurse of the prescribed class · under the Mental Health Act 1983, nurses entitled to exercise the power to detain a patient under section 5(4) are those who are registered as RN3, RN4, RN5, or RN6 on the UK Nursing and Midwifery Council's Register

O

observation · a two-way relationship between a service user and a nurse that is meaningful, grounded in trust, and therapeutic for the service user

opioids · synthetic opiates, usually with a long drug half-life, making them ideal for the treatment of dependence. Examples are methadone and buprenorphine

osteoarthritis · a form of arthritis involving the deterioration of the cartilage that cushions the ends of bones within joints

overdose · an event in which a person intentionally or accidentally ingests one or more substances at unsafe levels (more than the recommended levels for that person)

P

personal and professional development · keeping up to date with changes in practice and participating in lifelong learning and personal and professional development for oneself and colleagues through supervision, appraisal, and reflective practice

person-centred approach · term used to describe a way of being with clients that is non-directive and based on creating core conditions (respect, empathy, genuineness, and unconditional positive regard) as the main modality of treatment, rather than specific skills. Carl Rogers was the founder of this approach

physical intervention · safely immobilizing a person to prevent them from harming themselves, others, or damaging the therapeutic environment

positive reinforcement · the effect of reinforcement utilizing pleasure, whereby approach behaviour is increased

post-incident review · a reflective discussion within 72 hours of an incident to learn lessons, and support staff and service users

problem solving · a collaborative approach that helps people to manage their current problems in a systematic way; helps people to feel more in control of their difficulties and facilitates realistic appraisal of and practical solutions to problems

proportionality · not going beyond the necessary to achieve a desired outcome

psycho-education · specific information exchange to help service users access facts about illness/treatment that are clear and concise

psychosocial intervention (PSI) · specific interventions for people with psychotic experiences. To be a valid PSI, the intervention must be evidence based, person centred, and aimed at reducing the stress of an individual experiencing psychotic symptoms or their carers

R

randomized controlled trial · an experimental research design in which investigators randomly allocate eligible people into (e.g. treatment and control) groups to receive or not to receive one or more interventions that are being compared. The results are assessed by comparing outcomes in the treatment and control groups

rapid tranquillization · the use of medication to calm lightly a person to prevent them from harming themselves, others, or damaging the therapeutic environment

recovery · rebuilding a meaningful and valued life despite ongoing mental health problems

recovery approach · a personal process of tackling the adverse impacts of experiencing mental health problems, despite their continuing or long-term presence. It involves personal development and change, including acceptance that there are problems to face; a sense of involvement and control over one's life; the cultivation of hope; and using support from others

reflective practice · an approach in which you look at events in your practice and analyse them; involves thinking about your work in a structured way, sometimes with the help of a reflective journal, log, or diary

relapse prevention strategies · techniques to educate patients in recognizing their personal early signs of a previous disorder linked to a formal plan to undertake previously specified action to prevent a return of the disorder

relaxation techniques · help to reduce anxiety and stress; a useful way to maintain good mental health

retinopathy · disorders of the retina (nerve elements in the back portion of the eye that receive images) that can lead to impaired vision or blindness

risk · a hazard likely to cause loss or injury

S

seclusion · the supervised confinement of a patient in isolation to prevent them from harming others

self-efficacy · belief that one is capable of certain performance or of achievement of specific goals

self-harm · intentional self-poisoning or injury, irrespective of the apparent purpose of the act; includes poisoning, asphyxiation, cutting, burning, and other self-inflicted injuries

self-injury · an act that involves deliberately inflicting pain/and/or injury to one's own body, with or without suicidal intent

serious medical treatment · under the Mental Capacity Act 2005, defined as treatment that involves providing, withdrawing, or withholding treatment in circumstances where: (a) in a case where a single treatment is being proposed, there is a fine balance between its benefits to the patient and the burdens and risks it is likely to entail for him; (b) in a case where there is a choice of treatments, a decision as to which one to use is finely balanced; or (c) what is proposed would be likely to involve serious consequences for the patient

Skilled Helper Model · developed by Gerard Egan; uses stages in a problem-solving cycle to prompt and direct clients towards solutions for change

social inclusion · involvement in non-segregated (community) opportunities, relationships, roles, and facilities

stepped care · a model of treatment options to offer simpler and less expensive interventions in the first instance, and more complex and expensive options if the patient has not benefited with the aim of increasing efficiency and effectiveness. The model is 'self-correcting' where a systematic process of monitoring the results of treatments and decisions about treatment provision is conducted

substance misuse · a term commonly used to describe the presence of problems in an individual related to current or historical drug or alcohol use. There is no consensus about the meaning of this term (some will argue that any drug or alcohol use is misuse, whereas others differentiate between use and misuse)

suicidal ideation · suicidal thoughts and ideas are those with or without actual plans for acting on them. Suicidal ideation is common and important in risk assessment when accompanied by other risk factors

suicidal intent · the degree to which the individual wished to die at the time of the act

suicide · death following an act of self-harm

supportive therapy · any approach that focuses on the therapist's use of core relationship conditions to develop self-awareness in the patient

systematic reviews · rigorous secondary research method that locates, appraises, and synthesizes evidence from primary research studies to arrive at the best evidence for practice

T

therapeutic alliance · another term for the therapeutic relationship that perhaps more clearly emphasizes the notion of collaboration and partnership in resolving life problems

therapeutic relationship · a relationship in which at least one of the parties has the intent of promoting growth, development, maturity, improved functioning, and improved coping with life of the other

three systems theory · the understanding that human emotions consist of three separate but interlinked components: physical, cognitive, and behavioural

U

unconditional positive regard · the ability to respond to another so that they feel valued whatever they say, think, or feel

usual care · a range of **non-treatment** options (waiting list, inert control conditions) delivered to the patient in a randomized controlled trial

V

values-based practice · using theory and skills as a base for effective health care decision-making where different values are influencing the process

violence · physical force intended to hurt or injure others

W

working in partnership · developing and maintaining constructive working relationships with service users, carers, families, colleagues, lay people, and wider community networks. Working positively with any tensions created by conflicts of interest or aspiration that may arise between the partners in care

PART 1

Putting values into practice

Chapters

1 Introduction: mental health nursing past, present, and future

Patrick Callaghan

▼ Introduction

Mental health problems and disorders account for 13% of the burden of disease across the world, and in high income countries the estimate increases to 23%, with such problems and disorders being the most common cause of disability and premature death (World Health Organization [WHO] 2004). Since the publication of *Mental Health: New Understanding, New Hope* (WHO 2001a), there have been concerted efforts internationally to promote mental health, reduce the burden of mental health problems, and increase the social inclusion (see Chapter 9) of people living with such problems (WHO 2001b). In the UK, since the 1999 National Service Framework (NSF) for Mental Health (Department of Health [DH] 1999) and other NSFs (DH 2001, DH/Department for Education and Skills 2004), mental health has become one of the government's national health priorities (DH 2004b, 2006d). Within UK NHS mental health services, mental health nurses (MHNs) make up the largest proportion of the professional workforce, making them pivotal to the delivery of the NSF. Mental health nursing takes place in an increasingly wide variety of practice contexts, and rapid developments in mental health and social care policy, research, and service delivery within the past ten years have impacted significantly upon the work of MHNs.

There has been an increased emphasis on partnership working with service users and carers (NHS Executive 2000). The patient choice agenda is now central to service and care delivery (Care Services Improvement Partnership/National Institute of Mental Health in England 2005), and new roles, new ways of working, and new types of service have proliferated (DH 2003a–c, 2005b). Staffing challenges within mental health services, together with further opportunities to extend nursing roles, raise important issues as to the most effective use of the resource of MHNs (DH 2006a, Sainsbury Centre for Mental Health [SCMH] 2005).

Developments in the evidence base for practice and the increased availability of good practice and clinical effectiveness guidelines require MHNs to learn new knowledge and skills and adapt their practice accordingly (DH 2002, 2004a, National Institute for Health and Clinical Excellence [NICE] 2003, 2004a–c, 2005a,b).

Recent legislative changes in the UK as a whole, and England in particular, including the Disability Discrimination Act (Department for Work and Pensions [DWP] 1994, 2004), Human Rights Act (Department for Constitutional Affairs [DCA] 1998), Race Relations (Amendment) Act (DWP 2003), Mental Capacity Act (DCA 2005), and the revised Mental Health Act (DH 2007), will impact on MHN practice, with more legal and statutory duties. Equally important is the changing multicultural context of practice and the need for culturally sensitive services responsive to the needs of diverse populations (DH 2005a). Regarding the educational preparation of MHNs to respond to the many challenges and opportunities, there is clear evidence that, despite recent changes, current pre-registration programmes are still not preparing MHNs with the essential knowledge and skills needed to practise in current and future contexts (Bee et al. 2007, DH 2004c, 2006b, Jones and Lowe 2003, Musslewhite and Freshwater 2005).

To keep pace with and respond to this rapidly changing health care environment, MHNs must reflect upon their roles, and the values, attitudes, and knowledge (see Chapter 3) that underpin their practice.

In some respects mental health nursing is at a cross-roads and heading into uncharted and exciting territory. Recently the Nursing and Midwifery Council (NMC) launched a consultation document seeking views on a possible reform of pre-registration nursing education; new roles for MHNs are developing rapidly and there is now an abundance of nurse-led mental health services throughout the UK. Notwithstanding current and future developments in the profession, there are prevailing issues that appear to remain topical for MHNs, and some of these are explored in the next section.

Defining key values and models in mental health nursing

There is now a strong drive towards MHNs using a recovery approach in providing a values- and evidence-based approach to support good practice. This approach has undoubted promise and there are good practice examples of nurses using this approach to improve the care of people using mental health services; see Chapter 9 for a detailed discussion of recovery and social inclusion. It is important, however, that nurses demonstrate the necessary skills, competencies, and capabilities to underpin the values. The importance of working in partnership not only with users and their carers, but also with the wider communities and agencies with which users and their carers interact, is recognized. A values-based practice approach provides a set of key values that all MHNs should demonstrate. Recruitment and selection procedures for entry to mental health nursing education programmes should assess the extent to which people demonstrate these values. Arguably, nursing education programmes at the pre-registration level for mental health nursing must retain a strong focus on mental health so that nurses can realize these values in action. The demonstration of these values should be a pre-requisite for entry to education programmes; see Chapter 3 for an examination of values-based practice and how you may demonstrate these values in practice.

Ensuring equality and meeting diverse needs

Considering how MHNs can contribute to delivering a service that acknowledges and respects the differences between differing needs of service users is an important objective at the heart of serious debate about mental health nursing. MHNs can best contribute to equality through demonstrating capabilities in providing care that does not discriminate on the grounds of race, gender, sexuality, age, ability, and personal status. Use of a **values-based practice model** is a good starting point that should help facilitate the provision of such care; Linda Cooper addresses this in Chapter 3.

Psychological therapies

The issue of whether nurses should be trained in psychological therapies is aired frequently. It is important that MHNs continue to be trained in evidence-based psychosocial interventions where required, and should use these interventions in circumstances where they are needed, and where evidence indicates that they will improve outcomes for service users.

Nurses are likely to play an important role in delivering the high-intensity (cognitive behavioural therapy) interventions that the Department of Health in England requires to improve people's access to psychological therapies. Students should demonstrate capabilities in user-centred assessment, interviewing, and education, measuring problems and their impact using standard measures, forming and sustaining helpful therapeutic alliances with users, their carers, and other agencies, shared decision-making, case formulation, and working in partnership with users and their carers, families, and significant others. These issues are explored in some detail in Chapters 6, 7, 11, and 12.

MHNs should contribute to facilitating therapeutic environments where care is occurring, using evidence-based approaches such as those demonstrated by the Sainsbury Centre's Acute Solutions Project (SCMH 2006) and by Bowers and others' work on acute psychiatric wards in East London (Bowers et al. 2007). MHNs must have adequate support in using evidence-based psychosocial interventions; such support will include clinical supervision, and education and training in these interventions. Chapters 11 and 12 highlight the promise of two different types of psychological intervention that MHNs can use in their work to good effect.

Leadership and organizational issues

Effective leadership at the level of practice, policy, research, and education is needed to support MHNs. The links between leadership and practice must be coherent, and strengthened. There needs to be synergy between leaders in practice, education, research, and policy. Effective leadership can best be developed by leaders modelling their skills close to the point of care delivery, sound education and training, and effective supervision. This issue is further explored by Neil Brimblecombe in Chapter 22 on leadership and management.

Providing holistic care

The notion of providing holistic care features strongly in the mental health nursing literature. It is not always clear, however, what is meant by 'holistic care'. Nevertheless, the ingredients of holistic care are those that address the needs of service users, as defined by them, and, as agreed by service users, a system of care that promotes their recovery. Holistic care is also about an awareness of service users as people, first and foremost, with all that this represents; mental health needs are part of the person, not the sum of his or her life.

Helping to overcome social exclusion

There can be little doubt that being mentally ill is often a condition of social exclusion. Getting to the bottom of what includes or excludes people socially can be a daunting task. MHNs can help to promote social inclusion by enabling people to work or engage in productive occupation, and to use and maintain supportive social contacts. In Chapter 9, Julie Repper and Rachel Perkins describe how mental health nursing students can demonstrate the competencies and capabilities they require to foster service users' recovery and social inclusion. The 'Moving People' campaign (http://www.movingpeople.org.uk) illustrates how socially excluded people can become more included.

Increasing patient choice

The issue of patient choice is high in the government's priorities for the NHS. It is arguably the most challenging part of its agenda. MHNs can best promote service user choice by helping people to access information to enable them to make decisions about what services to choose.

Mental health nursing is at its best when services users and carers report a high level of satisfaction with care; service users report that MHNs meet their reasonable expectations; the values, attitudes, and beliefs of MHNs lead to practice that promotes people's health and well-being through clear teaching and demonstration of skills; MHNs are able to demonstrate the competencies and capabilities people need (see next page); and the public image of mental health nursing is positive. The goals to which most of us aspire, and which are fundamental to our own quality of life—health, paid productive occupation, social support, safe, secure shelter, and freedom from fear, discrimination, and prejudice—are central to the lives of people with mental health problems. Arguably, the task of mental health nursing is to enable people living with mental illness to achieve these goals; the task of this book is to ensure mental health nursing students are competent and capable of contributing to these goals when they graduate, irrespective of where they practise. The next part of this chapter outlines the contributors' approaches to this challenging task.

Review of mental health nursing

In April 2005, the Chief Nursing Officer (CNO) for England announced a major review of mental health nursing. The final report, published in 2006 (DH 2006a), made recommendations for current and future practice and education. Promoting

the recovery of people using mental health services is at the core of the CNO review. A similar review was conducted in Scotland and reported in 2006 (Scottish Executive 2006). Like the English review, it also has recovery at its heart. Despite some of the differences in health and social care policy and health outcomes for people using services in both countries, the reviews of mental health nursing cover similar ground in their focus on recovery, developing capabilities for the mental health nursing workforce, preparing students with the best education for practice, and highlighting the importance of leadership and support. In England, the publication of the *Review of Mental Health Nursing* was followed by subsequent publications of good practice guidance for pre-registration MHN education (DH 2006b) and a 'self-assessment toolkit' for Mental Health Trusts to assess progress in implementing the review recommendations (DH 2006c).

Much has changed since the last (UK-wide) review of mental health nursing in 1994 (DH 1994); we now have devolved government in the different countries of the UK, mental health sits near the top of the health care agenda, a National Service Framework set standards for the delivery of care, a Care Quality Commission monitors how services are meeting these standards, and nurse consultants have appeared, as have a mental health tsar, revised Mental Health Acts, and the integration of health and social care. The term 'serious untoward incident' (SUI) has entered the lexicon of mental health. Service users and carers are, in theory, at the heart of care. MHNs are now prescribing medication, working with colleagues who are also service users, and there is finally a drive to address diversity issues in service delivery. These reviews took place in the context of work on new roles for new and existing professionals, and reviews of nursing education by the NMC.

It is tempting to be cynical with the announcement of yet another government review. Reasonable people ask whether these reviews change anything. The evidence following the recommendations made in the 1994 review suggests that they can lead to changes: shifting the focus of mental health services onto people with so-called severe and enduring mental illness; championing new psychosocial intervention (PSI) roles for nurses; increasing the number of liaison mental health services in emergency departments; working in partnership with service users and user choice; educators and service providers working in partnership in the delivery of nursing education; and the accreditation of prior learning for entry to pre-registration programmes. Whether or not you agreed with these recommendations at the time, these issues are now part of mainstream mental health and seem, 15 years on, almost routine.

The reviews of mental health nursing in England and Scotland involved the formation of expert advisory groups that included service users and carers, students, clinicians, academics, the NMC, managers, and representatives from professional organizations. The reports of the reviews in Scotland and England have provided the impetus for this book.

Best practice competencies and capabilities for pre-registration mental health nurses

The best practice competencies and capabilities for pre-registration MHNs, which are the focus of this book, were developed following extensive consultation with MHNs in practice, MHN academics, researchers, managers, service users, carers, and students. They are mapped against previous work by the NMC in setting learning outcomes for pre-registration nursing programmes, the Essential Shared Capabilities for mental health practice, and the National Occupational Standards for Mental Health, published by the DH in England, and competencies for mental health practice, developed by Skills for Health. If mental health nursing students have acquired the best practice competencies and capabilities by the time they graduate, they should be fit for practice as registered nurses. The three categories of best practice competencies and capabilities that mental health nursing students require at the point of registration, as reported in the CNO Review of Mental Health Nursing in England, are shown in Box 1.1. The detailed knowledge and performance criteria for each of the competencies, and the respective NMC learning outcome to which they refer, are shown in the original report. You can access this report at http://www.dh.gov.uk/en/Publicationsandstatistics/Publications/PublicationsPolicyAndGuidance/DH_4135647.

How this book can help you to develop your skills

Mental Health Nursing Skills is designed to show you how you can acquire, develop, and demonstrate the best practice competencies and capabilities described in the CNO Review of Mental Health Nursing in England, and those addressed in the Scottish Review of Mental Health Nursing, in your interactions with service users.

The approach taken in this book is to teach the core skills that service users need from mental health nurses, mapped to the competencies and capabilities recommended in the reviews of mental health nursing, including the Ten Essential Shared

Box 1.1 Best practice competencies and capabilities for pre-registration mental health nurses in England (DH 2006b)

Putting values into practice
Values

Promote a culture that values and respects the diversity of individuals, and enables their recovery.

Improving outcomes for service users
Communication

Use a range of communication skills to establish, maintain, and manage relationships with individuals who have mental health problems, their carers, and key people involved in their care.

Physical care

Promote physical health and well-being for people with mental health problems.

Psychosocial care

Promote mental health and well-being, enabling people to recover from debilitating mental health experiences and/or achieve their full potential, supporting them to develop and maintain social networks and relationships.

Risk and risk management

Work with individuals with mental health needs in order to maintain health, safety, and well-being.

A positive, modern profession
Multidisciplinary and multi-agency working

Work collaboratively with other disciplines and agencies to support individuals to develop and maintain social networks and relationships.

Personal and professional development

Demonstrate a commitment to the need for continuing professional development and personal supervision activities, in order to enhance knowledge, skills, values, and attitudes needed for safe and effective nursing practice.

Capabilities, NMC skills clusters, Skills for Health, the National Occupational Standards for Mental Health, and the Knowledge and Skills Framework. Each chapter in this book is mapped against the best practice competencies and capabilities; Table 1.1 shows you where in the book the competencies and capabilities are

Table 1.1 Mapping the best practice competencies and capabilities of mental health nursing to each chapter

Best practice competency and capability	Chapters
Putting values into practice	2: Service users' expectations and views of mental health nurses 3: Values-based mental health nursing practice 4: Evidence-based mental health nursing practice 5: Caring: the essence of mental health nursing 8: Working in partnership 9: Recovery and social inclusion
Improving outcomes for service users	6: Interpersonal communication–Heron's Six Category Interventions Analysis 7: Forming, sustaining, and ending therapeutic interactions 10: The essence of physical health care 11: Fostering guided self-help 12: Behavioural activation 13: Medication management 14: Legal, professional, and ethical issues 15: Risk assessment and management 16: Safe and effective observation of patients 17: Recognition and therapeutic management of self-harm and suicidal behaviour 18: Prevention, recognition, and therapeutic management of violence 19: Working with people with substance misuse problems
A positive, modern profession	20: Interagency and interprofessional working 21: Personal and professional development 22: Leadership and management

addressed. A tour at the beginning of the book explains the learning features and accompanying website.

Mental health nursing education: the pre-registration period

The minimum exit qualification for nursing education will be a degree. Before this comes to pass, an Equality Impact Assessment may be necessary to ensure that moving towards a degree does not hinder attempts to widen access to nursing for under-represented groups. In addition, the question of how nursing programmes will be funded, should they become all degree, will need to be considered.

The profession may also need to consider additional means of providing nursing students with practice experience; Client Attachment, for example, in which students are attached to clients instead of wards, shows some promise (Turner et al. 2004). There might need to be an increase in the number of roles linking education and practice where MHN education is delivered. It is important that there is a strong practice infrastructure to support the 50% of the curriculum that is delivered in practice. Strong partnerships between universities, Strategic Health Authorities, commissioners, and service providers are needed to deliver effective mental health nursing education.

Mental health nursing education: the post-registration period

At the time of writing this book, the Department of Health in England is consulting on the nature of post-registration education. In relation to the issue of what systems need to be in place to support MHNs to develop their knowledge and skills after initial qualification, there is promise in an internship period of at least one year after qualification. During this year, newly qualified nurses will have provisional registration. Once they have demonstrated further capabilities through formative assessment, whilst working under supervision, they can achieve full registration status. It is hoped that such an approach will lead to nurses being better able to deliver the care that service users need, and which contributes to their recovery as defined by them.

MHNs need protected time dedicated to research and development. Again, strong partnerships between universities, Strategic Health Authorities, commissioners, and service providers are needed to deliver the systems needed to support MHNs to develop their knowledge and skills after initial qualification. In Chapter 21, Sara Owen and Clare Fox explore in detail some of the personal and professional development issues of importance to MHNs.

Conclusion

Mental Health Nursing Skills has been written with you, the mental health student nurse, in mind. It addresses directly best practice competencies and capabilities that you will find indispensable when you move from being a student nurse to a registered nurse. The book is designed to provide relevant information based upon the best available evidence that will show you how to demonstrate that you are a MHN with the competence and capability to enable the service users for whom you care to recover from their experiences, or better manage their experiences, so that they feel more part of society.

Web links to key strategic documents

Chief Nursing Officer's Review of Mental Health Nursing. http://www.dh.gov.uk/en/Publicationsandstatistics/Publications/PublicationsPolicyAndGuidance/DH_4133839

The Ten Essential Shared Capabilities for mental health practice. http://www.dh.gov.uk/en/Publicationsandstatistics/Publications/PublicationsPolicyAndGuidance/DH_4087169

NMC Essential Skills Clusters for Pre-registration Nursing Programme. http://www.nmc-uk.org/aFrameDisplay.aspx?DocumentID=3663&Keyword=

NMC Guidelines for Mental Health and Learning Disabilities Nursing. http://www.nmc-uk.org/aFrameDisplay.aspx?Docu-mentID=521

Rights, Relationships and Recovery: The Report of the National Review of Mental Health Nursing in Scotland. http://www.scotland.gov.uk/Publications/2006/04/18164814/0

References

Bee, P., Playle, J., Lovell, K., Barnes, P., Gray, R., and Keeley, P. (2007). Service user views and expectations of UK-registered mental health nurses: a systematic review of empirical research. *International Journal of Nursing Studies* 45(3), 442–57.

Bowers, L., Whittington, R., Nolan, P., et al. (2007). *The City 128 Study of Observation and Outcomes on Acute Psychiatric Wards*. London: HMSO.

Care Services Improvement Partnership/National Institute for Mental Health in England (2005). *Our Choices in Mental Health: A Framework for Improving Choice for People Who Use Mental Health Services and Their Carers*. London: Department of Health.

Department for Constitutional Affairs (1998). *Human Rights Act*. London: HMSO.

Department for Constitutional Affairs (2005). *Mental Capacity Act*. London: HMSO.

Department of Health (1994). *Working in Partnership: A Collaborative Approach to Care. Report of the Mental Health Review Team*. London: HMSO.

Department of Health (1999). *National Service Framework for Mental Health*. London: DH.

Department of Health (2001). *National Service Framework for Older People*. London: DH.

Department of Health (2002). *Mental Health Policy Implementation Guide: Adult Acute Inpatient Care Provision*. London: DH.

Department of Health (2003a). *Fast-forwarding Primary Care Mental Health 'Gateway Workers'*. London: DH.

Department of Health (2003b). *Mental Health Policy Implementation Guide – Support, Time and Recovery Workers*. London: DH.

Department of Health (2003c). *Mental Health Policy Implementation Guide – Community Development: Workers for Black and Minority Ethnic Communities*. London: DH.

Department of Health (2004a). *National Mental Health Workforce Strategy*. London: DH.

Department of Health (2004b). *The National Service Framework for Mental Health—5 Years On*. London: NHS Executive.

Department of Health (2004c). *Organising and Delivering Psychological Therapies*. London: DH.

Department of Health (2005a). *Delivering Race Equality in Mental Health Care: An Action Plan for Reform Inside and Outside Services and the Government's Response to the Independent Inquiry into the Death of David Bennett*. London: DH.

Department of Health (2005b). *New Ways of Working for Psychiatrists: Enhancing Effective, Person-centred Services Through New Ways of Working in Multidisciplinary and Multiagency Contexts. Final Report 'But Not the End of the Story'*. London: DH.

Department of Health (2006a). *From Values to Action: the Chief Nursing Officer's Review of Mental Health Nursing*. London: DH.

Department of Health (2006b). *Best Practice Competencies and Capabilities for Pre-Registration Mental Health Nurses in England: The Chief Nursing Officer's Review of Mental Health Nursing*. London: DH.

Department of Health (2006c). *Self-assessment Toolkit. From Values to Action: The Chief Nursing Officer's Review of Mental Health Nursing*. London: DH.

Department of Health (2006d). *Our Health, Our Care, Our Say: A New Direction for Community Services*. London: DH.

Department of Health (2007). *The Mental Health Act 2007*. London: HMSO.

Department of Health/Department for Education and Skills (2004). *National Service Framework for Children, Young People and Maternity Services: Executive Summary*. London: DH.

Department for Work and Pensions (1994). *Disability Discrimination Act*. London: HMSO.

Department for Work and Pensions (2003). *Race Relations Act 1976 (Amendment) Regulations 2003*. London: HMSO.

Department for Work and Pensions (2004). *Disability Discrimination Act*. London: HMSO.

Jones, J. and Lowe, T. (2003). The education and training needs of qualified mental health nurses working in acute adult mental health services. *Nurse Education Today* 23(18), 610–19.

Musslewhite, C. and Freshwater, D. (2005). Workforce planning and education: mapping competencies, skills and standards in mental health. *Nurse Education Today* 26(4), 277–85.

National Institute for Health and Clinical Excellence (2003). *Schizophrenia: The Management of Symptoms and Experiences of Schizophrenia in Primary and Secondary Care*. London: NICE.

National Institute for Health and Clinical Excellence (2004a). *Depression: Management of Depression in Primary and Secondary Care*. London: NICE.

National Institute for Health and Clinical Excellence (2004b). *Self-harm: The Short-term Physical and Psychological Management and Secondary Prevention of Self-harm in Primary and Secondary Care*. London: NICE.

National Institute for Health and Clinical Excellence (2004c). *Eating Disorders: Core Interventions in the Treatment and Management of Anorexia Nervosa, Bulimia Nervosa and Related Eating Disorders*. London: NICE.

National Institute for Health and Clinical Excellence (2005a). *Depression in Children and Young People: Identification and Management in Primary, Community and Secondary Care*. London: NICE.

National Institute for Health and Clinical Excellence (2005b). *The Short-term Management of Disturbed/ Violent Behaviour in Psychiatric In-patient Settings and Emergency Departments*. London: NICE.

NHS Executive (2000). *The NHS Plan. A Plan for Investment, a Plan for Reform*. London: DH.

Sainsbury Centre for Mental Health (2005). *Acute Care 2004: A National Survey of Adult Psychiatric Wards in England*. London: SCMH.

Sainsbury Centre for Mental Health (2006). *The Search for Acute Solutions*. London: SCMH.

Scottish Executive (2006). *Rights, Relationships and Recovery: The Report of the Review of Mental Health Nursing in Scotland*. Edinburgh: Scottish Executive.

Turner, L., Callaghan, P., Eales, S., and Park, A. (2004). An evaluation of the introduction of a pilot client attachment scheme in mental health nursing education. *Journal of Psychiatric and Mental Health Nursing* 11, 414–21.

World Health Organization (2001a). *Mental Health: New Understanding, New Hope*. Geneva: WHO.

World Health Organization (2001b). *Mental Health Global Action Programme*. Geneva: WHO.

World Health Organization (2004). *Global Burden of Disease*. Geneva: WHO.

2 Service users' expectations and views of mental health nurses

John Playle   **Penny Bee**

▼ Introduction

The primary role of mental health professionals and services is to meet the defined health needs of the individuals they serve, ultimately service users (SUs) and their carers. Whilst this is a rather obvious statement, it can as a core principle easily get lost in the design and delivery of care. As with any public service there are often many different competing agendas, political, professional, and economic, that may lead to the importance of SU views and expectations lacking the priority they deserve. However, there is a growing recognition that the involvement and views of SUs and carers is an important principle and quality measure. It is vital that mental health nurses (MHNs) work together in partnership with SUs based on a clear understanding of their needs and negotiated expectations. At a wider level it is important to take a systematic approach to reviewing the evidence base related to SUs' expectations and views of MHNs in order to advance understanding of the contribution that MHNs can make to the modernization of mental health care provision.

This chapter is based on a systematic review of existing UK research into these factors that was commissioned by the UK Department of Health (DH) to inform the Chief Nursing Officer's Review of Mental Health Nursing in England (DH 2006a) and the National Review of Mental Health Nursing in Scotland (Scottish Executive 2006). The review examined all available UK research evidence since 1994 that reported on SUs' views, expectations, and satisfaction with MHNs. The 1994 date limit was chosen to coincide with the last published UK MHN review. This chapter will provide you with a brief overview of key findings. The full report submitted to the DH is available from the authors, and full details of the methods used are provided in Bee et al. (2008). Owing to the extensive sources included in the original review, only exemplar references are used here to support the summary offered.

Learning outcomes

By the end of this chapter you should be better able to:

1 Identify the importance of SU views and expectations of MHNs

2 Describe key SU expectations and views of MHNs based on a systematic review of evidence

3 Outline implications for practice, education, and the development and delivery of mental health nursing services.

Background

The UK National Service Framework (NSF) for Mental Health (DH 1999) identified the need to ensure adequate SU involvement in the development, delivery, and evaluation of mental health services, indicating that the expectations and experiences of SUs are a recognized marker of service performance. Within the UK, registered MHNs make up the largest proportion of the National Health Service (NHS) mental health workforce and have a pivotal role in the delivery of the NSF for mental health (DH 1999).

The importance of engaging SUs in all aspects of health care has been increasingly recognized in the UK, with the NHS experiencing a general shift towards a more consumerist model in which consumer satisfaction has become an important objective of health care and a key quality indicator. The involvement of SUs is a core policy recommendation as part of a drive for people-centred services and increasing public involvement (DH 2000, 2001, 2003).

Before the rise of the consumer movement and a user orientation in UK Government policy, the assessment of service satisfaction amongst mental health SUs had been largely neglected. Clinicians and researchers alike believed that lack of insight amongst many SUs may ultimately compromise the validity of their self-reported views (Noble et al. 1999). However, much of this concern has subsequently been discounted, with clear evidence that SUs do have important, valid, and useful opinions about their care (Noble et al. 1999, 2001). Reynolds et al. (1999) argue that, irrespective of the methods adopted, SUs ultimately remain the most appropriate individuals to inform nurses about the quality of their care.

To date, research examining SU views of MHNs has examined several constructs including attitudes, preferences, and expectations. Early studies revealed predominantly negative views of MHNs as impersonal, indifferent, controlling, threatening, and possessing a low empathetic sensitivity to the experience of others (Reynolds 1988, Sloane 1993). More recently, studies have been extended to examine the match between SU preferences and views of their professional and non-professional caregivers (Shumway 2003, Swartz et al. 2003).

Prior to the systematic review summarized here, only two previous systematic reviews of mental health service provision provided data relating to SU views of MHNs. The first (Noble et al. 1999, 2001) reported that SUs' expectations had previously been assessed in a variety of settings with findings indicating that SUs expected professionals to influence their mental health positively using a range of interventions. Where expectations remained incongruent with services received, poorer clinical outcomes were more likely to be present. A subsequent update to this work (Noble and Douglas 2004) reported that SUs sought to establish good relationships with their service providers that included at their core an adequate exchange of information and clear pathways for communication. The second review by Quirk and Lelliott (2001) focused on adult mental health acute inpatient environments and reported similar findings. It concluded that, although the duration of nurse–patient contact may have declined within acute inpatient settings, the quality of the relationship between the MHN and SU continued to be identified as the most important aspect of care received. Much of the evidence on which this conclusion was based came from a direct examination of SU views. SUs' attitudes towards, and beliefs about, mental health care have been linked to the initial uptake of services and subsequent treatment withdrawal, indicating that SU satisfaction is not only an important measure *per se* but also an influential factor on other outcomes (Briteen 1998).

Modern mental health nursing has become a topic of considerable debate, with different and often opposing theories of practice being developed. Despite some fundamental differences in their approach, all emphasize the nature, boundaries, and attitudinal basis of MHN–SU interactions. The core of mental health nursing practice has long been recognized as necessitating the maintenance of a discrete relationship between MHNs, SUs, and their families/carers. Despite this consensus, however, factors that specifically impede or facilitate this interaction have not been fully identified. Professional theorists have previously been criticized for relegating the expertise of SUs, with SU accounts of their needs and experiences being accorded much less privilege than those espoused in the professional domain (Repper 2000). Good reasons therefore exist for conducting a systematic review of SUs' expectations of and opinions about their care.

Key findings from the review

A total of 14 649 potentially relevant studies were identified through an in-depth literature search, with 13 921 being discarded because they did not meet one or more of the review inclusion criteria. Following in-depth review of the remaining 728 studies, 131 met criteria for inclusion. A further 12 reports identified from non-academic sources meant a final total of 143 studies were included in the review, equating to a total sample of more than 36 793 SUs. Most views related to MHNs working within adult mental health settings, with only one study explicitly focused on services for the elderly and a further eight studies of child and adolescent services. Distinctions were made between residential services, requiring 24-hour MHN–SU relationships, and non-residential or mixed/unspecified services, in which SUs experience more intermittent MHN contact. SU representatives were invited to comment on the findings of the review as they emerged.

What do service users expect from mental health nurses?

A large number of studies report on the range of skills, qualities, and responsibilities that SUs deem essential to effective mental health nursing. Central to this are SUs' views of key factors contributing to a high-quality MHN–SU relationship. Studies across settings reveal two core categories of response. The first relates to opportunities for nursing contact, the second to the content and quality of the resulting interaction.

Desire for nursing contact—opportunities, content, and quality

A key theme arising from many studies is a requirement by SUs for continuity of care, a concept grounded in the consistency and regularity of their interactions with MHNs (Adam et al. 2003, Kai and Crosland 2001). In relation to this, SUs highlight the potentially damaging impact of high staff turnover, high staff sickness, and the increasing tendency for services to rely on bank/agency nurses, perceived as having less investment in patient care. The main consequence of this kind of 'conveyer belt' approach is that SUs often experience only a passing relationship with their named nurse, which is seen as de-motivating as well as being associated with a potentially increased risk of relapse (Higgins et al. 1999). Kai and Crosland (2001) reported high staff turnover and repeated reviewing of case histories by different staff to be particularly frustrating for SUs, with other studies reporting similar findings, suggesting that continually disclosing personal problems to different nurses may undermine the entire MHN–SU relationship (Watts and Priebe 2002).

In addition to wanting stable relationships with their MHNs, SUs also highlight a desire to spend distinct and increasing amounts of time with them. Time for MHN–SU interaction is valued as an opportunity to talk through problems, enabling SUs to express emotion and identify potential solutions to their problems, particularly during periods of severe illness (Barker et al. 1999, McLaughlin 1999). One evaluation of acute mental health services (Godfrey and Wistow 1997) reported regularity of contact, coupled with a high-quality relationship, as key to enabling staff to respond effectively to deteriorations in mental health. Another reason for the desire for increased MHN contact is associated with a more constant SU need for social inclusion (Street 2004). Bonner et al. (2002) reported that, although SUs think nurses should dedicate more time to discussing difficulties, they also believe a key aspect of care should focus on opportunities for more general communication. In describing types of support wanted from MHNs, study participants refer to the benefits of what might be described as less clinical interventions such as having someone to 'visit for a cup of tea', 'watch a bit of telly', or 'go for a walk with them' (Barker et al. 1999, Meddings and Perkins 1999).

In discussing their perceptions of MHNs, some SUs refer directly to a perceived duality of nursing roles. One small-scale survey by Barker et al. (1999) concluded that SUs want nurses to be '*both ordinary and professional*'. A range of other studies confirm that SUs consistently conceptualize a good MHN as having both 'professional' and 'lay' qualities including warmth, empathy, and compassion (Edwards 2000, Goodwin et al. 1999). Across all types of service setting, SUs repeatedly report the essential components of a therapeutic relationship in terms of nursing knowledge and skills (what a nurse should know and do) and personal attributes (what a nurse should be like as a person). Both of these aspects are reported as highly influential on the nature of the relationship and its therapeutic benefit.

Expectations of nursing knowledge and skills

In a number of studies SUs suggest that, in terms of diagnosing and explaining mental health problems, MHNs are perceived to be the professional 'experts' and in this context are expected to have the necessary skills, confidence, and training to identify problems and offer solutions. One acute inpatient study (MacGabhann 2000) found that SUs believe in the nurses and want them specifically to show insight and understanding, and respond effectively to deteriorations in mental health. From a number of studies, SUs typically perceive clinical skills as being helpful, and attribute some value to the ability of MHNs to deliver psychological interventions as a result (Callaghan et al. 2002, Wakefield et al. 1998). They perceive counselling and talking therapies as particularly beneficial, emphasizing the need for nurses to have the ability to listen to SUs and to understand their points of view. Several studies suggest that professional listening skills are key to SUs' perceptions of an effective MHN, their experiences of being understood being variously described as helpful, powerful, and reassuring (Wood and Pistrang 2004). The use of such skills by MHNs is seen as fostering the well-being of the most vulnerable of SUs, as well as supporting the vast majority of SUs in exploring their identity, purpose, and self-worth.

Despite the high value attributed to talking therapies within the literature, several studies suggest that SUs see the role of MHNs as extending beyond the use of such formal therapies and including working to reduce stigma, providing structure and safety (Beech and Norman 1995, Edwards 1995), preventing feelings of isolation, and providing practical support including liaising with other services (Hayward et al. 2004, Rose and Muijen 1998). Indeed, many studies present this type of multifaceted support as one of the most important and desirable aspects of mental health nursing. Irrespective of setting, SUs indicate a desire for MHNs to engage in a broad range of activities including providing assistance with finances, improving patients' personal hygiene, and helping SUs to develop social skills.

Requirements for collaborative care

SUs' desire for MHNs to work together with them to address psychosocial problems is just one feature of a commonly held desire for collaborative care. Studies suggest that regardless of treatment setting, the ultimate aim of most SUs is to possess sufficient ability and self-confidence to enable them to function more independently (Williams et al. 1999). There is a repeated desire for relationships with staff that, whilst built on the foundations of professional knowledge, allow for the expression of more individual concerns. SUs report a clear wish to participate in the planning of their treatment, including identifying different ways in which they can help themselves and open discussions about the range and implications of different interventions (Callaghan et al. 2002, Pollock et al. 2004). A smaller number of studies also highlight a desire by SUs to include family and carers in consultations (Cutting and Henderson 2002).

The available evidence suggests that SUs require a variety of information related to their illness, the social and legal implications of care, features of care environments, and the identification of other organizations that may be of help. Some studies conclude that to be fully effective, such information should be provided in written format as well as verbally, maximizing exchange of advice and providing invaluable opportunities for clarification (Pollock et al. 2004). The interpretation of medical terminology is seen by SUs as key responsibility of MHNs, as well as having a mediating role with medical staff. Where relevant information is withheld, SUs are much more likely to perceive MHNs as impersonal and paternalistic, with potentially negative consequences for treatment adherence (Chiesa et al. 2000).

Nursing attributes—professional and personal

Although the 'professional skills' of MHNs are frequently reported as important to SUs, their usefulness is seen as being mediated by more personal aspects of the MHN–SU relationship, including the ability of MHNs to display warmth, **acceptance**, and understanding. One large study reported that, although SUs want experienced and well trained staff and services that are need-specific, they also seek relationships with professionals that engender a sense of belonging (Mental Health Foundation 2000). Many other studies included in the review reported similar findings.

Although some small-scale studies indicated a desire by SUs to be cared for by professionals with similar characteristics, such as age, ethnicity, and gender, it is unclear whether it is these characteristics *per se* that are seen as important, or SUs' perceptions of the ability of the nurse to understand their own situation. Secker and Harding's (2002) study of black African-Caribbean clients found that staff were able to build close relationships with clients not because they were black, but because they offered ordinary opportunities for warmth, friendship, and understanding. Other studies indicate that SUs are more likely to judge professional caregivers in terms of maturity and life experience rather than actual age (Buston 2002, Edwards 2000). The importance of MHNs possessing positive personal qualities is one of the most frequently emergent categories from SU responses in studies reviewed, with a set of common expectations that include at their centre a desire for empathy, respect, and compassion. More negative and unhelpful characteristics identified by SUs as undesirable nursing attributes include:

- being dismissive
- being judgemental
- trivializing symptoms
- adopting an essentially paternalistic or coercive approach.

Baker (2002) found that the extent to which SUs perceive MHNs as approachable may ultimately represent the key distinction between MHNs who are regarded highly and those who are not. Other studies confirm that a lack of perceived barriers between SUs and MHNs provides a greater sense of social acceptance and exerts considerable influence on the quality of the recovery process and its psychosocial outcomes (Adam et al. 2003, Barker et al. 1999, Breeze and Repper 1998).

Service user satisfaction with and views of mental health nurses

Service user satisfaction

Many of the studies reviewed present at least some data relating to SUs' perceived levels of satisfaction with MHNs. These include quantitative studies in which SU satisfaction was assessed according to predefined criteria, but also qualitative studies in which detailed SU views were collected via open-ended questioning. Whilst some provide a generic indication of SU satisfaction, others report more specific opinions relating to particular aspects of care. In all studies SU views varied depending upon the setting, with lower levels of satisfaction being much more common in inpatient than non-residential services.

General indicators of satisfaction

The findings from quantitative surveys generally indicate that SUs hold MHNs in high regard. Where satisfaction has been measured by a questionnaire developed in collaboration with SUs, findings suggest that the majority of respondents are satisfied with their care (Blenkiron and Hammill 2003, Lelliott et al. 2001, Macpherson et al. 2005). Hill et al.'s (1996) study of over 1500 SUs reported that community MHNs were rated as 'very helpful' by almost half of the survey group. Two other user-led studies (Rose 2001, Rose et al. 1998) reported the proportion of satisfied SUs to be between 42% and 73%. Qualitative findings from studies also confirm that SUs hold community MHNs in predominantly positive regard, with the vast majority of SUs reporting staff as supportive, helpful, and understanding. One study rated community MHNs as the most helpful members of the multidisciplinary team (Warne and Stark 2004).

In contrast, only one quantitative study assessing SU satisfaction with MHNs within inpatient settings reported similar levels of satisfaction (Rogers and Pilgrim 1994). Almost 60% of the 475 SUs in this study reported that they were either '*satisfied*' or '*very satisfied*' with their nursing care, 32.4% of participants ranking the helpfulness of their nurse as higher than that of psychiatrists and fellow patients. However, open-ended comments from a range of qualitative studies demonstrate a more mixed picture. For example, whilst one small-scale study reported respondents as universally experiencing 'good' relationships with 'helpful nurses' (Breeze and Repper 1998), another study concluded that such positive interactions were '*the exception rather than the rule*' (Secker and Harding 2002).

Satisfaction with nursing contact

A number of studies suggest comparatively lower levels of satisfaction among inpatient SUs compared with those in the community, a finding that may partially be explained by SUs' tendency to perceive ward-based MHNs as inaccessible. Negative views of nurse availability arose more frequently than any other topic in the inpatient studies reviewed, and constituted the main criticism of inpatient care. Although quantitative assessments of nurse availability were few, the evidence suggests that most inpatients feel MHNs spend insufficient amounts of time with them. Ford et al. (1999) reported that, whilst 73% of SUs found talking to nurses helpful, only 57% felt that the amount of time spent with them was always or usually enough. A national user-led study of 343 inpatients reported

similar findings, with 57% of all SUs surveyed saying that they had inadequate contact with staff, and 82% reporting less than 15 minutes of interaction per day (Barker 2000).

A high level of dissatisfaction with this aspect of care is further confirmed by a large number of qualitative comments from a range of inpatient studies. SUs report finding it difficult to secure sufficient time with their named nurse, with the effect that many experience only a passing relationship with this person.

As for the reasons for this lack of contact, some SUs refer to problems created by high nursing workloads, identifying inadequate staff–patient ratios as a key factor limiting their nursing contact time. More frequently, however, SUs highlight a general lack of enthusiasm amongst staff that reduces opportunities for contact and often leaves SUs feeling undeserving of nursing care (Smith 2002). Other studies refer to nurses 'congregating in offices', reinforcing a view of ward staff as inaccessible, disinterested, and irritated by patient contact (Jones and Mason 2002). Although student nurses were viewed favourably for being more ward-centred, qualified nurses were more often seen as 'office-bound', with longer serving members of staff being perceived as particularly apathetic.

In comparison to inpatient studies, dissatisfaction with nurse availability arises much less frequently in studies in non-residential settings. Valentine et al.'s (2003) study of community MHNs reported that 87% of participants mostly or always felt that they received sufficient attention from nurses, with 70% reporting that their views and choices were mostly or always taken into account. Where negative views were reported in non-residential settings, they tended to relate less to a lack of staff contact and more to limitations of service provision, in particular difficulties associated with high staff turnover, non-24-hour services, and inadequate access to crisis care.

Satisfaction with nursing skills

Although many qualitative studies identify a lack of opportunities for MHN–SU interaction, most SUs none the less appear to hold nurses' listening skills in high regard. Community MHNs are viewed as being particularly competent, which some SUs attribute directly to their ability to combine genuine friendliness with a professional approach (Adam et al. 2003, Baker 2002, Hostick and Newell 2004).

Other criticisms of nursing competencies are none the less observed. In relation to the community treatment of auditory hallucinations, SUs in Coffey et al.'s (2004) study reported nurses to possess 'a limited clinical repertoire'. Other studies highlight a perceived lack of confidence, both in the nurses themselves and in their professional capabilities (Chiesa et al. 2000). When asked what they would most like to change about their professional caregivers, SUs variously cite:

* better one-to-one communication skills
* increased responsiveness and flexibility
* improved liaison within and between services.

Compared with these qualitative findings, most quantitative studies report a higher level of perceived satisfaction. The Verona Satisfaction Scale (VSS), used in a number of studies, measures satisfaction with three key aspects of staff-based care—'professional skills and behaviour', 'relatives' involvement in care' and 'provision of information'—each being rated on a five-point scale from 1 (terrible) to 5 (excellent). Parkman et al.'s (1997) study of 202 SUs across community and inpatient settings reported a moderate level of satisfaction across the three key variables of the scale, with mean levels of satisfaction 2.90–3.93. Other studies using the same scale found that SUs were more satisfied with 'professional skills and behaviour' and less satisfied with 'information provision' and 'relatives' involvement in care' (Ruggeri et al. 2000, Tyson et al. 2001). Other surveys, although often using non-validated scales, indicate poor transfer of knowledge between MHNs and SUs, particularly in terms of diagnoses and treatment options.

In a wide range of qualitative studies reviewed, SUs report particular dissatisfaction with their care coordinator or key worker, and confusion over nursing and multidisciplinary team roles. Powell et al. (1996) found that participants were unsure of their key worker's role and at least some had experienced difficulty in contacting this individual. Furthermore, almost all participants believed that their key worker had not provided them with sufficient information. An analysis of data obtained from residential and non-residential services highlights a clear need for improvement in this aspect of the MHN's role, in particular enhancing SUs' knowledge of their illness, their associated care packages, and other potentially relevant services.

Many studies suggest that a general lack of information from MHNs often prevents SUs from feeling adequately involved in their own care. Only a small number of studies concluded that SUs felt empowered by their MHN (Beech and Norman 1995, Rogers et al. 2004), with the vast majority reporting a perceived reluctance among MHNs to acknowledge SU views. MHNs were at times perceived to have coerced SUs into receiving treatment, with some SUs feeling intimidated by MHNs as a result.

Satisfaction with nursing attributes

Despite the difficulties reported by SUs in achieving collaborative care, most quantitative studies conducted within non-residential settings report a relatively high level of satisfaction with the attitudes of MHNs. The largest of these, a national study of 27 398 SUs (Healthcare Commission 2004), found that of those SUs who had seen a community MHN in the previous 12 months, 85% reported **definitely** being treated with respect and dignity, with a further 12% reporting that they had been treated with respect and dignity *to some extent*. In qualitative studies, community MHNs are variously described as '*friendly*', '*approachable*', or '*empathic*' (Reed et al. 2002, Shanley et al. 2001), and in Barker et al.'s (1999) study community MHNs were seen by SUs as the '*glue holding the service together*'. Indeed, only one study (Bailey 1997) explicitly reported SUs as experiencing difficulties in establishing trusting relationships with community MHNs, although it is acknowledged that this may have arisen from prior negative experiences of mental health staff whose approach was deemed unsatisfactory.

In contrast, studies of SU satisfaction with the attitudes of MHNs within inpatient settings remain much less conclusive. The MIND (2004) user-led study of 335 inpatients reported that only 20% of respondents felt they were treated with dignity and respect by hospital staff, 17% stating that they were **never** treated in this way. However, although the results of this study are undoubtedly of value, its reliance on an opportunistic sample of SU group members limits the generalizability of its results. Smaller studies that recruited samples from consecutive service referrals often present more positive findings. Two studies conducted within residential rehabilitation units (Spence et al. 1997, Valentine et al. 2003) found that 62–73% of SUs perceived staff as approachable, although Spence and colleagues (1997) concluded that further improvements in communication were still needed.

Qualitative studies of inpatient SUs reflect more negative findings. One study of the lived experiences of 60 black inpatients reported that participants frequently perceived staff as confrontational and condescending, with many MHNs demonstrating an autocratic use of power that failed to acknowledge the needs of the individual (Sainsbury Centre for Mental Health 2002). Other studies involving predominantly white samples have reported similar results (Bailey 1997).

▲ Conclusion

This review has shown that research has consistently identified a core set of views amongst SUs that are capable of informing current and future mental health nursing. Irrespective of the care setting, SUs typically expect MHNs to fulfil a multifaceted role that combines practical and social support alongside the delivery of more formal psychological interventions. SUs expect MHNs to possess and exhibit both specific clinical skills and more generic skills and attributes related to effective interpersonal communication.

There has traditionally been delineation between two, at times seemingly opposing, conceptualizations of mental health nursing (Repper 2000). Advocates of the first emphasize the interpersonal and relational aspects, viewing the process of mental health nursing as an activity in which attention is focused primarily on the quality of the relationship between the MHN and SU. The conditions and attributes of the relationship are seen as key influences on SU satisfaction, often with an implicit assumption that the demonstration of such conditions is in itself adequate for effective outcomes (e.g. Barker 1998, Barker and Reynolds 1996). Advocates of the second, often seen as opposing, view tend to place much greater emphasis on the value of specific treatments and interventions (Gournay 1995). At times it has been argued that this view can lack attention to the interpersonal and relational aspects of nursing (Repper 2000). Our systematic review suggests that SUs are unlikely to describe mental health nursing as relying solely on either one of these conceptualizations. Rather, it suggests that SUs draw on a number of different models of mental health nursing and in so doing expect MHNs to demonstrate sufficient skills and flexibility to fulfil a range of different roles. From a professional perspective, SUs expect MHNs to have the skills to recognize symptoms and deliver appropriate, effective interventions and treatment. Central to this is a clear expectation of open and adequate information, and a greater provision of choice and involvement in a collaborative care process. However, from the findings of this review, the extent to which such processes are viewed as successful by SUs appears to rest primarily with their perceptions of the MHNs' propensity to listen, empathize, and understand.

Despite the value that SUs attribute to professional or clinical skills, an equal, if not greater, emphasis is placed upon the more personal attributes of the MHN. This is not necessarily counter to a focus on the need for MHNs to use professional skills to deliver specific evidence-based interventions. As studies in this review suggest, for many SUs there is an almost taken for granted assumption, whether rightly or wrongly, that MHNs should be equipped with the skills and confidence to offer such interventions. However, it is clear that relationships built on respect, compassion, and warmth not only influence the effectiveness of more formal interventions but are seen by SUs as a key mediating factor, often seen as having considerable therapeutic value in themselves.

Based on the research reviewed, the current ability of MHNs to meet the expectations of SUs remains unclear. Studies that rely mainly on quantitative data frequently conclude that SUs hold MHNs in relatively high regard. However, a renowned problem with satisfaction-based questionnaires is their tendency to record consistently positive responses, and when qualitative approaches are adopted more wide-ranging experiences and views emerge. Many qualitative studies in this review suggest that lower levels of satisfaction are most likely to be expressed by users of inpatient mental health services.

The need for a shift in the focus and quality of inpatient care is well recognized and extensive literature exists to provide explanations for the perceived limited quantity, quality, and depth of interaction that inpatient SUs experience (Quirk and Lelliott 2001). Related factors identified in this review include the impact of rapid staff turnover, extensive use of bank/agency staff, and low staff morale. However, although some SUs do indeed attribute some negative experiences directly to such factors, many more identify negative personal attributes and behaviours amongst MHNs as key explanatory factors.

MHNs working in whatever setting clearly need to be equipped with both therapeutic clinical skills, including the ability to deliver a range of psychological interventions, and more generic skills, personal attributes, and values associated with SU-centred engagement, relationship building, and interpersonal communication. In addition to the increasing emphasis on underpinning practice with core, user-centred values (DH 2004), pre-registration MHN curricula have highlighted the importance of the development of effective interpersonal communication and personal attributes. However, the evidence from the studies reviewed here suggests that many SUs continue to highlight shortcomings in this aspect of care. The latest UK Chief Nursing Officer review (DH 2006a) re-emphasizes the importance of an appropriate value base for MHN practice, as well as the necessity for pre- and post-registration training to teach and assess appropriate interpersonal and relational skills systematically (DH 2006b). Whilst it is hoped that the refocusing of pre-registration education for MHNs will, over time, address these shortcomings, it is equally important to recognize that, unless the needs of already qualified MHNs and the systems within which they practice are addressed, little is likely to change.

This review has identified particular problems within inpatient settings where MHNs are often viewed by SUs as having negative attitudes, lacking enthusiasm, being confrontational, failing to demonstrate respect, and being inaccessible. These factors clearly have the potential to affect treatment adherence and outcomes negatively, and there is a need to address these issues through education and training. However, this review has also highlighted other factors related to the wider system of care that SUs acknowledge as both contributing to, and in some cases accounting for, such negative attitudes and behaviours among MHNs. It needs to be acknowledged that resource shortages and an increase in illness severity among SUs in inpatient settings has previously been implicated in placing undue pressure on inpatient staff, who have been shown to cope by creating barriers to therapeutic engagement by resorting to more custodial models of care. Unless actions to address these wider system issues are taken, further investment in training and education may be unproductive. SUs expect and desire consistent relationships with MHNs who are equipped with both professional skills and the appropriate personal values to enable meaningful interactions. In order to achieve this, the environments, resourcing, and systems of care within which MHNs operate must be conducive to the meeting of SUs' needs.

Acknowledgements

We are grateful to the rest of the team who contributed to the original systematic review that forms the basis for this chapter: Professor Karina Lovell, Pamela Barnes, Dr Richard Gray, Dr Philip Keeley.

✛ References

Adam, R., Tilley, S., and Pollock, L. (2003). Person first: what people with enduring mental disorders value about community psychiatric nurses and CPN services. *Journal of Psychiatric and Mental Health Nursing* 10(2), 203–12.

Bailey, D. (1997). What is the way forward for a user-led approach to the delivery of mental health services in primary care? *Journal of Mental Health* 6(1), 101–5.

Baker, J. (2002). The service and illness experiences described by users of the Mood Swings network. *Journal of Mental Health* 11(4), 453–63.

Barker, P. (1998). The future of the theory of Interpersonal Relations? A personal reflection on Peplau's legacy. *Journal of Mental Health and Psychiatric Nursing* 5, 213–20.

Barker, P. J. and Reynolds, B. (1996). Rediscovering the proper focus of nursing: a critique of Gournay's position on nursing theory and models. *Journal of Psychiatric and Mental Health Nursing* 3, 75–80.

Barker, P., Jackson, S., and Stevenson, C. (1999). What are psychiatric nurses needed for? Developing a theory of essential nursing practice. *Journal of Psychiatric and Mental Health Nursing* 6(4), 273–82.

Barker, S. (2000). *Environmentally friendly? Patients' Views of Conditions on Psychiatric Wards.* London: MIND.

Bee, P., Playle, J. F., Lovell, K., Barnes, P., Gray, R., and Keeley, P. (2008). Service user views and expectations of UK-registered mental health nurses: a systematic review of empirical research. *International Journal of Nursing Studies* 45, 442–57.

Beech, P. and Norman, I. (1995). Patients' perceptions of the quality of psychiatric nursing care: findings from a small-scale descriptive study. *Journal of Clinical Nursing* 4(2), 117–23.

Blenkiron, P. and Hammill, C. (2003). What determines patients' satisfaction with their mental health care and quality of life? *Postgraduate Medical Journal* 79(932), 337–40.

Bonner, G., Lowe, R., and Rawcliffe, D. (2002). Trauma for all: a pilot study of the subjective experience of physical restraint for mental health inpatients and staff in the UK. (Effects of incidents leading to restraint on patients and staff and their relationship.) *Journal of Psychiatric and Mental Health Nursing* 9(4), 465–73.

Breeze, J. and Repper, J. (1998). Struggling for control: the care experiences of 'difficult' patients in mental health services. *Journal of Advanced Nursing* 28(6), 1301–11.

Briteen, N. (1998). Psychiatry, stigma and resistance. *British Medical Journal* 317, 763–4.

Buston, K. (2002). Adolescents with mental health problems: what do they say about health services? *Journal of Adolescence* 25(2), 231–42.

Callaghan, P., Eales, S., Coats, T., Bowers, L., and Bunker, J. (2002). Patient feedback on liaison mental health care in A&E. *Nursing Times* 98(21), 34–6.

Chiesa, M., Drahorad, C., and Longo, S. (2000). Early termination of treatment in personality disorder treated in a psychotherapy hospital. Quantitative and qualitative study. *British Journal of Psychiatry* 177, 107–11.

Coffey, M., Higgon, J., and Kinnear, J. (2004). 'Therapy as well as the tablets': an exploratory study of service users' views of community mental health nurses' (CMHNs) responses to hearing voices. *Journal of Psychiatric and Mental Health Nursing* 11, 435–44.

Cutting, P. and Henderson, C. (2002). Women's experiences of hospital admission. *Journal of Psychiatric and Mental Health Nursing* 9, 705–12.

Department of Health (1999). *National Service Framework (NSF) for Mental Health*. London: DH.

Department of Health (2000). *The NHS Plan. A Plan for Investment, a Plan for Reform*. London: DH.

Department of Health (2001). *Involving Patients and the Public in Healthcare: A Discussion Document*. London: DH.

Department of Health (2003). *Building on the Best Choice, Responsiveness and Equity in the NHS*. London: DH.

Department of Health (2004). *The Ten Essential Shared Capabilities. A Framework for the Whole of the Mental Health Workforce*. London: DH.

Department of Health (2006a). *From Values to Action: The Chief Nursing Officer's Review of Mental Health Nursing*. London: DH.

Department of Health (2006b). *Best Practice Competencies and Capabilities for Pre-Registration Mental Health Nurses in England: The Chief Nursing Officer's Review of Mental Health Nursing*. London: DH.

Edwards, K. (1995). A preliminary study of users' and nursing students' views of the role of the mental health nurse. *Journal of Advanced Nursing* 21(2), 222–9.

Edwards, K. (2000). Service users and mental health nursing. *Journal of Psychiatric and Mental Health Nursing* 7(6), 555–65.

Ford, K., Sweeney, J., and Farrington, A. (1999). User views of a regional secure unit—findings from a patient satisfaction survey. *International Journal of Psychiatric Nursing Research* 5(1), 526–41.

Godfrey, M. and Wistow, G. (1997). The user perspective on managing for health outcomes: the case of mental health. *Health and Social Care in the Community* 5(5), 325–32.

Goodwin, I., Holmes, G., Newnes, C., and Waltho, D. (1999). A qualitative analysis of the views of in-patient mental health service users. *Journal of Mental Health* 8(1), 43–54.

Gournay, K. (1995). Mental health nurses working purposefully with people with serious and enduring mental illness: an international perspective. *International Journal of Nursing Studies* 32, 341–52.

Hayward, M., Ockwell, C., and Bird, T. (2004). How well are we doing? *Mental Health Today* October, 25–8.

Healthcare Commission (2004). *Patient Survey Report—Mental Health*. London: Healthcare Commission.

Higgins, R., Hurst, K., and Wistow, G. (1999). Nursing acute psychiatric patients: a quantitative and qualitative study. *Journal of Advanced Nursing* 29(1), 52–63.

Hill, R., Hardy, P., and Shepherd, G. (1996). *Perspectives on Manic Depression: A Survey of the Manic Depression Fellowship*. London: Sainsbury Centre for Mental Health.

Hostick, T. and Newell, R. (2004). Concordance with community mental health appointments: service users' reasons for discontinuation. *Journal of Clinical Nursing* 13(7), 895–902.

Jones, S. and Mason, T. (2002). Quality of treatment following police detention of mentally disordered offenders. *Journal of Psychiatric and Mental Health Nursing* 9(1), 73–80.

Kai, J. and Crosland, A. (2001). Perspectives of people with enduring mental ill health from a community-based qualitative study. *British Journal of General Practice* 51, 730–6.

Lelliott, P., Beevor, A., Hogman, G., Hyslop, J., Lathlean, J., and Ward, M. (2001). Carers' and users' expectations of services—user version (CUES-U): a new instrument to measure the experience of users of mental health services. *British Journal of Psychiatry* 179, 67–72.

MacGabhann, L. (2000). Are nurses responding to the needs of patients in acute mental health care? *Mental Health and Learning Disabilities Care* 4(3), 85–8.

Macpherson, R., Summerfield, L., Haynes, R., Slade, M., and Foy, C. (2005). The use of carers' and users' expectations of services (CUES) in an epidemiological survey of need. *International Journal of Social Psychiatry* 51(1), 35–43.

McLaughlin, C. (1999). An exploration of psychiatric nurses' and patients' opinions regarding in-patient care for suicidal patients. *Journal of Advanced Nursing* 29(5), 1042–51.

Meddings, S. and Perkins, R. (1999). Service user perspectives on the 'rehabilitation team' and roles of professionals within it. *Journal of Mental Health* 8(1), 87–94.

Mental Health Foundation (2000). *Rosalinde Caplin Project on Eating Distress*. London: Mental Health Foundation.

MIND (2004). *Ward Watch: Mind's Campaign to Improve Hospital Conditions for Mental Health Patients*. London: MIND.

Noble, L., Douglas, B., and Newman, S. (1999). What do patients want and what do we know? A review of patients' requests of psychiatric services. *Acta Psychiatrica Scandinavica* 100(5), 321–7.

Noble, L., Douglas, B., and Newman, S. (2001). What do patients expect of psychiatric services? A systematic and critical review of empirical studies. *Social Science and Medicine* 52(7), 985–98.

Noble, L. and Douglas, B. (2004). What users and relatives want from mental health services. *Current Opinion in Psychiatry* 17(4), 289–96.

Parkman, S., Davies, S., Leese, M., Phelan, M., and Thornicroft, G. (1997). Ethnic differences in satisfaction with mental health services among representative people with psychosis in South London: PRISM Study 4. *British Journal of Psychiatry* 171, 260–4.

Pollock, K., Grime, J., Baker, E., and Mantala, K. (2004). Meeting the information needs of psychiatric inpatients: staff and patient perspectives. *Journal of Mental Health* 13(4), 389–401.

Powell, R., Single, H., and Lloyd, K. (1996). Focus groups in mental health research: enhancing the validity of user and provider questionnaires. *International Journal of Social Psychiatry* 42(3), 193–206.

Quirk, A. and Lelliott, P. (2001). What do we know about life on acute psychiatric wards in the UK? A review of the research evidence. *Social Science and Medicine* 53(12), 1565–74.

Reed, J., Cantley, C., Clarke, C., and Stanley, D. (2002). Services for younger people with dementia: problems with differentiating needs on the basis of age. *Dementia* 1(1), 95–112.

Repper, J. (2000). Adjusting the focus of mental health nursing: incorporating service users' experiences of recovery. *Journal of Mental Health* 9(6), 575–87.

Reynolds, W. (1988). The influence of clients' perceptions of the helping relationship in the development of an empathy scale. *Journal of Psychiatric and Mental Health Nursing* 1, 23–30.

Reynolds, W., Scott, B., and Jessiman, W. (1999). Empathy has not been measured in clients' terms or effectively taught. *Journal of Advanced Nursing* 30, 1177–85.

Rogers, A. and Pilgrim, D. (1994). Service users' views of psychiatric nurses. *British Journal of Nursing* 3(1), 13–26.

Rogers, A., Oliver, D., Bower, P., Lovell, K., and Richards, D. (2004). People's understandings of a primary care-based mental health self-help clinic. *Patient Education and Counseling* 53(1), 41–6.

Rose, D. (2001). *Users' Voices: The Perspectives of Mental Health Service Users on Community and Hospital Care*. London: Sainsbury Centre for Mental Health.

Rose, D. and Muijen, M. (1998). 24-hour nursed care: users' views. *Journal of Mental Health* 7(6), 603–10.

Rose, D., Ford, R., Lindley, P., and Gawith, L. (1998). *The KCW Mental Health Monitoring Users' Group. In Our Experience: User-Focused Monitoring of Mental*

Health Services in Kensington and Chelsea and Westminster Health Authority. London: Sainsbury Centre for Mental Health.

Ruggeri, M., Lasalvia, A., Dall'Angnola, R., et al. (2000). Development, internal consistency and reliability of the Verona Service Satisfaction Scale – European Version. *British Journal of Psychiatry* 1777(suppl 39), 41–8.

Sainsbury Centre for Mental Health (2002). *Breaking the Circles of Fear: A Review of the Relationship Between Mental Health Services and African and Caribbean Communities*. London: Sainsbury Centre for Mental Health.

Scottish Executive (2006). *Rights, Relationships and Recovery: The Report of the National Review of Mental Health Nursing in Scotland*. http://www.scotland.gov.uk/Resource/Doc/112046/0027278.pdf

Secker, J. and Harding, C. (2002). African and African Caribbean users' perceptions of inpatient services. *Journal of Psychiatric and Mental Health Nursing* 9, 161–7.

Shanley, E., Watson, G., and Cole, A. (2001). Survey of stakeholders' opinions of community psychiatric nursing services. *Australian and New Zealand Journal of Mental Health Nursing* 10(2), 77–86.

Shumway, M. (2003). Preference weights for cost–outcome analyses of schizophrenia treatments: comparison of four stakeholder groups. *Schizophrenia Bulletin* 29, 257–66.

Sloane, J. (1993). Offences and defences against patients: a psychoanalytic view of the borderline between empathic failure and malpractice. *Canadian Journal of Psychiatry* 38, 265–73.

Smith, S. (2002). Perceptions of service provision for clients who self-injure in the absence of expressed suicidal intent (views of staff and people who self-injure on existing mental health services). *Journal of Psychiatric and Mental Health Nursing* 9(5), 595–601.

Spence, M., Valentine, G., and Kettles, A. (1997). Residents' perceptions of staff attitudes and their care:

problem areas and improvements. *Psychiatric Care* 4(4), 150–6.

Street, C. (2004). In-patient mental health services for young people—changing to meet new needs? *Journal of the Royal Society for the Promotion of Health* 124(3), 115–18.

Swartz, M. S., Swanson, J. W., Ryan Wagner, H., Hannon, M. J., Burns, J., and Shumway, M. (2003). Assessment of four stakeholder groups' preferences concerning outpatient commitment for persons with schizophrenia. *American Journal of Psychiatry* 160, 1139–46.

Tyson, P., Ayton, A., Al Agib, A., Bowie, P., Worrall-Davies, A., and Mortimer, A. (2001). A comparison of the service satisfaction and intervention needs of patients with schizophrenia and their relatives. *International Journal of Psychiatry in Clinical Practice* 5(4), 263–71.

Valentine, G., Jamieson, B., Kettles, A., and Spence, M. (2003). Users' involvement in their care. A follow-up study. *Journal of Psychosocial Nursing and Mental Health Services* 41(4), 18–25.

Wakefield, P., Read, S., Firth, W., and Lindesay, J. (1998). Clients' perceptions of outcome following contact with a community mental health team. *Journal of Mental Health* 7(4), 375–84.

Warne, T. and Stark, S. (2004). Service users, metaphors and teamworking in mental health. *Journal of Psychiatric and Mental Health Nursing* 11(6), 654–61.

Watts, J. and Priebe, S. (2002). A phenomenological account of users' experiences of assertive community treatment. *Bioethics* 16(5), 439–54.

Williams, B., Cattell, D., Greenwood, M., LeFevre, S., Murray, I., and Thomas, P. (1999). Exploring 'person-centredness': user perspectives on a model of social psychiatry. *Health and Social Care in the Community* 7(6), 475–82.

Wood, D. and Pistrang, N. (2004). A safe place? Service users' experiences of an acute mental health ward. *Journal of Community and Applied Social Psychology* 14(1), 16–28.

3 Values-based mental health nursing practice

Linda Cooper

'Values are at least as important as evidence in human affairs. People do not love, or share, or go to war primarily on the basis of evidence. Whenever any thing matters to us we act first because of our values. By treating values as evidence, and by revealing otherwise unperceived differences in our values, we can create more harmony, understanding and balance in our world.'

Seedhouse (2006)

▼ Introduction

Everybody's values are different. Life experiences shape our personal values, which in turn often provide a driving force (or motivation) for our behaviour. Despite this, it can be difficult to explain your values to others. By creating opportunities to explore and identify your values, you can help to clarify them. This is as true for mental health service users and carers as it is for all those seeking to provide mental health care.

I start with these assumptions, in the hope that they will encourage you in your practice to explore and understand your own values and the values of those with whom you are working. Through the process of exploration, sometimes you may discover that service users, carers, or those seeking to support them—be they, for example, an advocate, social worker, mental health nurse, occupational therapist, doctor, or a manager of services—have similar values to you. There will be times, however, when you discover that the values of those involved in the care process are different and potentially in conflict. When this occurs you may wonder what to do for the best. As an accountable professional mental health nurse, working to a professional code of conduct, you will need to bring a number of skills to bear on the decision-making process. These skills include awareness, reasoning, knowledge, and, in order to embrace difference and resolve conflict, skills in communication, negotiation, and working in partnership respectfully, with all parties (Woodbridge and Fulford 2004).

To assist with this process, this chapter will help you to explore the following questions and key ideas:

- What are values?
- How to identify your personal values

- How to identify and respect the values of others
- Why are values important in helping professions?
- How to develop and apply values to mental health nursing practice
- How to identify and resolve a conflict of values.

In essence, this chapter is concerned with the first category of the *Best practice competencies and capabilities for pre-registration mental health nurses in England, the Chief Nursing Officer's review of mental health nursing:* Putting values into practice. This requires students, at the point of registration, to identify and demonstrate their understanding of the key values and principles, and to apply this values base 'to promote a culture that values and respects the diversity of individuals and enables their recovery' (Department of Health [DH] 2006b).

Learning outcomes

By the end of this chapter you should be better able to

1 Explain what **values-based practice** means in modern mental health and social care

2 Explain the relationship of values-based practice to the ten Essential Shared Capabilities for mental health practice

3 Promote a culture that values and respects diversity

4 Promote the health and recovery of those who use mental health services

5 Deliver care based on an integration of values *and* best evidence.

These learning outcomes link with standards espoused in three key Nursing and Midwifery Council (NMC) publications (NMC 2004a,b, 2007).

What are values?

The first question often asked is:

> What is the difference between ideals, morals, principles, ethics, and values?

Table 3.1 gives us a definition of each of these terms.

Identifying your personal values

Before exploring the meaning of values-based practice in mental health, it may be useful to reflect on **your personal understanding** of the term 'values', by completing the activity in Box 3.1, adapted from Woodbridge and Fulford (2004)—you can also do this online.

In health care, values are closely associated with ethics (Seedhouse 2005, Woodbridge and Fulford 2003). Personal values, however, often include your wishes, preferences, standards, beliefs, and principles that guide your life choices. To explore your values is to discover your priorities at a personal level. In so doing, you find out what is really important to you.

The concept of 'values' is complex; as can be seen in Table 3.2, it means different things to different people, so can be difficult to define. It might be argued that professional values are a set of professionally validated moral principles on which to base mental health (nursing) practice. Examples of validating

Box 3.1 Personal understanding of the term 'values'

1 Take five minutes to list all the words/phrases that you associate with values.

2 Compare your list with those in Table 3.2 and notice similarities and differences.

organizations might be a professional body (e.g. NMC) or governmental bodies (e.g. DH, Welsh Assembly Government, or Scottish Government). These provide codes or frameworks that inform our professional engagement with mental health users and carers. One might expect that users' and carers' values may differ from professional values, as they are based on the unique importance each individual user (or carer) attaches to their personal wishes, desires, thoughts, feelings, needs, behaviour, and relationships.

In this context, 'values-based practice' involves professionals, users, and carers working together respectfully, to explore and understand personal values, resolve conflicts, and implement (where at all possible) agreed action(s).

Fulford (2004, p. 16) offers a definition of values-based practice as '*the theory and skills base for effective health care decision making where different (and hence potentially conflicting) values are in play*'. His definition invites the question:

> What is the theory and skills base for modern mental health nursing practice?

Table 3.1 Definitions (adapted from the *Oxford Dictionary of English* 2007)

Concept	Definition
Ideal	A concept or a thing as a standard for imitation
Morals	Concerned with the goodness or badness of human character or behaviour; distinguishing between right and wrong
Principle	Fundamental truth, or law, that forms the basis for reasoning or action. These can be formed from a collection of moral or ethical standards. Principles often underpin a policy or a personal code of conduct
Ethics	A set of moral principles
Value	The worth, desirability, importance, or emotional investment (either for or against) we attach to something

Table 3.2 Lists of word/phrases associated with values written by people with different perspectives of mental health (from Woodbridge and Fulford 2004, p. 14)

LIST 1 Delegates at a recovery conference	LIST 2 Trainee psychiatrists	LIST 3 Managers/Chief executives
Core beliefs	Concepts which govern ethics	What you believe in
Your perspective on the world	Right and wrong	Self-esteem
Principles—cultural, individual	Belief systems	Principles
Justice	Ideals and priorities	Integrity
Anything that's valued	Govern behaviour and decisions	Openness/honesty
Integral to being human	Community health—individuals, society, culture	Personal motivating force
Quality of life	Ideals	Primary reference point
Right to be heard	Morals	Ethics
Social values	Principles	Virtues
Self-respect	Standards	Sharing
Valuing neighbours	Conscience	Touchstones/bases
	Fluid/changeable	Willing to sacrifice for self-interested tenets

The evidence base

Policy that supports putting values into mental health practice

In the four countries of the UK, the policy context for putting values into practice is clearly in place. Taking forward the standards in the National Service Framework (NSF) for Mental Health (DH 1999), the National Institute for Mental Health in England developed its Values Framework (NIMHE et al. 2004) and Ten Essential Shared Capabilities for Mental Health Practice (DH 2004, NIMHE et al. 2004).

The NIMHE Values Framework is underpinned by three principles of values-based practice seen in Box 3.2.

Having established the principles, NIMHE set out ten essential shared capabilities for all professionals working in mental health care. The key essential shared capabilities for mental

health practice that specifically prescribe a professional value are shown in Table 3.3.

The evolution of a values base for mental health nursing practice

Mental health nursing has a history and character quite different from that of general/adult nursing. Peter Nolan (1993) reminds us that it has its origins in the asylum system, where the predecessors of today's nurses were first called 'keepers', then 'attendants', and had nothing much to do with organized, professional nursing at all.

Commissioned reviews of mental health nursing provide significant markers in the history of the profession. There have been three reviews of mental health nursing in England in the past 50 years. Following devolution in the UK, the Scottish Executive (2006a) and the Northern Ireland Government

Box 3.2 The three principles of the NIMHE Values Framework

1 **Recognition:** NIMHE recognises the role of values alongside evidence in all areas of mental health policy and practice.

2 **Raising awareness:** NIMHE is committed to raising awareness of the values involved in different contexts, the role/s they play and their impact on practice in mental health.

3 **Respect:** NIMHE respects diversity of values and will support ways of working with such diversity that makes the principle of service user centrality a unifying focus for practice. This means that the values of each individual service user/client and their communities must be the starting point and key determinant for all actions by professionals.

From NIMHE et al. (2004)

(2006) also published reviews of mental health nursing. At the time of writing, Wales is undertaking a 'mental health nursing stock-take'. Examination of these reviews gives a history, context, and understanding to the evolution of a values base for mental health nursing.

In 1968, the Ministry of Health published *Psychiatric Nursing: Today and Tomorrow*. The professional aspirations of mental health nursing are often underpinned by the claim that nurses possess an occupationally distinct constellation of knowledge and skills related to the formation and maintenance of helpful interpersonal relations with people experiencing psychological distress. This claim, and the idea that nurses exercise this particular set of skills and knowledge in the context of their everyday interactions (as opposed to, for example, the context of formal therapy), also underpins much mental health nursing theory, including that associated with the post-war North American nurse, Hildegard Peplau. In a report that is otherwise notable for its lack of reference to either theory or research, it is significant that reference is made to her work, which focuses on the primacy of the therapeutic relationship between the nurse and the service user (Peplau 1952).

Some 26 years later, *Working in Partnership: A Collaborative Approach to Care* (Mental Health Nursing Review Team 1994) was commissioned by the then Secretary of State for Health, chaired by Professor Tony Butterworth of Manchester

Table 3.3 Linking the values framework with specific Essential Shared Capabilities (ESC) for mental health practice (Department of Health 2004)

Respecting diversity	ESC 2
Working in partnership with service users, carers, families, and colleagues to provide care and interventions that not only make a positive difference but also do so in ways that respect and value diversity, including age, race, culture, disability, gender, spirituality, and sexuality	
Practising ethically	ESC 3
Recognizing the rights and aspirations of service users and their families, acknowledging power differentials and minimizing them whenever possible. Providing treatment and care that is accountable to service users and carers within the boundaries prescribed by national (professional), legal, and local codes of ethical practice	
Challenging inequality	ESC 4
Addressing the causes and consequences of stigma, discrimination, social inequality, and exclusion on service users, carers, and mental health services. Creating, developing, or maintaining valued social roles for people in the communities they come from	
Promoting recovery	ESC 5
Working in partnership to provide care and treatment that enables service users and carers to tackle mental health problems with hope and optimism, and to work towards a valued lifestyle within and beyond the limits of any mental health problem	

University, UK. Forty-two recommendations were made, which suggests that the review team were of the opinion that much had to be done to place mental health nursing on a surer footing. At the start of their report, the Working in Partnership team declared (p. 9) their:

> 'belief that the work of mental health nurses rests on their relationship with people who use mental health services'.

Both the 1968 and 1994 reviews advanced the claim that the particular value of mental health nursing rests on the capacity of its practitioners to form and maintain helpful relationships with the people for whom they care. Like its predecessor, *Working in Partnership* draws attention to the value of nurses' use of interpersonal skills to forge helpful therapeutic relationships, but in addition challenges the profession to:

> 're-examine every aspect of its policy and practice in the light of the needs of people who use services'.

This 're-examination' should involve nurses: forging more equal and collaborative relationships with service users; working more effectively as team members; paying greater attention to the importance of care provision for ethnicity, gender, and sexuality; and paying additional attention to the needs of marginalized and poorly served groups including older people and children, the homeless, and those living with HIV/AIDS.

Working in Partnership is particularly strong on the skills expected of mental health nurses; this is not surprising, as at the time of its publication a common criticism was that many nurses lacked the practical ability to provide effective care and treatment for people with severe mental health problems (White 1993). 'Values' get a mention, but are not considered in a systematic way. Thus, the report stated (p. 17) that:

> 'it is the combination of these particular skills, together with the values and practice common to the nursing profession as a whole, which provides the unique expertise of mental health nurses'.

Surprisingly (in the light of current thinking), these values were not made explicit.

The recent Chief Nursing Officer's review of mental health nursing in England, *From Values to Action* (DH 2006a), and the Scottish Review of Mental Health Nursing, *Rights, Relationships and Recovery* (Scottish Executive 2006a), both emphasize the important role of values in mental health nursing.

'Values' now seem to be a standard part of the lexicon of authors of professional reviews, and not just the authors of this most recent review of mental health nursing. The words 'value', 'values', 'valued', and 'value-based', for example, appear together in the recent reviews of the work of psychiatrists (Royal College of Psychiatrists et al. 2005) and a review of social work services in Scotland (Scottish Executive 2006b).

Recovery approach: values and principles

The idea of 'recovery' from mental illness has gained significant ground in recent years (Repper and Perkins 2003). Recovery refers to more than obtaining relief from distressing symptoms; rather, the modern usage of recovery has come to mean a broadly based, positive approach to care, which includes the promotion of social inclusion, citizenship, choice, and hope. Deegan (1988, p. 136), a service user, captures the essence of recovery values:

> 'The role of recovery is not to become normal. The goal is to embrace the human vocation of becoming more deeply, more fully human'.

This stance suggests that professional mental health nursing practice is about supporting and empowering the service user to become 'the architect of their own recovery'. To facilitate this process with congruence, you, as the practitioner, have to believe (and convey the belief to others) that recovery, through self-management, is possible. Rethink, a UK mental health charity, gives us a clear sense of what self-management means to service users:

> 'Self management is something we all do. It is whatever we do to make the most of our lives by coping with our difficulties and making the most of what we have. Applied specifically to people with a schizophrenia diagnosis, it includes the ways we cope with, or manage, or minimise the ways the condition limits our lives, as well as what we do to thrive, to feel happy and fulfilled, to make the most of our lives despite the condition.'

> Martyn 2002, p.3

Valuing the principle of equality

In order to facilitate recovery in a values-based approach to mental health nursing practice, we must pursue the value pursuit of equality. From a policy point of view, this figured strongly in the recent Chief Nursing Officer's review *From Values to Action* (DH 2006a), and represents a continuation from *Working in Partnership* (Mental Health Nursing Review Team 1994), which also recognized the need for mental health practitioners and services to adopt more sophisticated and sensitive approaches to meeting the needs of *all* sections of the community.

Valuing the principle of evidence-based practice

It is of central importance that mental health nurses should ground their activities in knowledge of 'what works'. Evidence-based practice is widely thought to be solely about evidence derived from clinical research trials. It is not. You can read more about evidence-based practice in Chapter 4 of this book. Sackett et al. (2000, p. 6), writing about 'evidence-based medicine', define it as the integration of best research evidence *with* clinical judgement *and* patient values:

> '*By patient values we mean the unique preferences, concerns and expectations each patient brings to a clinical encounter and which must be integrated into clinical decisions if they are to serve the patient*'.

It is noteworthy that medical colleagues affirm the principle of bringing both an evidence *and* a values base to bear on your practice. Woodbridge and Fulford (2004) call this applying the 'two feet' principle—the idea being that care decisions are more grounded if both 'feet' (the one foot being values and the other evidence) are used to strengthen the reasoning underpinning the care stance proposed. If this principle is not applied in practice, care based on 'values without evidence' could be viewed as resulting from solely subjective or intuitive clinical decisions, whereas care based on 'evidence without values' could result in an objectively 'right' care intervention that lacks empathy or consideration of the service user's rights, relationships, and choices regarding the perceived impact the proposed 'evidence-based' care might have on their quality of life and recovery.

Box 3.3 Key areas to improve users' and carers' experience of mental health services (adapted from Thurgood 2004)

Values and relationship-building interventions of workers
- A needs-led, client-centred approach
- Flexibility, responsiveness, and creativity
- Optimism and hope—viewing clients positively
- Perseverance, patience, and realism
- Seeing the client as an expert and being willing to compromise and negotiate
- Advocacy and challenging oppressive practice
- Positive risk-taking
- Choice and the sharing of good information
- Cultural sensitivity and anti-discriminatory practice
- Honesty, genuineness, trust, and respect

Values and organization of service to support the values and relationship-building interventions of workers
- Commitment to engagement
- Service users' involvement
- Effective teamwork
- Staff support and development
- Leadership
- Joint working across agencies
- Resources

Skills to improve the service user experience

Thurgood (2004) notes that the values and relationship-building interventions of workers need to inform, and be informed by, the values and organization of the service to support these interventions, the implication being that service models adopted by organizations need to actively promote key areas in order to improve the users' and/or carers' experience of mental health services (Box 3.3).

The Sainsbury Centre for Mental Health has published an excellent workbook for values-based practice in mental health care, entitled *Whose Values?* (Woodbridge and Fulford 2004). The workbook is highly recommended as a supplementary learning tool, as it is practical, skills-focused, and uses examples of service user experience to support your further development. The practice example in Box 3.6 is taken from this workbook. A commentary is provided on care given, using the authors' ten indicators (or pointers) of values-based practice in mental health care. The skills and pointers are listed in Boxes 3.4 and 3.5. Intentional use (Egan 2006) of these skills (or pointers) is required of the mental health nurse who is seeking to ensure that values underpin practice.

Box 3.4 Skills required of a values-based practitioner: the first four pointers

1 *Awareness*: of the values present in a given situation. This is an essential first step. Careful attention to language is one way of raising awareness of values.

2 *Reasoning*: using a clear reasoning process to explore the values present when making decisions.

3 *Knowledge*: of the values and facts relevant to the specific situation.

4 *Communication*: combined with the previous three skills, this is central to the resolution of conflicts and the decision-making process.

From Woodbridge and Fulford (2004, p. 20), with kind permission from the Sainsbury Centre for Mental Health

Box 3.5 Pointers of good process in values-based practice

5 *User-centred:* The first source for information on values in any situation is the perspective of the service user concerned.

6 *Multidisciplinary:* Conflicts of values are resolved in values-based practice not by applying a 'pre-prescribed rule' but by working towards a balance of different perspectives (e.g. multidisciplinary team working).

7 *The 'two feet' principle*: All decisions are based on facts and values (evidence and values working together).

8 *The 'squeaky wheel' principle*: We only notice values when there is a problem.

9 *Science and values*: Increasing scientific knowledge creates choices in health care, which introduces wide differences in values.

10 *Partnership*: In values-based practice decisions are taken by service users and the providers of care working in partnership.

From Woodbridge and Fulford (2004, p. 20), with kind permission from the Sainsbury Centre for Mental Health

✖ Practice Example

John: Part 1

> **Box 3.6** Starting with evidence as a basis for practice
>
> *John's experience*
>
> *John is an 18-year-old man who has recently been diagnosed as having schizophrenia by a local psychiatrist. John started experiencing psychotic symptoms from the age of 14 years and has been seen by a psychiatric service which works across child and adult care. His mother, Maggie, has been referred by her GP to the practice counsellor as he believes Maggie is depressed. John's father, Malcolm, has told his wife he wants to move out of the family home. John is an only child. John's community psychiatric nurse (CPN) has invited Maggie and Malcolm on two occasions to a group meeting for carers of people who have a diagnosis of schizophrenia. The meetings are intended to be both educational and supportive. John's parents have not attended on either occasion.*
>
> From Woodbridge and Fulford (2004, p. 86), with kind permission from the Sainsbury Centre for Mental Health

The research and policy evidence base would suggest that family work (involving Malcolm, Maggie, *and John*) would be more likely to be successful in this situation. The National Institute for Clinical Excellence (NICE 2002) guidance for schizophrenia indicates that there is strong evidence that family work reduces relapse rates during treatment, and for up to 15 months after treatment has ended. The benefits are maximized if the family meets for more than ten planned sessions over at least a six-month period.

The mental health nurse who knows this evidence (and works within an organization whose service model promotes family work in psychosis) is more likely to recommend this intervention to John and his family. It is important that, wherever possible, care is recommended and explored with (rather than imposed on) service users; otherwise it may not be perceived by the service user as having positive meaning for their recovery. Unless there is a shared commitment (between the user and those prescribing health

and social care) regarding the purpose of a care intervention, it is difficult for the service user to feel motivated to engage with the intervention.

> **Box 3.7** Bringing together evidence with values-based practice
>
> *It is a few months later and John has received a visit from the CPN.*
>
> *John was a grade-A student and did well in GCSEs. He was expecting to do well in A levels but over the last year he has found it increasingly difficult to concentrate. He has found out that, after discussions between his teacher and his parents, he is to be moved to a college to study on a course with people with special needs.*
>
> *John hasn't been sleeping very well, and says he has intrusive images of torture and death during the night. He says no one is listening to him and he is desperate for help. His parents are distressed by his behaviour and feel helpless. John recently smashed a pane of glass in his bedroom door with his head during the night.*
>
> *John's mother is tearful during the interview and she mentions that John's father is temporarily moving out of the house.*
>
> *John's care plan includes risk assessment; antipsychotic medication with night sedation when necessary; and a referral for social skills training. John's CPN will visit again next week to monitor his progress. John's mother has been prescribed antidepressant medication.*
>
> From Woodbridge and Fulford (2004, p. 87), with kind permission from the Sainsbury Centre for Mental Health

John: Part 2

The authors pose the questions: what is being valued in this care plan *and* what meaning does it have for John?

From a values perspective these are important questions. It is desirable to be curious about practice as this process can reveal the negative impact (often unintentional, but nevertheless un-thought through) that some care can have on users and carers. It seems that medical intervention, with the hope of a reduction of symptoms (and thereby risk), is being valued in John's care plan. You do not know, however, whether these are John's primary concerns. It is also notable that he has been excluded from most decisions that affect him. Examples from the account include: the move to a special needs school; the invitation by the CPN to his parents (not John) to attend appointments to discuss the experience of mental distress in the family; the commencement of antipsychotic medication; and the referral to social skills training. These decisions appear to be based on the values of his parents and involved professionals (in this example, teachers, psychiatrist, and CPN).

It would be reasonable (and compassionate) to assume that all these events will have given rise to concerns that John needs to express. Furthermore, these changes require John to make major adjustments to his life and identity. As a mental health nurse who believes in the value of user-centred care, you may find yourself wondering: *what are John's values?* We do not know, because the approach taken in Part 2 is not user-centred.

Table 3.4 Applying the ten pointers of values-based practice to John's experience

Values-based practice: 10 pointers	Does this apply?	Evident in John's care?	What was evident in John's care?	Why is it important to base John's care on key values?
1. Awareness	Yes	No	It is questionable whether those involved in John's care were aware that their values dominated.	Once the mental health nurse is aware of the values present in a situation, she or he can choose to redress the balance and explore John's needs and concerns (and thereby discover his values).
2. Reasoning	Yes	No	Values are not explored. Decisions are made on the assumption that others know what is best for John. He is then expected to be compliant.	If values of all parties were transparent, this could form a basis on which to discuss with John the benefits and costs to him of a proposed intervention.
3. Knowledge	Yes	Yes	The evidence base for family intervention (NICE 2002) may have been known, but other values, traditions, or service models dominated the care.	Knowledge of the evidence base for family intervention (or its inclusion in a care pathway) may enable a mental health nurse to discuss the benefits, and explore concerns, with the family.

»

Table 3.4 Continued

4. Communication	Yes	No	Communication with John appears to be minimal. Prescriptive (practitioner-centred) interactions dominate over facilitative (user-centred) interactions (Heron 2001).	Drawing on pointers 1, 2, and 3, the mental health nurse can ask John what he wants to achieve, explore his concerns, and in so doing establish his priorities and work towards agreeing a plan of care.
5. User-centred	Yes	No	The care plan was not user-centred. The danger is that this conveys a negative message to John.	If John had been involved from the beginning, a whole different set of possibilities may have been discovered. Respecting and engaging with John will give a positive message.
6. Multidisciplinary	Yes	Yes	Psychiatrist, CPN, and teachers involved but no evidence of their discussing John's care with one another. This process may have revealed and resolved differences in values.	Active multidisciplinary working would facilitate a thoughtful consideration of the whole package of care and the psychosocial impact on John.
7. 'Two feet'	Yes	No	Care decisions appear to be based on facts and pre-prescribed rules regarding the appropriate care response. There is little awareness of the values operating in this situation and their impact on John.	Care based on evidence without regard to John's values is unbalanced and likely to be ineffective.
8. 'Squeaky wheel'	Yes	Yes	John feels desperate (hence the smashed window pane) that no one is listening to him.	He needs to feel others are hearing his desperation and doing something that he agrees to try or finds helpful.
9. Science and values	Yes	No	John's right to a choice has been ignored.	The key here is John's choice.
10. Partnership	Yes	No	Service providers have dominated John's care.	Service providers need to take the lead in working with John and his family, and support them in identifying goals and coping strategies.

Conclusion

Modern mental health nursing promotes **evidence and values** to inform service models, delivery, practice, and education. Values are embodied in the Ten Essential Shared Capabilities for the Whole of the Mental Health Workforce. These have been strengthened and emphasized by recent mental health nursing reviews and the development of good practice competencies for pre-registration mental health nurses in England and Scotland.

Building on these principles, in consultation with service users, NHS Education for Scotland (2007) has led a consultation on *A National Framework for Pre-Registration Nursing Programmes in Scotland*. This new framework represents a further development of the values in the English and Scottish reviews in that it has a strong emphasis on implementing the core values of rights and recovery underpinned by collaborative relationships with service users and carers based on best available evidence. Meanwhile, in conjunction with *Modernising Nursing Careers* (Department of Health 2006c), the NMC (2007) is undertaking a branch review of pre-registration nursing in which options such as generalist nursing and/or specialist mental health pre-registration programmes are being considered for implementation in 2015. This presents both a challenge and an opportunity for change. Whatever the outcome of these consultations, it is vital that pre-registration education continues to provide nurses with the capabilities to improve practice, standards, and outcomes for mental health service users and carers driven by evidence and values-based approaches. Applying the ten pointers of values-based practice in your work with service users and their carers should enable you to deliver the care that people need and want, and that promotes their recovery.

Acknowledgements

We wish to thank the Sainsbury Centre for Mental Health for permission to reproduce case studies and to adapt material from their excellent workbook by Kim Woodbridge and Bill Fulford (2004) *Whose Values? A Workbook for Values-based Practice in Mental Health Care* in Chapter 3.

We are also grateful to Ben Hannigan for sharing work he has undertaken as part of the Values Group at Cardiff University, for use in Chapter 3.

Website

You may find it helpful to work through our short online quiz and scenario intended to help you to develop and apply the skills in this chapter. These can be found at our online Resource centre:

www.oxfordtextbooks.co.uk/orc/callaghan

References

Deegan, P. E. (1988). Recovery: the lived experience of rehabilitation. *Psychosocial Rehabilitation Journal* 11, 136–8.

Department of Health (1999). *National Service Framework for Mental Health: Modern Standards and Service Models*. London: DH.

Department of Health (2004). *The Ten Essential Shared Capabilities. A Framework for the Whole of the Mental Health Workforce*. London: DH.

Department of Health (2006a). *From Values to Action: The Chief Nursing Officer's Review of Mental Health Nursing*. London: DH.

Department of Health (2006b). *Best Practice Competencies and Capabilities for Pre-registration Mental Health Nurses in England: The Chief Nursing Officer's Review of Mental Health Nursing*. London: DH.

Department of Health (2006c). *Modernising Nursing Careers—Setting the Direction*. London: DH.

Egan, G. (2006). *The Skilled Helper: A Problem Management and Opportunity Development Approach*. Belmont, CA: Brooks/Cole.

Fulford, K. W. M. (2004). Ten principles of values-based medicine. In: *The Philosophy of Psychiatry: A*

Companion (ed. J. Radden), pp 205–36. New York: Oxford University Press.

Heron, J. (2001). *Helping the Client: A Creative and Practical Guide*. London: Sage.

Martyn, D. (2002). The Experience and Views of Self-management of People with a Schizophrenia Diagnosis. London: Rethink. http://www.rethink.org/recovery/self-management [accessed 11 Nov 2007].

Mental Health Nursing Review Team (1994). *Working in Partnership: A Collaborative Approach to Care*. London: HMSO.

Ministry of Health (1968). *Psychiatric Nursing: Today and Tomorrow*. London: HMSO.

National Institute for Clinical Excellence (2002). *Schizophrenia: Core Interventions in the Treatment and Management of Schizophrenia in Primary and Secondary Care*. London: NICE.

National Institute for Mental Health in England, Sainsbury Centre for Mental Health, and the National Health Service University (2004). The national framework of values for mental health. In: *The Ten Essential Shared Capabilities. A Framework for the Whole of the Mental Health Workforce*. London: DH.

NHS Education for Scotland (2007). *A National Framework for Pre-Registration Nursing Programmes in Scotland. Vol. 1 & 2 Draft for Consultation*. Edinburgh: NES.

Nolan, P. (1993). *A History of Mental Health Nursing*. London: Chapman and Hall.

Northern Ireland Government (2006). *The Bamford Review of Mental Health and Learning Disability Services in Northern Ireland*. Belfast: NIG.

Nursing and Midwifery Council (2004a). *The NMC Code of Professional Conduct: Standards for Conduct, Performance and Ethics*. London: NMC.

Nursing and Midwifery Council (2004b). *Standards of Proficiency for Pre-registration Nursing Education*. London: NMC.

Nursing and Midwifery Council (2007). *Essential Skills Clusters (ESCs) for Pre-registration Nursing Programmes*. London: NMC.

Oxford Dictionary of English (2007). Oxford: Oxford University Press.

Peplau, H. (1952). *Interpersonal Relations in Nursing*. New York: G. P. Putnam.

Repper, J. and Perkins, R. (2003). *Social Inclusion and Recovery: A Model for Mental Health Practice*. Edinburgh: Baillière Tindall.

Royal College of Psychiatrists, National Institute for Mental Health in England, and Modernisation Agency Changing Workforce Programme (2005). *New Ways of Working for Psychiatrists: Enhancing Effective, Person-centred Services Through New Ways of Working in Multidisciplinary and Multi-agency Contexts. Final Report 'but not the end of the story'*. London: Department of Health.

Sackett, D. L., Staus, S. E., Scott Richardson, W., Rosenburg, W., and Hayes, R. B. (2000). *Evidence-based Medicine: How to Practice and Teach EBM*. Edinburgh: Churchill Livingstone.

Scottish Executive (2006a). *Rights, Relationships and Recovery: The Report of the National Review of Mental Health Nursing in Scotland*. Edinburgh: Scottish Executive.

Scottish Executive (2006b). *Changing Lives: Report of the 21st Century Social Work Review*. Edinburgh: Scottish Executive.

Seedhouse, D. (2005). *Values-based Decision Making for the Caring Profession*. Chichester: Wiley.

Seedhouse, D. (2006). http://www.vide.co.nz/personal.asp [accessed 3 Jan 2008].

Thurgood, M. (2004). Engaging clients in their care and treatment. In: *The Art and Science of Mental Health Nursing: A Textbook of Principles and Practice* (ed. I. J. Norman and I. Ryrie), pp 655–9. London: Open University Press.

White, E. (1993). Community psychiatric nursing 1980 to 1990: a review of organization, education and practice. In: *Community Psychiatric Nursing: A Research Perspective* Vol. 2 (ed. C. Brooker and E. White), pp 1–26. London: Chapman and Hall.

Woodbridge, K. and Fulford, K. W. M. (2003). Good practice? Values-based practice in mental health. *Mental Health Practice* 7(2), 30–4.

Woodbridge, K. and Fulford, K. W. M. (2004). *Whose Values? A Workbook for Values-based Practice in Mental Health Care*. London: Sainsbury Centre for Mental Health.

Evidence-based mental health nursing practice

Patrick Callaghan   Paul Crawford

▼ Introduction

This chapter is concerned with the second category of Best Practice Competencies and Capabilities for Pre-registration Mental Health Nurses in England (Department of Health 2006), that of **improving outcomes for service users**. This requires students at the point of registration to demonstrate their understanding of the principles of research and their application to the evidence base for practice, and to show that they can assess, plan, implement, and evaluate evidence-based care under supervision.

During the Qing dynasty in eighteenth century China, several scholars developed an interest in gaining knowledge from a type of methodology that they called *kaozheng*. This has been translated as 'practising evidential research', and was based on painstaking evaluation of data according to high standards of rigour and precision. The aim of *kaozheng* scholars was to base their studies not on speculation, but in hard facts (Spence 1991). This is an early example of the philosophy driving much **evidence-based practice** (EBP) today.

The use of informed, up-to-date, high-quality evidence underlies every nursing interaction. Mental health nurses are increasingly called to account for their own practice in terms of evidence, and students need to master the skills of evaluating published **evidence** and guidelines, understanding the research process, and utilizing these to deliver best practice. The concept of the individual as a self-governing entity responsible for his or her own education, development, and EBP is central to a number of initiatives that promote quality of care and service delivery, especially Clinical Governance (Brown and Crawford 2003). EBP has been embraced by health services as the antidote to ritualistic and 'outdated' practice, inappropriate variations in care delivery, and ineffective and wasteful service provision.

In this chapter we will describe the origins of EBP, examine contested issues about EBP, and show you how to evaluate published evidence.

Learning outcomes

By the end of this chapter you should be better able to:

1 Demonstrate an understanding of the origins of evidence-based practice

2 Describe the contested issues about evidence-based practice

3 Evaluate published evidence

4 Demonstrate your critiquing skills in academic work

5 Use evidence in practice.

What is evidence-based practice?

In beginning to identify criteria against which to evaluate published evidence, you need to appreciate that there are two main models (or paradigms) for gaining knowledge of the world: **positivism or quantitative research,** and **interpretivism or quantifiable research**. Positivism seeks to establish universal laws and views knowledge as reducible to observable positive facts and numbers and the relations between them—it goes forth and quantifies (numbers-based research). Interpretivism seeks to understand the social world as actively constructed by human beings who are continuously making sense of or interpreting our social environments—it goes forth and qualifies (words-based research) (Brown et al. 2003).

Adopting one or other of these approaches, or combining them, shapes how we go about gathering knowledge. The choice taken by researchers will say something about their values and beliefs about the nature and utility of evidence. Unfortunately, over many years there have been heated debates about which is the best kind of research and what constitutes valid 'evidence' (Crawford et al. 2002), and objections have been raised to hierarchies of evidence. Indeed, many practitioners have complained that EBP demotes the evidence of clinical experience, or what has been called practice-based evidence (PBE), or 'overrules' the preferences of clients and patients.

Research then is not a single, straightforward entity—it is a competitive field in which particular accounts of 'what is what', 'what causes what', or 'what relates to what' are contested and preferred. Furthermore, the continuum of confidence in research can run from the idea that we can build knowledge 'upon a set of firm, unquestionable…indisputable truths' (Hughes and Sharrock 1997)—so-called foundationalism—to an emphasis of the provisional nature of knowledge or, indeed, the impossibility of arriving at any truths at all—so-called anti-foundationalism. In beginning to critique research, a key starting point is to identify the underlying paradigm of any given study and to be aware of the researcher's 'take' on, or 'framing' of, evidence. This requires 'philosophy' skills from the student, identifying the kinds of thinking and wisdom behind attempts to gain knowledge of the world.

There is considerable variation in how the concept of EBP is defined and described (e.g. Coyler and Kamath 1999, McKenna et al. 2000). However, a useful definition that captures the range of views is shown in Box 4.1. The pursuit of EBP comprises several components, which are shown in Box 4.2.

Gray (1997) argues that patient care decisions are based on evidence, values, and resources. He goes on to state that the optimum use of resources will be evidence based. According to Gray (1997), the evidence-based decision-maker requires several skills, as shown in Box 4.3.

In assessing the quality of any evidence, Gray suggests the following helpful questions:

1 Is this the best type of research method to address the question?

2 Is the research of adequate quality?

3 What is the size of the beneficial effect and of the adverse effect?

Box 4.1 Definition of evidence-based practice

'Evidence-Based Practice is the process by which nurses make clinical decisions using the best available research evidence, their clinical expertise and patient preferences, in the context of available resources.'

DiCenso et al. (1998, p. 38)

Box 4.2 The components of evidence-based practice (von Degenberg 1996)

- Clinical guidelines
- Patient and public choice
- Information on epidemiology
- Success or failure of certain interventions
- Evidence-based purchasing, reflecting audit outcomes and performance measures
- Health service management
- Organizational audit
- Financial audit and guidelines
- Education and training
- Curricula based on best available evidence

Box 4.3 Skills required of an evidence-based decision-maker

- An ability to define criteria such as effectiveness, safety, and acceptability
- An ability to find articles on the effectiveness, safety, and acceptability of a new test or treatment
- An ability to assess the quality of evidence
- An ability to assess whether the results of research are generalizable to the whole population from which the sample was drawn
- An ability to assess whether the results of the research are applicable to a 'local' population

Gray (1997, p.2)

---

4 Is the research generalizable to the whole population from which the sample was drawn?

5 Are the results applicable to a 'local' population?

6 Are the results applicable to this patient?

However, answering these questions requires a sound understanding of how to evaluate published evidence. We will now move on to this issue. It is not possible here to review all the arguments and counter-arguments about the philosophical 'seeding' of research or what stands as 'best' evidence (see Brown et al. [2003] for a wide-reaching analysis), but rather to adopt a fairly mainstream position in presenting foundational skills in evaluating or 'critiquing' evidence. To do this we will indicate how to judge both the quantitative and qualitative evidence that is put before us or we seek out.

Critiquing or judging research

There are two main approaches to critiquing research: individual and collegial. Individual critiquing is when a student or practitioner independently reviews published research papers, whereas collegial critiquing is conducted by groups of reviewers working together. The latter has evolved in response to the daunting task of reviewing large amounts of research and the need to facilitate practitioners in using research findings as part of EBP. Collegial critiquing can be formal and programmatic, as with the Cochrane Collaboration, the Centre for Reviews and Dissemination at York University, and through bodies such as the Department of Health and Royal College of Nursing, which produce guidelines for practice based on best available evidence. But collegial critiquing can also be informal and involve groups of practitioners joining forces to review and evaluate research relevant to their own area of clinical practice.

Whether you take an individual or informal, collegial approach, the skills of 'critiquing' can begin only when the student/practitioner or group of students/practitioners have developed sufficient knowledge of the research process itself. Even then, such skills are generally developed over time and through regular practice. With sufficient background knowledge and comprehension, a series of questions can be applied to any piece of research, rather as evidence may be examined in a courtroom context. The correct questions should elicit the strengths and weaknesses of the research; assess how such research relates to professional or clinical practice; and discriminate or differentiate between quantitative and qualitative research as part of the 'philosophy' skills outlined above previously.

Evaluation is concerned with examining each of the key components to research papers and 'making a value judgement on what is reported' or 'weighing what was done against accepted practice by researchers' (Parahoo 2006). The components that need to be 'weighed' are as follows: abstract; research question; literature review; methodology; sample; data collection; data analysis; results; discussion; and recommendations for practice or further research.

In Box 4.4 we now consider the kinds of questions that we may skilfully deploy for each of these categories in making a general critique of any research paper, before going on to look specifically at **quantitative** and **qualitative** research.

Box 4.4 General tips on evaluating published research-based evidence

Abstract

Does the abstract provide a clear summary of the research paper, including the research question and methods applied?

Are the key findings and the conclusions stated?

Research question

Does the research paper identify a question or hypothesis?

Is the question or hypothesis followed through into the conclusion?

Were the chosen methods appropriate to the question at hand?

Literature review

Is the literature comprehensive and up-to-date?

Are gaps in the literature identified?

Does the literature review support the case for further research?

Methodology

Does the research paper indicate the research approach it is taking?

How relevant is the methodological framing of the research?

Are the best methods applied to answer the research question?

Sample

Is the sample size included?

Is the sample size appropriate to the aims of the research?

Are the characteristics of the sample described?

Is the response rate stated?

Data collection

What method was used to collect data?

What is the validity and reliability of the method?

Data analysis

Does the research paper state how the data were analysed?

Were these methods appropriate?

Discussion/Conclusion

Does the paper provide a balanced account or discussion of the findings?

Box 4.4 *Continued*

Were the limitations of the research indicated?

Do the conclusions match the findings?

Were recommendations reasonable or credible?

Evaluating quantitative research

You are likely to be quite new to the process of evaluating published research-based evidence. To help you in this challenging task, and because there are several different designs within quantitative research, we recommend that you use a checklist to help you conduct your evaluation. Checklists to help you evaluate different types of quantitative research design are widely available. In Table 4.1 we summarize many different checklists and signpost you to websites where you should find these to save and print off. In addition to the resources listed in Table 4.1, the *British Medical Journal* (BMJ) published a series of *How to read a paper* articles between 19 July and September 1997 (BMJ, Volume 315), written by Professor Trisha Greenhalgh, widely respected in the EBP field. This series provides excellent advice on how to read and understand papers reporting various types of research. We also recommend that you look at these articles.

Table 4.1 Checklists for evaluating quantitative research papers

Research design	Checklist	Source of checklist
Randomized controlled trial (RCT)	Revised CONSORT statement (Moher et al. 2001)	www.consort-statement.org/Statement/revisedstatement.org
Clustered RCT	CONSORT-PLUS (Campbell et al. 2004)	www.consort-statement.org
Non-randomized evaluations	TREND (Des Jarlais et al. 2004)	www.consort-statement.org
Observational studies in epidemiology	STROBE	www.strobe-statement.org
Studies testing diagnostic accuracy	STARD initiative (Bossuyt et al. 2003)	www.consort-statement.org/Initiatives/newstard
Meta-analysis and systematic reviews of literature	QUOROM	www.consort-statement.org/Evidence/evidence.html#quorom
Evaluating ethical probity of study	ASSERT	www.assert-statement.org
Cohort study	12 questions to help you make sense of a cohort study	Critical Appraisal Skills Programme http://www.phru.nhs.uk/Pages/PHD/CASP.htm
Case control study	12 questions to help you make sense of a case control study	Critical Appraisal Skills Programme http://www.phru.nhs.uk/Pages/PHD/CASP.htm
Economic evaluations	10 questions to help you make sense of economic evaluations	Critical Appraisal Skills Programme http://www.phru.nhs.uk/Pages/PHD/CASP.htm

Evaluating qualitative research

There are multiple approaches to qualitative research, and the skilled practitioner will need to build up knowledge of these to assist in the critiquing process. For example, there are language-oriented approaches such as Conversation Analysis or Discourse Analysis; a range of descriptive/interpretative approaches such as phenomenology and ethnography; and theory building as in Grounded Theory. All such approaches, according to Tesch (1990) share the following:

'A concern with meanings and the way people understand things. Human activity is seen as a product of symbols and meanings that are used by members of the social group to make sense of things. Such symbols and meanings need to be analysed as a 'text'—to be interpreted rather like a literary critic interprets a book.'

Qualitative research tends to involve interviews, observation, action research, or documentary analysis. Box 4.5 outlines questions that can help you make sense of published qualitative research.

Whittemore et al. (2001) and Jorgensen (2006) advocate the following as primary criteria for evaluating qualitative research:

- Credibility
- Authenticity
- Criticality
- Integrity.

Credibility (Lincoln and Guba 1985) relates to whether the results of the research reflect the experience of the participants in a believable way. Confidence in the themes derived by researchers from interviews or focus groups is strengthened when findings are discussed subsequently with participants. This enables refinements and corrections in the light of feedback, thus addressing the challenge *'of preserving participants' definitions of reality'* (Daly 1997, p. 350) through a process of participant validation. **Authenticity** is evident when researchers retain a reflective awareness of their preconceptions and also the possibility of being surprised by findings. The criteria of **criticality** and **integrity** relate to the potential for many different interpretations to be made, dependent on the assumptions and knowledge background of the investigators. This calls for researchers to review emerging themes and to establish their credibility, plausibility, and resonance with experiences beyond the confines of the original study (Horsburgh 2003). Thus, the resulting organization of data is both plausible and rigorously defensible in terms not only of

Box 4.5 Indicative questions for evaluating published qualitative research`

- Were the aims of the research clearly stated?
- Is a qualitative methodology appropriate and justified in this case?
- Were theory and methods sound?
- Did the researchers include the context of the study?
- Were details of sampling provided?
- Was the sample sufficiently diverse to promote transferability?
- Is it clear how the data were collected?
- Was there a clear description of analysis?
- Were multiple methods used (triangulation) so as to test the validity of data and analysis?
- Did a second researcher conduct a separate analysis to test the reliability of both data and analysis?
- Did the researchers critically evaluate their own influence on the research process?
- Did the researchers 'return to the field' and check out their interpretation of the data with participants?
- Do the findings clearly relate to the research question?
- Can the findings be applied in other kinds of setting?
- Is the study relevant or important?
- Does it have implications for practice?

the authors' interpretation but also that of participants and fellow researchers. You can also find helpful guidelines on how to evaluate a qualitative research paper on the Critical Appraisal Skills Programme website (http://www.phru.nhs.uk/Pages/PHD/CASP.htm).

Tips on how to demonstrate skills in evaluation when writing assignments

As a student mental health nurse you will be asked to write assignments where you are asked to evaluate ideas, arguments, or positions people take in written work. Here are some tips on how you can demonstrate skills in evaluation:

1   Compare and contrast arguments using set criteria.

2   Look for evidence supporting arguments that authors make.

3   Think of some alternatives to these arguments.

4   Cite the source of your alternatives.

5   Justify your arguments (e.g. from clinical observations, your reading of other research).

6   Judge the position being taken, not the person taking it.

7   Separate facts from opinions—your own and others'.

8   Think about what you believe, and why you believe this.

9   Identify all possible sources of material that you can draw upon in forming your argument.

10 State the criteria against which you have made your judgement.

Opportunities and obstacles in the pursuit of evidence-based practice

We know that multiple factors can conspire to inhibit the appearance of EBP (Crawford et al. 2002, Ray 1999). It is important that the student and practising mental health nurse appreciate that EBP is not a step-by-step unproblematic process of reviewing or evaluating journal research papers and then applying the evidence in practice. Alongside the kind of stepwise process of judging the quality of a piece of research discussed previously, both student and practitioner will need to utilize skills, not least those around creating partnerships, in achieving the necessary conditions for accessing and evaluating evidence in the first place and then for making good use of this evidence in practice. In other words, there needs to be a strategy for sustainable EBP. In Table 4.2 we outline some of the opportunities and obstacles in the pursuit of EBP.

Table 4.2 Opportunities and obstacles in the pursuit of evidence-based health care (Miles et al. 2000, Renfrew 1997)

Opportunities	Obstacles
Improved care	'Top down' driven
Directing resources cost-effectively	Conflicting evidence
Advancing care	Disseminating and implementing evidence
Improved research	Lack of available evidence
Increased professionalism	Cross-cultural validity
Development of clinical guidelines	Inadequate managerial support
Partnerships in care	Reliance on particular types of evidence
'Doing the right things and doing things right'	Lack of time to retrieve and read evidence
Drawing upon expert knowledge	Research literacy of clinician
	Lack of time
	Poor access to information
	Conflicting ideologies

You will need to work flexibly and creatively to promote EBP in the face of such obstacles. Box 4.6 gives four tips on how to overcome these obstacles.

Disseminating, diffusing, and implementing the best available evidence

So far we have examined the origins of EBP, described the contested issues arising from it, and shown you how to evaluate published evidence. For the final part of this chapter we want briefly to consider the most effective methods for getting research into practice—the most formidable challenge in EBP. The overall aim of generating evidence is to improve the quality of mental health nursing, in order to improve people's health outcomes (CRD 2001). However, this will happen only if the evidence generated gets into policy and practice.

First let us consider what is meant by dissemination, diffusion, and implementation, and what purpose this serves (Box 4.7).

Dissemination is '*The process through which target groups become aware of, receive, accept and utilize information*' (CRD 2001, p. 67).

Diffusion is '*A passive process by which information is spread to an audience*' (Granados et al. 1997, p. 221).

Implementation is '*Activities aimed at improving the compliance of the target group with the recommendations about changes in clinical practice and health policy*' (Granados et al. 1997, p. 224).

There is a wealth of literature showing the factors that are linked to the dissemination and implementation of evidence. This literature is both theoretical and empirical. The Coordinated Implementation Model that Lomas (1993) proposed is a theoretical contribution to the evidence. Lomas identifies four factors that are central, in his view, to getting research into practice:

1 Quality of evidence (see Table 4.1 for checklists that help you to judge the quality of evidence)

2 Credible dissemination body (see Table 4.3 and Box 4.8 for factors that inhibit and enhance dissemination)

3 Overall practice environment (see Table 4.2 for a list of opportunities)

4 Obstacles to implementing EBP and external factors (e.g. how society views the evidence and its relationship to their lives; how the media report the evidence).

A good example of the latter is the report by Kirsch et al. (2008) into the effectiveness of antidepressant drugs. This paper was published and was the main news item in national news bulletins in the UK. Most of the media summarized the report to state bluntly that antidepressants in widespread use such as Prozac did not work according to unpublished studies. This, however, is not the key message of the study, which reports

---

Box 4.6 How to overcome the obstacles to evidence-based practice

1 Education and skills development: in searching and judging the literature (see text); utilizing or providing clinical supervision; promoting EBP as a multidisciplinary activity.

2 Promoting access to evidence: requesting computer access in the workplace to evidence-based information packages and guidelines on key clinical practices or interventions.

3 Negotiating time: requesting that EBP is viewed as a core, formal activity in clinical practice that requires dedicated time.

4 Networking and sharing: using 'partnership' skills in setting up or joining journal clubs or groups discussing EBP; conducting informal, collegial critiquing; networking across institutions and between Trusts and higher education providers; sharing literature reviews and empirical research conducted as part of higher education course with colleagues.

Box 4.7 The purposes of dissemination and implementation (CRD 2001)

Dissemination

Communications to:

- Raise awareness of research evidence
- Facilitate readiness to change
- Help consideration of practice alternatives

Implementation

Activities to:

- Increase adoption of research findings
- Facilitate changes in practice
- Reinforce and support changes in practice

the conditions under which the drugs work (but this was not how the media reported it). An important message from this paper and its reporting in the media is the difference in outcomes from reviews of research when you include published and unpublished studies. Unpublished studies are often hard to find and subsequently are excluded from reviews, but they often report negative findings. In many respects, what Lomas (1993) is suggesting makes sense. Nevertheless, it remains an untested model in the field of EBP. Help is at hand, though, in the form of an increasing body of work on the most effective interventions for getting evidence into practice. We will briefly consider this work. Table 4.3 shows how to introduce change

Table 4.3 Enabling and inhibiting change

Introducing effective change	Impediments to effective change
Opinion leaders	Unclear objectives
Audit	Inappropriate means, messages, communicators, populations, incentives, timescales, and resources
Feedback	Top-down approaches
Informal education	Hierarchical and autocratic initiatives
Clinical guidelines	Advantage of introducing change is not clear
Financial incentives	Proposed change is incompatible with current beliefs and working practices
Role modelling	Proposed change increases complexity of clinical practice
Reflection on action	Perverse incentives
Action learning groups	Distortions of perception of risk
Research awareness groups	*Lobbying by special interest groups*
Timing	Bureaucratic manoeuvring
Direct contact with staff	Poor reward systems
Concise policy documents	Uncertainty of science—policy-makers want certainty
Clear and compelling presentation style	Timing
Mass media	Peer pressure
	Lack of self-efficacy
	Information overload
	Opinion leaders with opposing views

effectively and the impediments to the change (Davies 1999, Granados et al. 1997, Joyce 1999).

Systematic reviews of literature are useful sources to a clinician with little time for reading as they often summarize a lot of literature in one paper. On the basis of a review of systematic reviews we are better informed as to effective methods of getting evidence into practice. See Box 4.8.

An example of evidence that has impacted directly on mental health care

Evidence generated from research has shown consistently that psychosocial interventions of low and high intensity help people to recover from disabling mental health problems. This evidence was carefully evaluated, and as a result the National Institute for Health and Clinical Excellence (NICE) has developed a range of guidelines in mental health recommending the use of psychosocial interventions for a range of mental health problems. For a range of guidelines see http://www.nice.org.uk/search/guidancesearchresults.jsp?keywords=mental%20health&searchType=guidance_finder&healthTopic=13.

Box 4.8 What works? Evidence-based methods of effective dissemination and implementation (Bero et al. 1997)

Consistently effective interventions

- Educational outreach visits
- Reminders
- Multifaceted interventions (e.g. two or more of audit and feedback, reminders, local consensus processes, marketing)
- Interactive educational meetings

Interventions of variable effectiveness

- Audit and feedback
- Local opinion leaders
- Local consensus processes
- Patient-mediated interventions

Interventions that have little or no effect

- Simply providing educational materials
- Didactic educational meetings

 ## Conclusion

We have seen that evidence-based mental health nursing is a fairly complex notion driven by a number of competing definitions and expectations. In order to pursue the evidence base for particular clinical practices and interventions it is vital that students and practitioners are first of all sufficiently knowledgeable about and comprehend the research process. It is here that the first, and perhaps foundational, 'philosophy' skills are developed—not least an ability to differentiate the paradigmatic status of a piece of research, whether it owes to positivism or interpretivism. Beyond formal, collegial critiquing such as the Cochrane Collaboration, individual and informal, collegial critiquing skills can be applied in judging or valuing the key components of published research papers through a series of 'testing' systematic questions. There is a range of questions that are typically applied in a general critique, and more refined sets of questions to pursue further the value of either quantitative or qualitative research. Yet critiquing skills are more than 'item spotting' for each valid criterion, or adopting a 'tick-box' mentality. They require an ability won by experience and practice to 'weigh' the evidence, and to do this in

partnership with others. For it is through 'partnership' skills—working with others—and 'negotiation' and 'resource' skills that barriers to EBP are overcome and real progress can be made. The premise that mental health nursing care should be based on the best available evidence is sound, but it is unclear at what point enough evidence is gathered to justify a clinical decision. The integration of clinical acumen with current best evidence will improve mental health nurses' competence and care. However, health problems are not neatly resolved by recourse to research trials and hierarchies of evidence. Questions relating to the care of patients are not all answered by science; health care is at the interface of many disciplines, and to understand fully the experience of health and ill health we need to draw from many types of evidence. In terms of getting evidence into practice, diffusion is the most common, but least effective, approach. Methods to disseminate and implement evidence need to be (inter)active processes; dissemination and implementation involve change, and this takes time, resources, pragmatism, and flexibility.

w Website

You may find it helpful to work through our short online quiz and scenario intended to help you to develop and apply the skills in this chapter. Please go to:

 www.oxfordtextbooks.co.uk/orc/callaghan

+ References

Bero, L. A., Grilli, R., Grimshaw, J. M., Harvey, E., Oxman, A. D., and Thomson, M. A. (1997). Closing the gap between research and practice: an overview of systematic reviews of interventions to promote the implementation of research findings. *British Medical Journal* 317, 465–8.

Bossuyt, P. M., Reitsma, J. B., Bruns, D E., et al. (2003). Towards complete and accurate reporting of studies of diagnostic accuracy: the STARD initiative. *Clinical Chemistry* 49(1), 1–6.

Brown, B. and Crawford, P. (2003). The clinical governance of the soul: 'deep management' and the self-regulating subject in integrated community mental health teams. *Social Science and Medicine* 56, 67–81.

Brown, B., Crawford, P., and Hicks, C. (2003). *Evidence Based Research: Dilemmas and Debates in Health Care*. Milton Keynes: Open University Press.

Campbell, M. K., Elbourne, D. R., and Altman, D.G. (2004). CONSORT statement: extension to cluster randomised controlled trials. *British Medical Journal* 328, 702–8.

Centre for Reviews and Dissemination (2001). *Undertaking Systematic Reviews of Research on Effectiveness. CRD Report 4*. York: University of York.

Coyler, H. and Kamath, P. (1999). Evidence-based practice. A philosophical and political analysis: some matters for consideration by professional practitioners. *Journal of Advanced Nursing* 29(1), 188–93.

Crawford, P., Brown, Anthony, P., and Hicks, C. (2002). Reluctant empiricists: community mental health nurses and the art of evidence based praxis. *Health and Social Care in the Community* 10(4), 287–98.

Daly K. (1997). Re-placing theory in ethnography: a postmodern view. *Qualitative Inquiry* 3(3), 343–65.

Davies, P. (1999). Introducing change. In: *Evidence-based Practice: A Primer for Health Care Professionals* (ed. M. Dawes), pp 203–18. London: Churchill Livingstone.

Department of Health (2006). *Best Practice Competencies and Capabilities for Pre-Registration Mental Health Nurses in England: The Chief Nursing Officer's Review of Mental Health Nursing*. London: DH.

Des Jarlais, D., Lyles, C., Crepaz, N., and the TREND Group (2004). Improving the reporting of the quality of nonrandomized evaluations of behavioral and public health interventions. *American Journal of Public Health* 94(3), 361–6.

DiCenso, A., Cullum, N., Ciliska, D. (1998). Implementing evidence-based nursing: Some misconceptions. *Evidence-Based Nursing* 1, 38–9.

Granados, A., Jonsson, E., Banta, H. D., et al. (1997). EUR-ASSESS Project Subgroup Report on Dissemination and Impact. *International Journal of Technology Assessment in Health Care* 13(2), 220–86.

Gray, J. A. M. (1997). *Evidence-based Health Care*. London: Churchill-Livingstone.

Horsburgh, D. (2003). Evaluation of qualitative research. *Journal of Clinical Nursing* 12(2), 307–12.

Hughes, J. A. and Sharrock, W. W. (1997). *The Philosophy of Social Research*, 3rd revised edn. London: Longman.

Jorgensen R. (2006). A phenomenological study of fatigue in patients with primary biliary cirrhosis. *Journal of Advanced Nursing* 55(6), 689–97.

Joyce, L. (1999). Development of practice. In: *Achieving Evidence-based Practice: A Handbook for Practitioners* (ed. S. Hamer and G. Collinson), pp 109–27. Edinburgh: Baillière Tindall.

Kirsch, I., Deacon, B. J., Huedo-Medina, T. B., Scoboria, A., Moore, T. J., and Johnson, B. T. (2008). Initial severity and antidepressant benefits: a meta-analysis of data submitted to the food and drug administration. *Public Library of Science Medicine* 5(2), 260–8.

Lincoln, Y. S. and Guba, E. G. (1985). *Naturalistic Inquiry*. Newbury Park, CA: Sage.

Lomas, J. (1993). Retailing research: increasing the role of evidence in clinical services for child birth. *The Millbank Quarterly* 71, 439–75.

McKenna, H., Cutcliffe, J., and McKenna, P. (2000). Evidence-based practice: demolishing some myths. *Nursing Standard* 14(16), 39–42.

Miles, A., Hampton, J. R., and Hurwitz, B. (ed.) (2000). *NICE, CHI and the NHS Reforms: Enabling Excellence or Imposing Control*. London: Aesculapius Medical Press.

Moher, D., Schultz, K. F., and Altman, D. (2001). The CONSORT statement: revised recommendations for improving the reporting of parallel group randomised controlled trials. *Lancet* 357, 1191–4.

Parahoo, K. (2006). *Nursing Research: Principles, Process and Issues*, 2nd edn. London: Macmillan.

Ray, L. (1999). Evidence and outcomes: agendas, pre-suppositions and power. *Journal of Advanced Nursing* 30(5), 1017–26.

Renfrew, M. (1997). The development of evidence-based practice. *British Journal of Midwifery* 5(2), 100–4.

Spence, J. (1991). *The Search for Modern China*. New York: Norton.

Tesch R. (1990). *Qualitative research: Analysis types and software tools*. New York: Faimer Press.

von Degenberg, K. (1996). Clinical guidelines: improving practice at the local level. *Nursing Standard* 10(19), 37–9.

Whittemore R., Chase S. K., and Mandle, C. L. (2001). Validity in qualitative research. *Qualitative Health Research* 11(4), 522–37.

(5) Caring: the essence of mental health nursing

Theo Stickley   Gemma Stacey

▼ Introduction

This chapter explores the concept of caring in mental health nursing and locates the art of caring in twenty-first century practice. First we examine the language of 'caring' in health care settings, and identify the core ethical principles and values that underpin the concept of care. We then describe and explain the skills associated with a caring approach to mental health practice.

Learning outcomes

By the end of this chapter you should be better able to:

1 Consider the concept of caring in terms of the language of caring and its ethical underpinnings

2 Demonstrate an awareness of the relevance of caring to contemporary mental health nursing practice when working with people towards their recovery from mental health problems

3 Display the interpersonal and intrapersonal skills required to adopt a caring approach to practice

4 Transfer these skills into your mental health nursing practice.

The concept of caring in mental health nursing practice

The evidence supports the healing power of caring and argues that nurses develop this healing approach by mobilizing hope, confidence, and trust between themselves and the person with whom they are working (Benner 1984). If the nurse is able to develop a relationship of confidence and trust with the person, not only will healing occur, but the person's spiritual and emotional needs can also be addressed more effectively (Stoter 1995). The following section provides the historical and theoretical justification for caring to remain the essence of mental health nursing practice when working with people towards their recovery from mental health problems.

The ethics of caring

In a moment of crisis a caring practitioner will be physically present, acknowledge the need to be there, and offer solidarity, consolation, and support (Nouwen et al. 1982). Such practical expressions of care are at the heart of mental health nursing practice. Adopting a caring approach is thought to be related to a series of learned or behavioural reactions. However, at times caring for others can run against the grain of our normal behavioural expectations. Therefore, it also involves moral choices. One of the guiding choices or reasons for caring is altruism (Eisenberg and Miller 1987), in which there is planned, deliberate, and voluntary behaviour in support of another person that is not given with the expectation of any reward or punishment. In this context, caring for another can be seen as the nurse making informed, altruistic decisions that empower the person with whom they are working (Dietze and Orb 2000).

The moral choices we make in adopting a caring approach require the mental health nurse to justify their actions in the context of wider questions such as:

• How does the action taken agree or conflict with my other moral values?

• How has the action taken enhanced the choice and well-being of the person with whom I am working?

What are considered reasonable actions will vary from person to person or from situation to situation. There are some common principles that should underlie a caring approach, and these are, of course, supported by the Nursing and Midwifery Council (NMC) Code of Professional Conduct (Downie and Calman 1994, p. 50):

1 One ought not to harm physically or psychologically (non-maleficence).

2 One ought to give positive help to people wherever necessary (benevolence or beneficence, and compassion).

3 One ought to treat people fairly or equally (justice).

4 One ought to produce the greatest happiness for the majority (utility).

When attempting to adopt a caring approach to practice, the principles given above tend to encourage you to base your actions on duty and obligation, rather than your care and compassion for the person with whom you are working. Such obligations need to be understood, interpreted, and applied by you. This means they are inseparable from your character, and from the moral qualities and values you possess. Considering caring as a moral quality or value that you hold allows you to view caring for another as a complex situation in which the moral character, the role of emotion, and the significance of the relationship between you and the person with whom you are working should be fully acknowledged.

The language of care: 'caretakers' or caring nurses?

The word 'care' is perhaps one of the most over-used words in mental health practice. Not only does the word crop up in health settings, it appears in other contexts too; for example, we tell people to 'Take care' when we leave them, or we sometimes ask people, 'Would you care for a cup of tea?'. The building where you work or study may even have a 'caretaker', someone who takes care of the premises. As with any word, when it is used so much in so many contexts, it can easily lose its meaning. For example, is there much difference between caring for a building and caring for a person? We would argue that there is a huge difference, and unless we understand the meaning of 'care', and put that meaning into practice, we might as well become caretakers of buildings rather than people.

The word care originates from the Anglo-Saxon *caru*, which implies 'anxiety' or 'worry'. One who cares therefore contains a tension regarding the object of care. As a mental health nurse (the 'care-taker' of vulnerable people), you are inevitably caught up in the tricky business of human relationships. We discuss some of the implications for this kind of work in practice later in the chapter. We also argue that you need

skills to implement care, to complement your moral values and character.

History of care

For as long as humans have existed, they have cared for one another. Care is more easily accomplished with members of one's family. Societies, since the Middle Ages at least, have recognized the need to care for vulnerable members. This has usually focused upon orphans, the poor, the sick, the widowed, the elderly, and the mad. More often than not, social care was provided by religious orders according to the culture of any particular country. In the UK, the first record of institutional care being offered to the mad was in the fourteenth century in London at a Christian order named St Mary of Bethlehem, later to become known as 'Bedlam'. This heralded a period that later became known as 'the great confinement', where across Europe people who were deemed to be insane were locked up in asylums. Whilst such people were previously known as 'holy fools' or 'village idiots', they had now become identified as socially unacceptable and were to be removed. Many vulnerable people, however, did not receive care, but ended up in prisons or labouring in workhouses (Porter 2002).

It was not until the nineteenth century that asylums came under the auspices of medical practitioners. During the Victorian era, several philanthropists and parliamentarians forced a change in mental health care with the building of humane asylums. This era became known for its 'moral treatment' of the insane. The York Retreat, founded in 1796, has become the best known example of providing moral treatment, although, as Digby (1985) observed, it was not so much the activities that were provided that were considered curative, but the provision of such by people who genuinely cared and provided good therapeutic relationships. Such 'retreats' were designed to be homely and comforting, based upon the model of the family. Unfortunately, by the middle of the twentieth century it was usual for the Victorian-built asylums to house approximately 1000 people. In such environments, the potential for therapeutic caring diminished.

In the 1950s a psychiatric nurse theorist emerged whose work was to have a profound impact upon the development of the role and definition of the mental health nursing profession. Her name was Hildegard Peplau. In 1952, Peplau wrote her book, *Interpersonal Relations in Nursing,* which clearly identified a relational model for mental health nursing. She placed great emphasis upon the nurse–client relationship and was clearly influenced by the then current developments in humanistic psychology. Peplau gave mental health nursing a theoretical base from which mental health nurses could give a meaningful rationale for caring.

In the subsequent decades, mental health nursing developed as a profession with a theoretical cornerstone of caring through interpersonal relating. Upon this cornerstone was built a multifaceted paradigm incorporating counselling, communication, and interpersonal skills.

Consistent with the Rogerian theory of the discrete nature of the therapeutic relationship (Rogers 1951), mental health nursing care occurs **within** the relationship of the mental health nurse and the client. This is the very essence of mental health nursing practice. It is at the point where mental health nursing practice meets counselling and therapy practice: the 'work' is 'within' the relationship. Caring is central to the nurse–patient relationship and should be within the boundaries of the therapeutic relationship.

It is impossible to dissociate mental health care and the person-to-person relationship. The mental health nurse cannot avoid being in a relationship with his or her client. The relationship exists whether or not it is therapeutic, and whether or not the client or mental health nurse is conscious of its therapeutic efficacy (or otherwise). Generally speaking, the emphasis upon caring within human relationships has been maintained throughout the mental health nursing literature, but notably through Peplau (1952), Altschul (1985), Watkins (2001), and Barker (2003).

The contemporary context of caring

The government has developed a set of capabilities called the **Essential Shared Capabilities** (ESCs). These provide a framework for the whole of the mental health workforce across the National Health Service (NHS) and Social Care, and the statutory and non-statutory sectors (Department of Health [DH] et al. 2004). What is identified within this framework is the need for values-based practice (see Chapter 3).

As mentioned above, a key value associated with mental health practice, when working with people towards their recovery, is adopting a caring approach. Several contemporary models of nursing practice have emerged, including: the recovery and social inclusion model (Repper and Perkins 2003); the strengths perspective (Rapp 1998, Rapp and Goscha 2005); the tidal model (Barker and Buchanan-Barker 2004), and the wellness recovery action plan (Copeland 1997). It is recommended that you familiarize yourself with these models through further reading.

At the foundation of each of these models is the importance of maintaining the belief that every individual has the potential to change and grow, given the right therapeutic conditions. It is evident that each of these models has been informed by humanistic theory which stresses the significance of genuineness, empathy, and acceptance (Rogers 1961). None of these conditions can be achieved without the presence of authentic care for the person with whom you are working. A caring approach therefore represents the foundation for the therapeutic relationship which can act as a vehicle towards recovery.

Skills for caring in mental health nursing practice

Mental health nursing is primarily about human relationships. Sometimes, we can think this view is challenged by the fact that nurses need to spend so much time on the bureaucratic demands of the job. Some nurses who work in inpatient settings often complain about the lack of staff which prohibits nurses from forming good human relationships with their clients. These are very real problems that cannot be ignored; nevertheless, the primary objective of mental health nursing should be to form therapeutic human relationships. Everything else should be secondary. Mental health nurses need to develop a caring attitude (*caru*) in order to 'care'. Often, when we are stressed and working in an area that is under-resourced, our duty to 'care' can become draining and we feel exhausted carrying this therapeutic *caru* for our clients. This is why mental health nurse educators pay so much attention to self-awareness—what we referred to earlier as 'intrapersonal', literally, the relationship we have with ourselves. It is through self-awareness that we need to take our anxieties and exhaustion to our supervision sessions. Sadly, we often become tired and overwhelmed not just because of this commitment to caring, but also by the fact that our services become stretched and we do not have the resources to provide the care needed.

This kind of caring, therefore, is complicated. It is far easier on human skills and emotions to be a caretaker of buildings than it is to become a caregiver of vulnerable people. To become a human caretaker can be exhausting. There are, however, skills that can be developed to enable 'care in action'. The historical and theoretical foundations of mental health nursing emphasize the importance of interpersonal and intrapersonal skills that are essential for building therapeutic relationships. At the heart of these relationships is a caring approach, which can be communicated to the people you work with through the use of basic **interpersonal** and

intrapersonal communication skills, as introduced in the following section.

Interpersonal skills for caring

The basic interpersonal skills that communicate a caring approach are listed below. Each of these skills will be described and explained, and exercises are given for you to practise them. We suggest that you conduct these practical tasks with your fellow students and take turns to adopt the various roles outlined in the tasks. This will give you an opportunity to experience the skill in a safe environment where it is OK to make mistakes before practising in your placements. We also suggest you take the opportunity to reflect upon adopting each of the roles as a way of enhancing your understanding of how it feels to be placed in the varied positions within the interaction.

- Non-verbal communication
- Open questioning
- Clarifying
- Reflecting content
- Reflecting feeling
- Using silence.

When all the skills are being used together, the mental health nurse provides the proper, respectful conditions for personal growth to take place. The kind of environment and space that is created is caring and therefore therapeutic. By employing these skills in individual work you may be able to provide an effective way of truly listening to the client, and in doing so communicate your genuine care for the person. The skills are designed to communicate compassionate and empathic understanding. Therefore, not only does the client benefit from being offered these conditions, but the worker can also learn to develop empathic understanding in the process of exercising the skills.

All of the skills identified need to be practised. This cannot be emphasized enough. One of the best ways to practise these skills is to create role-play scenarios. In the Practice Scenario box we have included a number of such scenarios that might be useful.

✖ Practice scenarios to develop your skills

To practise skills for caring using these scenarios it is useful for three people to work together: a client, a helper, and an observer. The observer's role is to sit to one side and silently make notes about the skills the worker is using. The observer should give the worker feedback at the end of the session. When using these scenarios, ten minutes is usually allowed for practice. Once the skills have been learned they can be exercised in mental health practice areas.

A Client

You are Amanda, aged 28. Having experienced many abusive relationships you went into prostitution and began to use drugs and alcohol regularly. You were admitted to an acute ward after getting drunk one night. You have been detained under a section of the Mental Health Act, but you do not know why you are there and feel very angry that your freedom has been curtailed.

A Nurse

You have been asked to talk with Amanda, who is 28. She has been detained under Section 2 of the Mental Health Act. You know nothing about her past, other than that she has a history of drink and drugs. She was admitted to an acute ward after claiming to be the Virgin Mary and running around a local park with few clothes on.

B Client

You are Bev, aged 22. You have been admitted to the acute ward after a serious attempt on your life. You have now been an inpatient for six weeks. It is totally impractical for you to go back to your parents as you have a very destructive relationship with them. You have got no ideas for your future. Everything seems hopeless.

B Nurse

You have been asked to spend time with Bev, who is 22. She was admitted to the acute ward after a serious attempt on her life. She has now been an inpatient for six weeks. You are under a great deal of pressure to discharge her into a women's hostel.

C Client

You are Catelin, aged 25. You know you have a thing about food and eating, but do not know why everybody keeps talking to you about this. You now weigh six stones, although you think you are fat. You live at home with your parents, who you

»

» believe, infantilize you with their bossy, patronizing attitudes. Your parents have been threatening to get you admitted to an acute psychiatric ward.

C Nurse

You have been asked to visit Catelin in the community. Aged 25, she has been anorexic since she was 15. Her parents are considerate, caring people who are at a total loss as to what to do with their daughter. They have asked if she can be admitted to hospital.

D Client

You are Debbie, aged 22. You live in a flat on your own in the city. You came to the city to university but dropped out after you started hearing voices. The voices were disturbing and you have since been treated with medication. You cannot go home as you have a very difficult relationship with your parents. You try to do voluntary work but feel very sluggish with the medication.

D Nurse

You are visiting Debbie, aged 22. She lives in a flat on her own in the city. She came to the city to university but dropped out after she started hearing voices. The voices were disturbing and she has since been treated with

neuroleptics. She cannot go home as she has a very difficult relationship with her parents. You have encouraged Debbie to do voluntary work but you think she is deliberately sabotaging these opportunities for some reason and not helping herself enough.

E Client

You are Eve, a 22-year-old music graduate. You are quite a quiet person; you have been described as 'a bit of a loner'. Before coming to university your parents split up, both finding new partners. You are the youngest of three children and your older siblings all live in different parts of the country. You now feel very isolated. Most of your university friends have got jobs and moved away; you haven't worked since you graduated and you've been socially isolated. At university you experimented with many different kinds of drugs. You smoke cannabis regularly. A few months ago you started feeling very paranoid. You mentioned this to the GP, who has referred you to mental health services.

E Nurse

This is your first meeting with Eve, who you know is a 22-year-old music graduate. She has been referred to your community team by her GP. The referral letter said little, but mentioned the word paranoid.

The six skills for attentive listening and communicating care

Non-verbal communication

In establishing a caring relationship, our non-verbal communication is of utmost importance. Much of the communication that takes place between people is non-verbal. When we meet someone for the first time, we automatically make judgements about them, and this is invariably communicated non-verbally. It is important that we have the self-awareness to be aware of our non-verbal communication at all times.

Sadly, there are many stories of people being admitted to a ward for the first time who are then left alone. At this critical moment it is imperative that a person is warmly greeted and a member of staff dedicated to sitting with the person. From the outset the worker needs to create a therapeutic space with the client.

We have developed an acronym (SURETY) to help facilitate this therapeutic space.

S Sit at an angle to the client

U Uncross legs and arms

R Relax

E Eye contact

T Touch

Y Your intuition

Compare the two photographs in Figure 5.1. Assuming this sort of positioning may seem common sense, but it is not. You need to practise awareness of body language when working with clients.

Sit at an angle to the client—If we sit directly opposite somebody who is feeling vulnerable in any way, this position may be interpreted as confrontational. If we sit exactly next to a person (as in a waiting room), the position is not personal. If, however, we sit at a slight angle, it creates a non-confrontational, comfortable seating arrangement, ideal for one-to-one work.

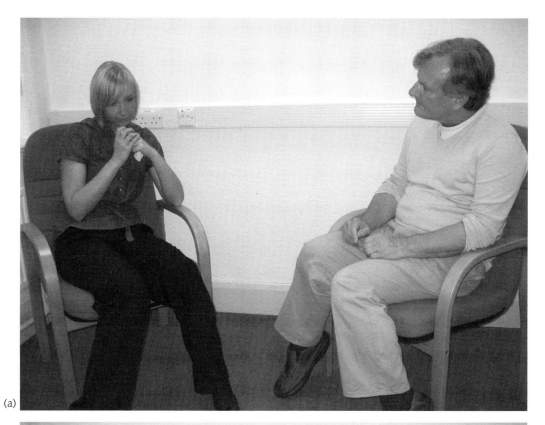

(a)

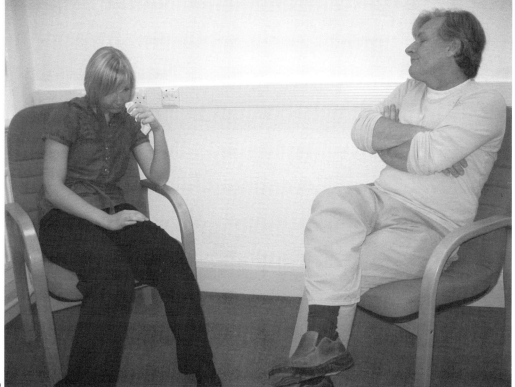

(b)

Figure 5.1 Comparisons of (a) effective and (b) ineffective non-verbal communication.

Uncross legs and arms–Research into non-verbal communication has shown that crossed arms and legs communicate defensiveness. Depending on the whole body position, crossed arms and legs may also communicate that we are not interested or in some way superior. If we deliberately uncross arms and legs, we communicate that we are open and receptive to what the person is saying.

Relax–In spite of the prescriptive nature of this method of deliberate non-verbal communication, it is most important that the listener learns to relax in the assumed position. It may feel awkward at first to practise this position, but it is worth it—and, furthermore, it works!

Eye contact–Retaining appropriate eye contact is a powerful way of communicating respect and that you are paying attention. Eyes that wander to windows or the clock are sure to be read as loss of interest or attention.

Appropriate eye contact is very different to staring. Staring is insensitive and intrusive. Appropriate eye contact breaks on occasions. It is always important to have eye contact at the ready if a client is distressed and perhaps looking down. If they momentarily look up and your eyes are not waiting for them, there can be a loss of trust.

The practice of eye contact is not universal. If a practitioner is asked to work with a client from a different culture (especially of the opposite gender), the worker would do well to find out about the cultural rights and wrongs, including the use of eye contact.

Touch–Again, the appropriate use of touch is not universal and cultural sensitivity is essential. Gushing hugs or kisses are not appropriate in mental health care, although sensitive use of touch is often essential, especially when working with troubled children, adolescents, or older people. Respectful use of touch can communicate compassion, love, empathy, and understanding. Conversely, inappropriate use of touch can be abusive.

On occasion you may be required physically to restrain somebody from harming themselves or others. This should never be conducted in a punishing way. This form of physical contact should be implemented in the most respectful manner. You will find further information and guidance on how to restrain safely in Chapter 18. See also National Institute for Health and Clinical Excellence (NICE) Guideline 25 on managing violence (NICE 2005). Our litmus test for judging the respectful use of restraint is: at a later time would the service user appreciate the manner in which he or she was restrained?

Your intuition–Our final point with non-verbal communication is the need for workers to trust their intuition. There are no universal guidelines for every situation, but as the practitioner grows in confidence so they should learn to trust their intuition.

Asking open questions

A closed question is one that elicits a yes or no answer. An open question invites the client to think, explore, and talk freely. Examples of open and closed questions are shown in Figure 5.2.

Look closely at Figure 5.2 and you will see that closed questions usually begin with: do, did, or are. Open questions usually begin with: how, when, what, and tell. Can you think of more? In one-to-one work, we usually avoid using the word 'why'. Often, when people are in distress, being asked 'why' can be infuriating—people often do not know 'why'.

Clarifying

When we need to clarify some factual information it is fine to ask closed questions: *'Did you say your husband was George?'.*

A woman has been admitted to a ward
having taken a large overdose.
The worker is conducting an assessment.

Open Questions	Closed Questions
• How were you feeling when you overdosed?	• Did you really want to die?
• Tell me about your home life?	• Do you live alone?
• What do you do for a living?	• Do you work?
• How are you feeling now?	• Are you feeling suicidal?

Figure 5.2 Examples of open and closed questions.

Unfortunately, however, assessments often sound like a tick list of information giving and receiving, and little time is given to open exploration.

Clarifying is essential if we are muddled about factual information. People are generally happy to clarify if we have misheard or made a wrong assumption.

Reflecting content

Reflecting back to the person the content of what they are saying has a number of effects:

- It demonstrates you are listening.
- It ensures accuracy.
- It communicates empathetic understanding.
- It creates dialogue.

Some examples are included in the Practice Example box. These responses may not be perfect and there is no absolute right or wrong. What you are attempting is to avoid being judgemental and to focus on being reflective.

Reflecting feeling

Reflecting feeling is the same as reflecting content, but there also needs to be a focus on the person's feelings. These may be communicated verbally or non-verbally; for examples see the Practice Example box.

Silence

The use of silence in **attentive listening** and communicating care is essential. Whilst silence is common between people who are intimate, it is often considered uncomfortable in normal conversation (Box 5.1). Working therapeutically with service users needs to be more than normal conversation and the use of silence has to be practised.

In using attentive listening skills for individual work it is necessary to allow adequate pauses between the service user speaking and your next response/intervention. See the scenarios in the Practice Example box.

Generally speaking we recommend a pause of five seconds before making an intervention. Now when you practise your skills, count to five in your mind before making your next intervention. If you can introduce this very simple skill into your work, it will have an immediate impact on the style and tone of the session. From the outset we have argued for the significance of respect in the caring relationship. The use of silence is a way of communicating that respect. Silence conveys a number of messages:

Box 5.1 Pause for thought

- How often do you experience silence?
- How do you feel?
- Why not sit in silence now for ten minutes?
- This is often very difficult to achieve—have you noticed?
- The world was a much quieter place years ago, before technology brought us recorded music and mobile phones!

- The person is important to you.
- You have time for the person.
- This interaction is more than a normal conversation.
- Your interventions are considered.
- It is OK to be with the person without feeling the need to do something.

Using the skills in practice

Whenever you are given the opportunity to work with a service user, we believe that it is necessary to employ interpersonal skills such as those presented in this chapter. It is not enough just to rely on personality or charm. The work of building, sustaining, and ending therapeutic relationships is complex and, if it is to be therapeutic, relationship building takes time, patience, and skill (see also Chapter 7). Our critics may accuse us of oversimplifying all of the skills needed for working in caring relationships. What we assert is that if the practitioner masters the skills in this chapter their work will be greatly enhanced. It may be helpful to access the 'transferring skills into your practice' self-assessment provided on the website to help you to prepare, plan, implement, and evaluate the use of these skills in your placement.

Intrapersonal skills for caring

Working in mental health is a privileged and very important social role. There is much emotional and psychological distress all around us. Workers are not immune from mental health problems either. At times, we all need somebody who will offer us the human qualities to provide a caring relationship. When we are in practice, this support should come from our supervisor, who themselves

✖ Practice Example: Reflecting Content

1 Service user
'I don't know why I've been sent here to talk to you.'

1 Student nurse
'You don't know why you are here.'

2 Service user
'Everything I do is rubbish.'

2 Student nurse
'You're feeling useless.'

3 Service user
'I don't know what's the matter with me. The doctor says one thing, my son says something else, and I don't know what to do.'

3 Student nurse
'You're getting conflicting advice and you are unsure what to do.'

4 Service user
'It's not my fault I got behind with my payments, the bills all came at the same time.'

4 Student nurse
'Your bills all came at once and that's the reason you got behind with your payments.'

5 Service user
'Why do people always target me? Why me?'

5 Student nurse
'You think you are being targeted.'

6 Service user
'I had a terrible holiday. Everything went wrong, just typical of my life.'

6 Student nurse
'Your holiday wasn't good and that's typical of your life.'

✖ Practice Example: Reflecting Feeling

Once again we stress the need for practising these skills. They are quite straightforward in principle but take a long time to develop. Do not underestimate the effectiveness of using skills of reflection. As people feel listened to and empathically understood, trust will inevitably develop and the service user will be able to begin to engage with you.

Examples of reflecting non-verbal feelings
'You had tears in your eyes when you said that.'
'You sounded angry when you said that.'
'You sound sad.'
'You look very tense.'
'I can see your fists are clenched.'

'You look afraid.'
'You look really pleased about that.'

Examples of reflecting feelings communicated verbally
For this, use the same expressions as before but this time add the reflection of feelings:
'… and you sound confused'
'… and you sound sad'
'… and you sound worried'
'… and you look angry'
'… and you look frightened'
'… and you sound despairing'

has had experience in mental health work and training in supervisory skills. On occasion, it may be necessary for mental health nurses to receive counselling or psychotherapy. It is perfectly understandable that people who work with others who are distressed or disturbed may be affected in some way. In fact, it would be strange if the nurse were unaffected by this demanding work.

Promoting caring in mental health

Mental health promotion strategies often ignore the significance of human relationships. Sometimes in the literature it is difficult to find the things that are most important to human existence, for example our need for love and affection. It is

✖ Practice Example: Pausing

Scenario without a pause
Service user: 'I don't know why I've been sent to talk to you.'
Student nurse: 'You don't know why you are here.'

Scenario with a pause
Note the dialogue changes:
Service user: 'I don't know why I've been sent to talk to you.'

[Pause]
Service user: 'Maybe it's for my own good.'
[Pause]
Student nurse: 'You don't know why you are here but maybe it's for your own good.'
The first pause allows the service user to think for themselves. The second pause allows you to reflect back.

highly likely that this is one of the most neglected areas in statutory health care provision. Many of the people we work with, certainly in secondary care locations, have experienced loneliness and rejection. This may have been from families, friends, or society in general. The kind of caring that we are promoting in this chapter is closely related to the person's need for positive human relationships. We are not advocating that you create friendships with service users; rather, that you should create relationships that communicate care. These have similar qualities to friendship relationships, but they are not the same. Friendships are dependent and reciprocal: a caring nurse–client relationship acknowledges the power dynamics and that the relationship will never be equal.

You need to promote opportunities for service users to form positive relationships that are not dependent upon you. The qualities that service users find in caring relationships should really be found in intimate relationships. In this respect, although our caring should be genuine, it should also be temporary.

Mental health promotion often uses theoretical language for what we are asserting here, for example 'social networks', 'social capital', or 'social inclusion'. People who use our services want the same as you and me: love, affection, and sexual pleasure. Good mental health promotion will acknowledge this and support people in getting these needs, desires, and wishes met.

▲ Conclusion

We have argued that communicating care towards another is not a natural emotional response, and neither is it a set of principles or reasoned justifications. Rather, it is part of a wider human experience. It requires both emotional and thoughtful response, but often leads to tension. The values of the nurse are not always in line with those of the service user or of the health care institution or system within which they are

working. Therefore, caring often requires taking sides and making decisions that are justified by adopting a compassionate response to the person with whom you work (Dietze and Orb 2000). We feel opportunity lies in accepting caring as more than a principle or ingredient of mental health nursing practice, but as part of the core that underlies every therapeutic interaction.

w Website

You may find it helpful to work through our short self-assessment exercise and scenario intended to help you to develop and apply the skills in this chapter. Please go to:

 www.oxfordtextbooks.co.uk/orc/callaghan

✛ References

Altschul, A. (1985). *Psychiatric Nursing: A Concise Nursing Text,* 6th edn. London: Baillière Tindall.

Barker, P. (2003). *Psychiatric and Mental Health Nursing: The Craft of Caring.* London: Arnold.

Barker, P. and Buchanan-Barker, P. (2004). *The Tidal Model: A Guide for Mental Health Professionals.* London: Brunner-Routledge.

Benner, P. (1984). *From Novice to Expert. Excellence and Power in Clinical Nursing Practice.* Menlo Park, CA: Addison-Wesley.

Copeland, M. E. (1997). *WRAP: Wellness Recovery Action Plan™.* West Dummerston, VT: Peach Press.

Department of Health, National Health Service University, Sainsbury Centre, and National Institute for Mental Health in England (2004). *The Ten Essential Shared Capabilities – A Framework for the Whole of the Mental Health Workforce.* London: DH.

Dietze, E. and Orb, A. (2000). Compassionate care: a moral dimension of nursing. *Nursing Inquiry* 7, 166–74.

Digby, A. (1985). *Madness, Morality, and Medicine: A Study of the York Retreat, 1796–1914.* New York: Cambridge University Press.

Downie, R. S. and Calman, K. C. (1994). *Healthy Respect: Ethics in Health Care,* 2nd edn. Oxford: Oxford University Press.

Eisenberg, N. and Miller, P. (1987). Empathy, sympathy and altruism: empirical and conceptual. In: *Empathy and its Development* (ed. N. Eisenberg and J. Strayer), pp 292–316. Cambridge: Cambridge University Press.

National Institute for Health and Clinical Excellence (2005). *Violence: The Short-term Management of Disturbed/Violent Behaviour in In-patient Psychiatric Settings and Emergency Departments.* Clinical Guideline 25. London: NICE.

Nouwen, H. J., McNeill, D. P., and Morrisson, D. A. (1982). *Compassion: A Reflection on the Christian Life.* London: Darton, Longman and Todd.

Peplau, H. E. (1952). *Interpersonal Relations in Nursing.* New York: G. P. Putnam.

Porter, R. (2002). *Madness: A Brief History.* Oxford: Oxford University Press.

Rapp, C. A. (1998). *The Strengths Model.* New York: Oxford University Press.

Rapp, C. A. and Goscha, R. (2005). *The Strengths Model: Case Management with People with Psychiatric Disabilities.* New York: Oxford University Press.

Repper, J. and Perkins, R. (2003). *Social Inclusion and Recovery: A Model for Mental Health Nursing Practice.* London: Baillière Tindall.

Rogers, C. R. (1951). *Client-Centred Therapy.* Boston: Houghton & Mifflin.

Rogers, C. R. (1961). *On Becoming a Person: A Therapist's View of Psychotherapy.* London: Constable.

Stoter, D. J. (1995). *Spiritual Aspects of Health Care.* London: Mosby.

Watkins, P. (2001). *Mental Health Nursing: The Art of Compassionate Care.* Oxford: Butterworth-Heinemann.

PART 2

Improving outcomes for service users

Chapters

6 Interpersonal communication – Heron's Six Category Intervention Analysis

Jean Morrissey

▼ Introduction

This chapter is concerned with the second category of Best Practice Competencies and Capabilities for Pre-registration Mental Health Nurses in England (Department of Health [DH] 2006), that of **improving outcomes for service users**. This requires students at the point of registration to demonstrate a range of effective and appropriate communication and engagement skills with individuals who have mental health problems, their carers, and the key people involved in their care.

Communication underlies everything we do, on a daily basis as well as in our professional practice. In mental health nursing, communication is a fundamental component of all therapeutic interventions and is essential for the delivery of quality nursing care. The knowledge and interpersonal skills that a mental health nurse conveys are important aspects of helping the person who is experiencing mental health problems as well as facilitating the development of a positive nurse–service user relationship. According to Peplau (1988), the **therapeutic relationship** serves as the foundation for all interventions provided to service users and is in itself a powerful intervention. Hence, in the therapeutic relationship, communication is an interpersonal and interactive process that aims to affect a positive change and involve the service user in decision-making about his or her care.

Traditionally the views of mental health service users have received minimal attention, but in recent years it has been acknowledged that service users are the experts, with an invaluable experience of how mental illness can impact on their life (Barker and Buchanan-Barker 2004, Repper and Perkins 2003). Involving mental health service users is therefore an essential component of high-quality mental health services. Several initiatives have recently promoted the concept of patient-centred communication and service user involvement as central to the delivery of quality health care and service delivery (DH 2002, 2004, NHS Modernisation Agency 2003). These initiatives were in response to the concerns raised about the quality of interactions between nurses and service users, and their therapeutic value (DH 1999, Sainsbury Centre for Mental Health 1998). Evidence suggests that, in practice, the therapeutic contact time between nurses and service users is minimal, and that when interactions do occur *'they are neither purposely therapeutic nor theoretically informed'* (Cameron et al. 2005, p. 65; Gijbels 1995, Robinson 1996a,b, Whittington and McLaughlin 2000). More recently, the Chief Nursing Officer's review of mental health nursing (DH 2006) recommended that mental health practice needs nurses who can offer more skilled, effective therapeutic communication. Acquiring new skills and learning how to use them effectively should facilitate an improvement in mental health nurses' knowledge and skill base so that they can deliver best practice in a variety of clinical situations. This chapter describes Heron's (2001) model of communication—Six Category Intervention Analysis—, illustrates how each category can be used in clinical practice, and examines some of the factors that may influence the therapeutic outcome of each category.

Learning outcomes

By the end of this chapter you should be better able to:

1 Describe Heron's Six Category Intervention communication framework

2 Demonstrate an understanding of how Heron's Six Category Intervention framework can be used in clinical practice

3 Identify factors that may influence the application of Heron's Six Category Intervention

4 Use Heron's Six Categories in practice.

What is Six Category Intervention Analysis?

Six Category Intervention Analysis is a communication/counselling framework developed by John Heron in 1975 at the Human Potential Research Project, University of Surrey (Heron 1975). It is a way of classifying a huge range of skills under six types of intervention that include six kinds of purpose or intention. As a therapeutic framework it provides a practical tool for mental health nurses to monitor, select, and review their communication skills and interactions with service users, their carers, and the key people involved in their care. All six categories can be used in a wide range of communication encounters whereby one person (the mental health nurse) is the **listener** and the facilitator, and the other person (the service user) is the **talker**—the one who is dealing with some issue that needs the time, attention, and service of another human being. The aim of this helping relationship is to offer some kind of enabling service and skill that is grounded fundamentally in a patient-centred attitude.

As a communication/counselling framework, each of the six categories and the respective interventions that fall under each category are **theoretically neutral**, that is, they are not aligned with any particular theoretical perspective of psychology or psychotherapy, for example a humanistic approach, cognitive behavioural therapy, and others (Heron 2001). Nevertheless, the Six Category system can be used as an analytical tool to compare and contrast the therapeutic practice of different theoretical approaches. Similar to other psychotherapeutic approaches, the quality of the nurse–service user relationship is central to the therapeutic use and outcome of each of the six categories. Sensitive and skilled use of verbal and non-verbal communication can offer the necessary core conditions of all therapeutic relationships with service users, including genuineness, respect, empathetic understanding, and openness (Rogers 1957).

Authoritative and facilitative interventions

The Six Categories and their designations are classified into two main groups: Authoritative and Facilitative. **Authoritative or directive** interventions are so called because in each case the practitioner is taking a more overtly assertive or directive role. When using authoritative interventions, the emphasis is more on what the mental health nurse is **doing** to or with the service user; they include prescriptive, informative, and confronting interventions.

Facilitative interventions are less obtrusive and the role of the practitioner is more discreet. The emphasis is on the **effect** of the intervention on the service user, and interventions may be cathartic, catalytic, or supportive.

What is an intervention?

An intervention is an identifiable piece of verbal and/or non-verbal behaviour that is part of the nurse's service to the service user. There is no set way of stating an intervention; it can have many verbal forms. Although the six interventions refer mostly to the nurse's verbal skills, components of non-verbal behaviour, such as eye contact, gestures, and body language, are equally important in determining how the verbal interventions come across to the service user. Therefore, you should be mindful not only about what you say, but also about how it is expressed. Furthermore, it is important that verbal and non-verbal messages are congruent. For a more detailed coverage of verbal and non-verbal skills in clinical practice see Rungapadiachy (1999), Stevenson (2008), and Sully and Dallas (2005).

Intention

All six categories comprise a specific intention that determines the ultimate choice of intervention. Each intervention can be defined in terms of its intention: what it is that you want to achieve by your intervention. Table 6.1 outlines the Six Categories and their intentions.

It is important to remember that the authoritative categories are not more or less valuable or effective than the facilitative interventions; it all depends on:

- the nature of the nurse's role

- the particular needs of the service user at the time

- the content or focus of the intervention.

In practice, however, authoritative interventions have traditionally tended to be overused. Burnard and Morrison's (1988, 1989, 1991) studies of qualified nurses' perceptions of their own interpersonal skills using Six Category Intervention Analysis found that nurses generally perceived themselves to be more skilful in the authoritative than in the facilitative categories. Although authoritative interventions are not **bad** or **incorrect** *per se*, they can become ineffective and therefore non-therapeutic when they are used to the exclusion of facilitative interventions. Equally, the sole use of a facilitative approach can also lead to ineffective interventions and outcomes, because it excludes the use of the nurse's professional

Table 6.1 The Six Categories and their intentions (source Heron 2001)

	Aim	Example
Authoritative interventions		
Prescriptive	To direct the behaviour of the service user by demonstration, advice, suggestion, command	'I think you might feel better if you talk about why you are anxious about being discharged.'
Informative	To impart new knowledge or information to the service user by telling, informing	'These tablets may cause you to feel drowsy.'
Confronting	To raise the consciousness (awareness) of the service user about some limiting attitude, belief, or behaviour that he or she is unaware of by challenging, giving direct feedback in a supportive manner	'Are you aware that when you shout you frighten your family?'
Facilitative interventions		
Cathartic	To enable the service user to share, express, or discharge painful emotions (primarily grief, fear, and anger) by encouraging and supporting the person to express his or her feelings	'It's okay to be frightened about being in hospital.'
Catalytic	To enable the service user to learn and develop by self-direction, problem-solving, and self-discovery within the context of nurse–service user encounter, but also beyond it	'What do you think you could do to help yourself when you hear the voices?'
Supportive	To affirm the worth and value of the service user's person, qualities, attitudes, or actions by enhancing the self-esteem of the person by giving encouraging, validating feedback.	'You made a great effort to participate in the group.'

authority in an appropriate way. For example, in practice there may be occasions when it is part of your role and responsibility to guide or direct the service user's behaviour, provide information, and challenge them in order to meet the service user's needs at that particular time. However, as Heron (2001) points out, balancing authoritative and facilitative interventions is all about the appropriate use of power in clinical practice, that is:

1 Your power over the service user

2 The power the practitioner and the service user share with each other

3 The autonomous power within the service user.

All three forms of power need one another, and always in the right amount and according to the changing needs of the service user throughout the therapeutic encounter.

Applying Six Category Intervention Analysis in practice

Each of the six interventions is **value neutral**, that is, each intervention is neither more nor less significant and important than any other when used in an appropriate context. All six categories embrace patient-centred communication—*'communication which invites and encourages the patient to participate and negotiate in decision making regarding their own care'* (Langewitz et al. 1998, p. 230)—and, most importantly, are of any real value only if they are rooted in care and concern for the service user. Although the Six Categories are independent of one another and have a specific intention or purpose, there are also significant areas of overlap between them. Where such overlap occurs, the intervention is classified under the category that covers its primary purpose, as illustrated in the example below. The following Practice Example illustrates the use of all six interventions, although this particular interaction reflects a more facilitative approach (see also Box 6.1).

In learning how to use the Six Categories the nurse is acquiring a set of analytical and behavioural tools to select, monitor, and evaluate his or her own therapeutic interactions in terms of their therapeutic outcome. Each intervention can be evaluated only by testing it against the evidence in a practical context to determine whether the selected interventions elicited the desired result. In principle, each intervention can be checked, rechecked, amended, and modified by personal inquiry and in clinical supervision. For many nurses, it is not a question of starting from scratch with a whole new system. Many of the listed interventions identify and describe interventions that nurses will realize they have already been using, whereas other interventions will be new and enable nurses to extend their knowledge

---

✖ Practice Example

Service user
'I feel really down . . . it's been a terrible week.'

Nurse
'I am sorry to hear that you are feeling this way. Would you like to tell me more about it?' [**Catalytic**]

Service user
'I just can't cope anymore with the voices. They never stop.'

Nurse
'What are the voices saying to you? [**Catalytic**]

Service user
'They say I am a bad person . . . causing trouble for my family.'

Nurse
'It must be very difficult for you to cope with this.' [**Supportive**]

Service user
'I feel sad . . . my family try so hard to help me . . . I have let them down.'

Nurse
'It's okay to be sad.' [**Cathartic**]

Service user
Begins to cry . . . 'I don't know what to do.'

Nurse
'I notice that you have stopped taking your medication.' [**Confronting**]

Service user
'I want to take it, but it makes me put on so much weight.'

Nurse
'I know that must be very difficult and I can understand why you stopped taking your medication.' [**Supportive**]

Service user
'I am always hungry.'

Nurse
'Do you remember I told you that one of the side effects of your medication was an increase in appetite, which is causing you to put on weight?' [**Informative**]

Service user
'Yes . . . I just don't want to get fat.'

Nurse
'Yes, I understand that. However, I am concerned that if you don't take your medication the voices will get worse and you might become ill again. I want you to take your medication for the next week and then we can review it again.' [**Prescriptive**]

and skill base. Learning to use the Six Categories in practice can increase your confidence and efficacy. In practice, the skilled nurse aims to:

- be equally proficient in a wide range of interventions in each of the categories

- be able to move skilfully from one type of intervention to any other as the developing situation and purpose of the interaction require

- know what category she or he is using, and why, at any given time

- know when to lead and when to follow the service user

- know that the value of an intervention is a function of the total situation at the time and the purpose of the nurse's role in relation to the service user.

Factors that may influence the application of Six Category Intervention Analysis in practice

Given the uniqueness of each therapeutic relationship, every interaction with a service user will require different skills and interventions, based on the aim of the therapeutic communication, the context of the therapeutic encounter, the nurse's stage of professional development and level of competence, as well as the nature of the therapeutic relationship. As such, each interaction presents different learning opportunities and challenges that are often interchangeable and context dependent. However, in order to recognize the learning to be gained and the implications for practice, the nurse needs to reflect on the above and other potential factors, for example the timing of the interaction, the service user's well-being, the nurse's cognitive and affective state, and many more that may affect the therapeutic outcome and quality of the therapeutic alliance.

The questions in Box 6.1 are intended to be used as an aide-memoire rather than a definitive checklist to assist you in monitoring, reviewing, and evaluating your use of the six interventions in practice. These questions may also be useful when using a model of reflection, such as the Gibbs Reflective Cycle (Gibbs 1988).

Box 6.1 A guide to using Heron's six interventions in practice

Consider the following reflective questions:

- What was my **primary** intention during this interaction?

- Was my intention appropriate for this particular interaction and service user? If not, why not?

- What interventions did I use during this interaction?

- What was my intention in using these interventions?

- How did I use each category (intervention) in terms of: the timing of the intervention; amount—too much or too little; tone; body language?

- How competent did I feel using these interventions?

- Which interventions were effective and how do I know they were effective?

- What factors enhanced my application of the chosen categories?

- What components of the interaction were not effective and why?

- What components of the interaction were least effective and why?

- What factors hindered my application of the chosen categories?

- What would I do differently and why?

- What have I learnet from reflecting on this interaction?

- What am I aware of about my interpersonal communication that I was unaware of before reflecting on this interaction?

- What intervention do I need to develop in the future?

- What interventions do I tend to overuse?

- What interventions do I tend to underuse?

▲ Conclusion

In this chapter I have outlined the principles and practice of Heron's Six Category Intervention Analysis. For the developing practitioner, this communication framework provides a flexible and user-friendly tool to learn, acquire, and develop a range of interpersonal skills that can be used in various clinical encounters. However, it is not enough simply to learn the specific interventions; they must be applied in practice, whereby real learning takes place. As with all new learning, this will require time, practice, and a willingness to be open to inquiry and feedback about the usefulness of your therapeutic work in clinical practice. While I hope that this chapter is useful to you in developing your repertoire of communication skills and style of working, it is not intended to be the only source of learning. Notwithstanding, it provides a useful framework to identify and clarify what you are doing, when, how you are doing it, and, more importantly, how you know it was useful.

 ## Website

You may find it helpful to work through our short online quiz and scenario intended to help you to develop and apply the skills in this chapter. please go to:

www.oxfordtextbooks.co.uk/orc/callaghan

References

Barker, P. and Buchanan-Barker, P. (2004). *The Tidal Model: A Guide for Mental Health Professionals*. London: Brunner-Routledge.

Burnard, P. and Morrison, P. (1988). Nurses' perceptions of their interpersonal skills: a descriptive study using Six Category Intervention Analysis. *Nurse Education Today* 8, 266–72.

Burnard, P. and Morrison, P. (1989). What is an interpersonally skilled person? A repertory grid account of professional nurse's views. *Nurse Education Today* 9, 384–91.

Burnard, P. and Morrison, P. (1991). Nurses' interpersonal skills: a study of nurses' perceptions. *Nurse Education Today* 11(1), 24–9.

Cameron, D., Kapur, R., and Campbell, P. (2005). Releasing the therapeutic potential of the psychiatric nurses: a human relations perspective of the nurse–patient relationship. *Journal of Psychiatric and Mental Health Nursing* 12, 64–74.

Department of Health (1999). *Mental Health Nursing: Acute Concerns*. London: DH.

Department of Health (2002). *Mental Health Policy Implementation Guide: Adult Acute In-Patient Care Provision*. London: DH.

Department of Health (2004). *Getting Over the Wall. How the NHS is Improving the Patient's Experience*. London: DH.

Department of Health (2006). *Best Practice Competencies and Capabilities for Pre-registration Mental Health Nurses in England: The Chief Nursing Officer's Review of Mental Health Nursing*. London: DH.

Gibbs, G. (1988). *Learning by Doing: A Guide to Teaching and Learning Methods*. Oxford: Further Education Unit, Oxford Brookes.

Gijbels, H. (1995). Mental health nursing skills in an acute admission environment: perceptions of mental health nurses and other mental health professionals. *Journal of Advanced Nursing* 21, 460–5.

Heron, J. (1975). *Six Category Intervention Analysis*. Guildford: University of Surrey.

Heron, J. (2001). *Helping the Client—A Creative Practical Guide*, 5th edn. London: Sage.

Langewitz, W. A., Eich, P., Kiss, A., and Wossmer, B. (1998). Improving communication skills—a randomized controlled behaviourally oriented intervention study for residents in internal medicine. *Psychosomatic Medicine* 60, 268–76.

NHS Modernisation Agency (2003). *Essence of Care, Guidance and New Communications Benchmarks*. London: Department of Health.

Peplau, H. (1988). *Interpersonal Relations in Nursing*. Basingstoke: Macmillan Education.

Repper, J. and Perkins, R. (2003). *Social Inclusion and Recovery: A Model for Mental Health Practice*. London: Baillière Tindall.

Robinson, D. (1996a). Measuring psychiatric nursing interventions, communication on an adult psychiatric ward. *Nursing Times Research* 1, 13–21.

Robinson, D. (1996b). Observing and describing nursing interactions. *Nursing Standard* 13, 34–8.

Rogers, C. (1957). The necessary and sufficient conditions of therapeutic personality change. *Journal of Consulting Psychology* 21, 95–103.

Rungapadiachy, D. (1999). *Interpersonal Communication and Psychology for Health Care Professionals: Theory and Practice*. Oxford: Butterworth.

Sainsbury Centre for Mental Health (1998). *Acute Problems: A Survey of the Quality of Care in Acute Psychiatric Wards*. London: SCMH.

Stevenson, C. (2008). Therapeutic communication in mental health nursing. In: *Psychiatric/Mental Health Nursing: An Irish Perspective* (ed. J. Morrissey, B. Keogh, and L. Doyle), pp 109–22. Dublin: Gill & Macmillan.

Sully, P. and Dallas, J. (2005). *Essential Communication Skills for Nursing*. London: Elsevier.

Whittington, D. and McLaughlin, C. (2000). Finding time for patients: an exploration of nurses' allocation in an acute psychiatric setting. *Journal of Psychiatric and Mental Health Nursing* 7, 259–68.

Forming, sustaining, and ending therapeutic interactions

Jeanette Hewitt   Michael Coffey   Greg Rooney

▼ Introduction

Over 50 years ago, Hildegard Peplau (1952) identified the primacy of the nurse–patient relationship and the phases of this **therapeutic alliance** (Barker et al. 1999). Her work is still considered seminal and her broadly humanistic view of the nurse–patient relationship remains influential in current mental health nursing literature (Watkins 2001). The provision of the therapeutic relationship has been viewed as being fundamental to the care of mental health service users (Stickley 2002) and underpins success of all types of psychological therapy (Department of Health [DH] 2001b).

Evidence suggests a consistent relationship between the development of therapeutic relationships and improved outcomes for service users (Bambling and King 2001, Howgego et al. 2003), regardless of the type of psychological therapy employed (Hewitt and Coffey 2005). Studies of the expressed needs of service users show that the quality of relationships formed with mental health practitioners are associated with satisfaction with services generally (Barker et al. 1999, Bee et al. 2008), and that positive relationships are central to recovery (Repper 2002, Watkins 2001).

Effective counselling skills are seen as essential for the development of successful therapeutic relationships (Booth et al. 1996, Faulkner 1998). This relationship is defined primarily through the underpinning theory, the conditions seen as being necessary for therapeutic change, and the characteristics of the mental health practitioner. The humanistic or **person-centred approach** originates from the work of Carl Rogers (1902–1987), whose work was founded on the non-specific factors that constituted the therapeutic relationship. The practitioner's use of warmth, empathy, genuineness, and unconditional positive regard in the therapeutic encounter were seen as being necessary and sufficient conditions for change to take place (Mace 2002). This was articulated as a 'way of being' with the client that creates a climate for growth

and change through the therapeutic use of self (Nelson 1997, Watkins 2001).

This approach focuses on general factors in relationships with people and cuts across different psychological schools or techniques (Stiles et al. 1986). Barkham (2002) identified core elements as including an emotionally charged, confiding relationship with the helper and a healing setting in which the person expects that the practitioner will help them. Non-specific elements of the relationship include supportive factors such as using the therapeutic presence of the helper, the ability to facilitate catharsis, and perceived warmth (Barkham 2002). The bond between client and practitioner is created through trust, empathy, liking, support, respect, challenge, and valuing (Egan 2002). Goals are set with the mutual agreement and valuing of the outcomes of therapy, with a rationale that provides a plausible explanation of the person's problems and how they can be addressed by reciprocal action (Barkham 2002).

Rogers (1951) provides a theory of counselling that offers a 'way of being' based on a belief system, whereas Egan's (2002) 'transtheoretical approach' advocates a way of doing that is problem focused and goal driven. Both theories can inform how mental health nurses might work within a therapeutic relationship with a service user. By examining the essential underpinning theory, principles, and rationale of these two approaches, it is possible to explore why certain practices work and how these can contribute to the effective development of therapeutic relationships.

Learning outcomes

By the end of this chapter you should be better able to:

1 Demonstrate an understanding of the literature surrounding the nature, context, and importance of therapeutic relationships

2 Describe the person-centred approach and the **skilled helper model** of therapeutic relationships, including helping skills

3 Consider ways in which mental health nurses can apply their knowledge of therapeutic relationships to their own practice and begin to develop your own skills in this area.

The policy background

In recent years the pace of reform in mental health policy has been relentless (Jenkins et al. 2002). Contemporary health policy emphasizes performance improvement, increasing capacity with sharper market-style incentives whilst improving public health through partnership working between the statutory health services, local government, and communities (Baggott 2007). Previously, health policy tended to focus on **how** services were organized and on structural adjustment as the key to shaping service delivery (Glasby and Lester 2006). A welcome recent feature of policy is the increasing emphasis on users of services as experts in relation to health care planning and delivery (DH 2001a, Tilley and Ryan 2005). Emphasis has also been placed on the performance of individual practitioners, and in mental health the relationship skills of practitioners has been a key aspect of practice. The National Service Framework for Mental Health in England (DH 1999, p. 43) stated '*the quality of the relationship between patient and professional … can make as much as 25% difference in outcome*'. The Capable Practitioner Framework (Sainsbury Centre for Mental Health [SCMH] 2001) outlines ways in which mental health nurses and other professionals can develop and use therapeutic relationship skills, arguing that mental health professionals need to understand the fundamental importance of relationships to the social and psychological well-being of service users whilst recognizing the engagement difficulties that many mental health service users face. The framework recommends that professionals '*develop and sustain trusting relationships and constructive partnerships with people with complex needs who are unwilling to engage with services*' (p. 21). The themes of trust and engagement within therapeutic relationships are central to policies pertaining to working with users with complex needs (SCMH 1998), with African and Caribbean communities (National Institute for Mental Health in England 2003, SCMH 2001), where risk is a key issue (DH 2007), where drug misuse is a factor (National Institute for Health and Clinical Excellence 2007), and where medication management is an issue (DH 2008).

In the UK, the Nursing and Midwifery Council (NMC) and the Quality Assurance Agency for Higher Education (QAA) also recognize the centrality of therapeutic relationships to mental health nursing practice. The QAA (2001, p. 8) states that mental health nursing '*… is essentially a human activity which has as its core the relationship between the nurse and his/her client(s) and carers*'. In England, the Chief Nursing Officer's Review of Mental Health Nursing (DH 2006) recommends that all mental health nurses should be able to form strong therapeutic relationships with service users and carers. Recommendation 5 states that '*the relationship between the mental health nurse and service user needs to be positive, trusting, meaningful, therapeutic and collaborative, with mental health nurses having sufficient time in which to build, develop and sustain such relationships*' (p. 26). What is now beyond question is that those who use mental health services are seeking quality therapeutic relationships with mental health nurses and other professionals who recognize their interpersonal, emotional, behavioural, cognitive, and spiritual needs, and can facilitate service users to reach their maximum potential.

The evidence base

The person-centred approach

The central premise of the person-centred approach is that the therapeutic relationship is sufficient in itself for change to take place. Rogers (1957) proposed that the use of warmth, **empathy**, **unconditional positive regard**, and **genuineness**, in the immediate therapeutic encounter, are necessary and sufficient conditions for therapeutic gain. He argued that, for constructive psychological change to occur, certain core conditions should be in existence: the client's state of incongruence and the helper's congruence and experience of unconditional positive regard for the client. The helper should demonstrate empathic understanding of the client's frame of reference and communicate this, together with unconditional positive regard, at least to a minimal extent.

The central focus of Rogers' (1951) person-centred approach is facilitating increased self-awareness through the reflection of feelings. For mental health nursing, this means acknowledgement of the service user as the expert on their own problems, and that the nurse's role is as a source of reflection in the here and now experience (McLeod 1998). This resonates with contemporary mental health recovery approaches that assert that the user is the expert in their own care and recovery (Copeland 1997, DH 2001a). Within a Rogerian approach, service users are able to meet their internal valuing systems through the alliance, allowing them to experience rather than to deny and distort their feelings (Nelson-Jones 1997). Being heard and understood is vital to the process of making sense of inner feelings and perceptions (Barrett-Lennard 1993). By reflecting back feelings expressed, without judgement or reduction, the helper gives permission to the user to experience these emotions without fear of censure (Figure 7.1). Sensing acceptance or unconditional positive regard from mental health nurses is critical to clients seeking the recovery of psychological equilibrium (Cutcliffe and McKenna 2000).

At times, certain roles and responsibilities of mental health nurses may conflict with some of the core elements of the person-centred approach to relationships. Maslach and Jackson (1984) argue that the contradictory expectations of the practitioners in a counselling role may eventually lead to burnout and feelings of personal failure. Formally detained service users present mental health nurses with particular relationship dilemmas, in that they need to balance their duty of care with the service user's right to self-determination.

Truax (1966) is sceptical about the existence of a nondirective approach to psychological therapy, identifying cases where practitioners were shown subtly to reinforce some statements made by clients, whilst withdrawing regard when other statements were made. Sharing empathic highlights without interpretation may prove to be difficult for mental health nurses where service users' thoughts and feelings indicate serious mental health problems or where there is a perceived risk to the safety of others.

The Rogerian approach requires mental health nurses to develop empathic understanding of the service user's conceptual world and to communicate this awareness back to them (Rogers 1957). Rogers (1980, p. 142) described empathic listening as '… *entering the private perceptual world of the other and becoming thoroughly at home in it. It involves being sensitive, moment by moment, to the*

changing felt meanings which flow in this other person, to the fear or rage or tenderness or confusion or whatever that he or she is experiencing.'

The intimacy generated by entering the service user's world through empathy may, however, lead the mental health nurse to make inadequate distinctions between themselves and the service user, and is not without risk. Blurred emotional boundaries are detrimental to the service user, and self-awareness is an essential skill in maintaining boundaries in helping relationships. Mental health nurses may internalize the distress of service users through the process of advanced empathy, and resulting over-identification may ultimately lead to emotional exhaustion (Maslach and Jackson 1984). Caring for others may lead to feelings of anger and frustration, which can be misdirected into other affiliations (Jones 1997). To cope with feelings of guilt and inadequacy, mental health nurses may adopt defence mechanisms that are inappropriate and destructive. Self-awareness on the part of the mental health nurse is therefore essential in the development and maintenance of therapeutic relationships. Access to regular clinical supervision is one way to address some of these concerns.

Watkins (2001) notes the resemblance between what users stated mental health nurses contributed to their recovery and what Rogers (1957) identified as the necessary and sufficient conditions for change: a working alliance with a practitioner who is empathic, accepting, and genuine.

Egan's skilled helper model

Egan (2002) argues that the therapeutic relationship is characterized by support, challenge, and empathy. Similar to Rogers, Egan weaves positive psychology into the helping process, rather than focusing exclusively on pathology, and highlights the need for the helper to communicate genuineness and respect for the service user. However, he argues that the core conditions are not in themselves sufficient for change to occur,

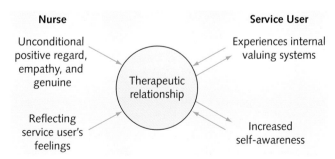

Figure 7.1 The Rogerian approach to therapeutic relationships in which the creation of a positive relationship enables the service user to reflect and increase self-awareness.

and focuses more on problem-solving with specific aims: to identify missed opportunities or unused potential. Whilst Rogers argues that change will naturally occur in the context of the therapeutic alliance, Egan proposes a model for action in which the service user is a partner in the process and is required to work through feelings of resistance to change.

Egan's model uses three stages in a fluid problem-solving cycle. In stage one, service users are helped to tell their stories, challenged to acknowledge blind spots, and helped to choose problems and/or opportunities to work on. This approach requires action from both the service user and the practitioner. Emphasis is on the service user taking responsibility within the relationship, whereas Rogers (1951) emphasizes the qualities of the practitioner. The focus of the relationship is on achieving valued outcomes for the service user through responding to wherever they wish to go, without preconceived ideas by the practitioner about where they ought to be (Egan 1998).

Stage two is about providing opportunities for service users to explore possibilities for a better future, identifying realistic, challenging, and solution-focused goals to address key problems and opportunities. Service users need to find incentives to facilitate commitment to their change agenda. In stage three, possible actions are explored, stimulating service users to think in different ways, with the practitioner assisting service users to choose best-fit strategies and to construct a plan of action. The stages are summarized in Figure 7.2.

Egan's model may appear somewhat mechanistic in comparison with the deeper messages implicit in Rogers' 'way of being'. Although it has been proposed as ideal for both counsellor training and workplace supervision therapy (Bimrose 2000, Reddy 1987), the novice practitioner can be tempted to value the strategy above the service user. Attempts to mould service users to the model are not advocated by Egan, but may prove to be the case in practice where time is limited.

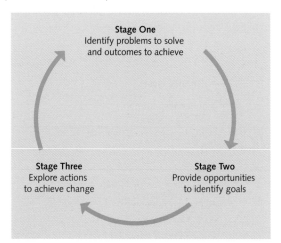

Figure 7.2 Egan's model of the skilled helper.

Considerable variations in success rates exist between practitioners of the same theoretical orientation (Luborsky et al. 1986), supporting the argument that therapeutic outcome is likely to be as related to the practitioner as to the type of therapy practised.

The nature of the client

In his theory of personality, Rogers (1959) argued that human beings have an actualizing tendency, which aims to develop, maintain, or enhance capacities in ways that increase autonomy. Personality change is possible and is a necessary part of growth (Rogers 1961). He identified the importance of self-concept as a means of defining self and asserted that where an experienced feeling fails to match self-concept this will be expressed in a distorted and inappropriate way. This state of incongruence results from conditions of worth, which were internalized in childhood in an attempt to gain the conditional love of parents (Merry 2000). The nature of the client in Rogers' theory is as one who experiences incongruence because of an external locus of evaluation leading to over-reliance on externally defined beliefs and further conditions of worth.

Egan's (2002) model views people as being likely to seek counselling because they are involved in problems arising through interpersonal or intrapersonal interactions. They may be experiencing conflict as a result of living within settings at home, work, or in the community. The problems they bring are viewed as reactions to living rather than an indication of underlying pathology. Deficiency in personal, social, and life-skills blocks them from making the most of opportunities and resources.

Helper skills

Rogers (1962) argued for a way of being that transcended the use of specific counselling techniques. Instead he identified the importance of bracketing off or suspending assumptions based on theoretical knowledge and experience. Empathy, for Rogers (1975), was thus not a skill but a way of being.

'To sense the client's inner world of private personal meanings as if it were your own, but without ever losing the "as if" quality, this is empathy.'

Rogers (1962, p. 419)

For Egan (2002), empathy is actually a communication skill made up of active listening, reflection with verbal and body messages, and mirroring the essence of meaning for the client (Nelson-Jones 1997). Egan's 'skilled helper' is in perpetual motion, probing, challenging, and looking for leverage (Bond et al. 2000), with empathic presence being transmitted through body language, attending, observing, and listening to service users' stories, behaviours, and feelings whilst highlighting key feelings and moods, using questions, and summarizing effectively.

The impact on the client

The person-centred approach uses counselling skills to increase self-awareness in the service user so that he or she may accept and act on internal evaluations. This allows them to experience and not fear their own feelings, leading to a greater sense of autonomy and personal value. Their skills and strengths, often hidden, may then be revealed through the therapeutic relationship (Rogers 1975).

The positive impact of the Rogerian approach on the service user has been attributed to the heightened sense of mastery the service user experiences over internal and external difficulties through their enhanced ability to name them (McLeod 1998). Grencavage and Norcross (1990) argue that it is the personal qualities of the practitioner that facilitate this change. The effectiveness of the therapy may be less to do with specific strategies and more to do with non-specific factors that do not seem to require the learning of elaborate techniques (Mace 2002). This would appear to support the assertion that, where mental health nurses and service users establish a meaningful alliance, the experience will be therapeutic for service users regardless of other psychological interventions used (Barkham 2002).

Rogers' (1961) view of human behaviour is that it is rational and that the core of a person's nature is essentially positive. Criticism of Rogers' theory includes scepticism regarding his view of human nature. He hypothesized that, where a person may learn to act on internal evaluations, these values will be valid for both self and others (McLeod 1998). This may be unrealistic and could lead to the breakdown of social relationships, where the person does not acknowledge the alternative reality of other beliefs. McLeod (1998) argues that the humanistic philosophy represents a positive view of the world that may deny the tragedy of human experience.

Egan (2002) asserts that helping is a social influence process and that psychological explanations alone are insufficient. Here, service users are helped through taking a pragmatic approach to problems in living. What is required are opportunities to manage social settings and systems more effectively (Connor 2000). Through shared use of Egan's model, decision-making is enhanced and actions become appropriate and effective with facilitation of creativity and imagination, allowing service users to think the unthinkable, leading to greater opportunities for change. Self-empowerment and insight are achieved through challenging blind spots (Egan 1998). As the

aim of the model is problem management, the result should be that the service user and mental health nurse are able to find and act upon appropriate solutions to problems.

Although there is little formal research validating Egan's model, it has been adopted in many different cultures, which may provide support for the model's universal understanding of human experience and capacity for change (McMahon 2000). Whilst problem-solving models are useful to help service users manage their current problems, they are often inadequate in addressing repeated underlying self-defeating behaviours (McLeod 1998). Although Egan (2002) includes identifying blind spots in his model of change, this may not focus sufficiently on underlying assumptions about self that are known and yet unchanging.

Forming relationships

An important principle of working with people with mental health problems is to establish realistic expectations from the outset (Repper et al. 1994). This enables the service user and the mental health nurse to reduce feelings of frustration and failure, which can envelop the process when working in this area. A cooperative approach is appreciated by people using services and can help in establishing the relationship.

Mental health professionals can struggle to actively engage service users, whether at home, hospital, or in other residential settings. Reasons for this may include services not providing the kinds of help valued by the service user. However, there are aspects of interaction that can help mental health nurses facilitate service user engagement with services, and with individual mental health professionals. *Keys to Engagement* (SCMH 1998) reported that many service users are suspicious of statutory services as a result of upbringing, life experiences, or attitudes. They may feel that services have little to offer, or they may have experienced negative staff attitudes, including racism. Mental health professionals may be too focused on immediate outcomes or on offering treatment with medication alone. Mental health nurses need to be able to meet service users on their own terms, wherever possible in their own environments. Onyett (1992) argues that service users need to place the mental health professional in context; knowing who they are, why they are there, and connecting with the mental health nurse as a person are fundamental when approaching the service user to commence a therapeutic relationship.

Not everyone wants to establish a therapeutic relationship, and the circumstances and context of the first contact can play an important role in these early stages. Mental health nurses need to persist without being intrusive or harassing to the service user. Initial rejection should not be seen as final and complete. Remember that many people need help but may not be familiar with ways in which to seek that help; this is a skill and it may have to be learned. Engagement with service users requires persistence, skill, imagination, and a respectful approach (Holloway et al. 1996, Onyett 1992).

Perhaps one of the most crucial tasks of working with service users with severe and enduring mental health problems is establishing contact and meaningfully engaging to facilitate later and ongoing work. Some may lack insight into their condition; others may be keen to put the experience behind them and feel they do not want the help that is offered. In some cases, lack of choice on these matters can compound the difficulties in forming a relationship with the mental health nurse. What does appear to be crucial is that the mental health nurse spends time getting to know the person as a whole person and not simply as a service user (Shattell et al. 2007).

Many people admitted to hospital are compelled to do so, and are sometimes required to take medication. They are also 'given' a primary nurse or key worker. They have no say in any of this and may resent the imposition. They may be frightened and fearful for their safety, especially if this is their first time in hospital. Being offered (or being told to take) medication you have never had before, or that you have had negative experiences of, can feel threatening. Noisy, busy admission wards can be a frightening experience—especially when you are not sure when you might be allowed to leave.

Mental health nurses need to be aware of this. Placing yourself in the shoes of the person you are working with may help you to gain an understanding of their experience. Approaching the person in an open, non-threatening, and friendly manner, making them comfortable in their surroundings, introducing them to others on the ward, and offering opportunities to talk and listen may all help to develop confidence in you and the team.

Trust is an essential component of establishing meaningful relationships with people generally, and people who are experiencing mental health problems are no different. As mental health nurses we should not automatically expect trust—we must work to achieve it. Establishing appropriate eye contact, being friendly and warm towards the person, and listening attentively to what they say will help to develop trust in you as a competent and caring mental health nurse. Engaging people who have previously rejected services, or who may be antagonistic toward services to the extent that they are likely to reject formal services, requires trust based on mutual respect. This means that mental health nurses must respect the views and rights of people using mental health services and that mental health nursing must be based on this principle rather than one of coercion.

Repper et al. (1994) investigated strategies used by mental health nurses, working as case managers, to establish therapeutic relationships with service users with serious mental health problems. Key areas of importance in the initial stages of the relationship identified by staff included the effectiveness of being able to demonstrate their usefulness to the service user—particularly important when service users were wary of their case manager. Repper et al. (1994) found the emphasis in the early stages of the therapeutic relationship was on achieving practical tasks, and this served to clarify the mental health professional's role and provided the foundations for the relationship.

Sustaining relationships

As discussed, contemporary mental health policy is driving mental health nurses and others to re-focus on the core elements of their work, in particular therapeutic relationships. This is in part the rationale behind initiatives to put in place protected nurse–service user time, particularly in acute inpatient units. For many mental health nurses working in the community, opportunities to spend time with service users are plentiful, although pressures of time may still limit this work. Given the recognized need to spend time with service users, many mental health nurses are concerned about how they should use the therapeutic relationship—what they should be talking about. We have argued elsewhere that sustaining a good-quality therapeutic relationship is necessary but not sufficient on its own to enable the types of change wanted by service users and desired by mental health nurses working with them (Hewitt and Coffey 2005). Mental health nurses should aim to address constructively the priorities for care expressed by service users. The processes of assessment in the initial stages of a relationship should be used and revisited periodically as a focus for the therapeutic relationship.

In classical treatments of the therapeutic relationship, service users bring problems and have the resources available to resolve them. More contemporary models place the emphasis on the strengths of the individual or their expressed needs for recovery as a means to achieving better outcomes (Rapp and Goscha 2006, Repper and Perkins 2003), with the role of the practitioner being to offer help in finding the way. However, in modern mental health services, many service users may be reluctant to engage, have few resources, and suffer from a complex of mental health and social needs that induce a sense of being unable to articulate the problem, or indeed to consider any possible ways of addressing it. Mental health nurses can facilitate opportunities to identify problems and find ways of addressing these with the person and their families to enable better future coping. The therapeutic relationship is the means to achieving change. However, the mental health nurse must do more than simply be available in the session with the service user. They must use the time

actively to involve, listen, and recruit the service user into addressing their problems. Where to start and what to focus on is, of course, entirely dependent upon the service user and the problems or challenges they are presented with. Many service users have clearly articulated priorities that should guide service provision, but for others helping them to prioritize their needs for care may be a useful first step. So, for instance, if someone is admitted to hospital because they

✖ Practice Example and Tips

Case

A young man, John, has been admitted to the ward where you work. He has never been in hospital before or had contact with mental health services. Recently he has had troubling experiences of voices, which prompted him to harm himself in the hope that this would help stop them. John is fearful and suspicious of help, and you, as his primary nurse, must reassure him and begin to engage him.

Based on this chapter what would you do?

Once you have finished this chapter, you can go online at

www.oxfordtextbooks.co.uk

to work through this scenario and read the authors' suggestions for forming, sustaining, and ending a therapeutic relationship with John.

Practice tips

You may find this a useful recap before going out on placement.

Establishing therapeutic relationships

- Use appropriate eye contact, be friendly, and listen attentively.
- Identify the service user's priorities for care.
- Establish realistic expectations from the outset.
- Facilitate service user engagement with services, demonstrate your usefulness, and achieve practical tasks to clarify your role.
- Foster an atmosphere of cooperation.
- Initial rejection should not be seen as final and complete—persist without being intrusive or harassing to the service user.

- Engage meaningfully in order to facilitate later and ongoing work.
- Spend time getting to know the person as a whole person and not simply as a service user.
- Offer opportunities to talk and listen.
- Do not automatically expect trust—nurses must work to achieve it.

Sustaining therapeutic relationships

1 Carry out a focused assessment to identify the service user's priorities for recovery.

2 If applicable, facilitate opportunities for the service user (and carers/family) to identify their needs for care and goals for recovery. Work in partnership to find ways of addressing these.

3 Use available time with the service user to address their expressed priorities for care.

4 Actively involve, listen, and recruit the service user into addressing their problems.

5 Use time to improve awareness and, if applicable, knowledge in order to promote recovery, self-management, or coping techniques.

6 Revisit the assessment and care plan periodically as a focus for the therapeutic relationship.

Ending therapeutic relationships

- Anticipate that the relationship will end at some point and discuss this with the service user.
- Discuss change in a positive manner.
- Promote self-management, connect with social supports and activities to enhance confidence.
- Evaluate the therapeutic relationship, addressing both the positive and negative elements from all perspectives.

have harmed themselves, then talking and listening time can be directed towards issues of their safety. In other circumstances the mental health nurse may wish to ascertain the level of knowledge the service user and their family have about their condition, and use the time in sessions to address deficits in knowledge about the illness and the treatments available. These are health-promoting tasks aimed at improving awareness and eventually self-management of the condition. Therapeutic relationships can only be strengthened and enhanced by such focused work.

As the relationship progresses, more involved work can focus on identifying and analysing problems in daily living, or with particularly bothersome symptoms such as distressing voices. Helping the service user to establish realistic goals for treatment, prioritizing which problems to address first, and developing structured problem-solving will all help develop and sustain the relationship, and encourage continuing engagement with addressing care needs. A useful approach is to seek support and supervision from experienced practitioners to enable the development of skills in this important area of practice.

Ending relationships

The types of therapeutic relationship that mental health nurses develop with service users will vary across settings, from individual to individual, and within the context of the wider mental health team, where others may be the primary professional involved. Some therapeutic relationships endure for many years, whereas others last just for the period of the assessment or intervention. In each case, however, mental health nurses must be oriented towards ending the relationship in a positive manner, as abrupt endings may lead to negative health outcomes. It has been shown that service users experience a range of feelings when therapeutic relationships are ended, including gratitude, regret, grief, and anxiety, particularly in relation to future continuity of care (Planavsky et al. 2001). Mental health nurses must anticipate that relationships will end at some point and engage with service users, and perhaps their family, in anticipatory dialogue about this. Attempts at promoting self-management, connecting with social supports, and enhancing confidence may help in easing anxieties about ending helping relationships (Forchuk et al. 1998). Formal evaluative discussions should usefully evaluate the experience of the relationship, addressing both the positive and negative elements from all perspectives. Demonstrating movement and change may enable both the service user and mental health nurse to move on with a sense of accomplishment and a focus on a future ripe with possibilities of further recovery. Handled well, endings can enable opportunities for enhanced outcomes.

▲   Conclusion

Mental health nurses require a working knowledge of counselling skills to enable the development of a therapeutic relationship with service users. Outcome studies and surveys of the expressed needs of service users confirm that meaningful therapeutic relationships with mental health practitioners are seen as necessary to recovery. In comparing the work of directive and non-directive theorists, it has been possible to explore the validity of a skilled helper framework and the uses of the therapeutic presence of the mental health professional. Using person-centred principles within the structure of a problem-solving cycle may prove to be the most practical approach to managing therapeutic relationships. Service users' experiences of therapeutic relationships suggest that in-depth personal knowledge and understanding of their experience by their mental health nurse is a necessary and valued factor contributing to their recovery. The mental health nurse will know the service user as a whole person and not simply as a recipient of services.

w   Website

You may find it helpful to work through our short online quiz and scenario intended to help you to develop and apply the skills in this chapter. Please go to:

   www.oxfordtextbooks.co.uk/orc/callaghan

✦ References

Baggott, R. (2007). *Understanding Health Policy*. Bristol: Policy Press.

Bambling, M. and King, R. (2001). Therapeutic alliance and clinical practice. *Psychotherapy in Australia* 8, 38–43.

Barker P., Jackson S., and Stevenson, C. (1999). What are psychiatric nurses needed for? Developing a theory of essential nursing practice. *Journal of Psychiatric and Mental Health Nursing* 6, 273–82.

Barkham, M. (2002). Common factors in psychological therapies. *Psychiatry* 1(3), 5–8.

Barrett-Lennard, G. (1993). The phases and focus of empathy. *British Journal of Medical Psychology* 66, 3–14.

Bee, P., Playle, J. F., Lovell, K., Barnes, P., Gray, R., and Keeley, P. (2008). Service user views and expectations of UK-registered mental health nurses: a systematic review of empirical research. *International Journal of Nursing Studies* 45, 442–57.

Bimrose, J. (2000). Careers counselling. In: *Handbook of Counselling and Psychotherapy* (ed. C. Feltham and I. Horton), pp 585–9. London: Sage.

Bond, T., Alred, G., and Hughes, P. (2000). Clinical practice issues. In: *Handbook of Counselling and Psychotherapy* (ed. C. Feltham and I. Horton), pp 152–70. London: Sage.

Booth, K., Maguire, P. M., Butterworth, T., and Hillier, V. F. (1996). Perceived professional support and the use of blocking behaviours by hospice nurses. *Journal of Advanced Nursing* 24, 522–7.

Connor, M. (2000). The skilled helper model. In: *Handbook of Counselling and Psychotherapy* (ed. C. Feltham and I. Horton), pp 393–8. London: Sage.

Copeland, M. E. (1997). *Wellness Recovery Action Plan (WRAP)*. West Dummerston, VT: Peach Press.

Cutcliffe, J. and McKenna, H. (2000). Generic nurses: the nemesis of psychiatric/mental health nursing? Part two. *Mental Health Practice* 3(10), 20–3.

Department of Health (1999). *National Service Framework for Mental Health*. London: DH.

Department of Health (2001a). *The Expert Patient: A New Approach to Chronic Disease Management for the 21st Century*. London: DH.

Department of Health (2001b). *Treatment Choice in Psychological Therapies and Counselling: Evidence-based Clinical Practice Guidelines*. London: DH.

Department of Health (2006). *From Values to Action: The Chief Nursing Officer's Review of Mental Health Nursing*. London: DH.

Department of Health (2007). *Best Practice in Managing Risk: Principles and Evidence for Best Practice in the Assessment and Management of Risk to Self and Others in Mental Health Services*. London: DH.

Department of Health (2008). *Medicines Management: Everybody's Business: A Guide for Service Users, Carers and Health and Social Care Practitioners*. London: DH.

Egan, G. (1998). *The Skilled Helper*, 6th edn. Pacific Grove, CA: Brooks/Cole Publishing.

Egan, G. (2002). *The Skilled Helper: A Problem-Management and Opportunity-Development Approach to Helping,* 7th edn. Pacific Grove, CA: Brooks/Cole Publishing.

Faulkner, A. (1998). *Effective Interaction with Patients*, 2nd edn. London: Churchill Livingstone.

Forchuk, C., Jewell, J., Schofield, R., Sircelj, M., and Valledor, T. (1998). From hospital to community: bridging therapeutic relationships. *Journal of Psychiatric and Mental Health Nursing* 5, 197–202.

Glasby, J. and Lester, H. (2006). *Mental Health Policy and Practice*. Basingstoke: Palgrave Macmillan.

Grencavage, L. M. and Norcross, J. C. (1990). Where are the commonalities among the therapeutic common factors? *Professional Psychology: Research and Practice* 21, 372–8.

Hewitt, J. and Coffey, M. (2005). Therapeutic working relationships with people with schizophrenia: literature review. *Journal of Advanced Nursing* 52(5), 561–70.

Holloway, F., Murray, M., Squire, C., and Carson, J. (1996). Intensive case management: putting it into practice. *Psychiatric Bulletin* 20, 395–7.

Howgego, I. M., Yellowlees, P., Owen, C., Meldrum, L., and Dark, F. (2003). The therapeutic alliance: the key to effective patient outcome? A descriptive review of the evidence in community mental health case management. *Australian and New Zealand Journal of Psychiatry* 37, 169–83.

Jenkins, R., McCulloch, A., Friedli, L., and Parker, L. (2002). *Developing a National Mental Health Policy*. Hove: Psychology Press.

Jones, A. (1997). A bonding between strangers: a palliative model of clinical supervision. *Journal of Advanced Nursing* 26, 1028–35.

Luborsky, L., Crits-Christoph, P., and Mellon, J. (1986). Advent of objective measures of the transference concept. *Journal of Consulting and Clinical Psychology* 54, 39–47.

Mace, C. (2002). The history of psychotherapy. *Psychiatry* 1(3), 1–3.

Maslach, C. and Jackson, S. E. (1984). Burnout in organisational settings. In: *Applied Social Psychology Annual 5: Applications in Organizational Settings* (ed. S. Oskamp), pp 173–201. London: Sage.

McLeod, J. (1998). *An Introduction to Counselling*, 2nd edn. Buckingham: Open University Press.

McMahon, G. (2000). Assessment and case formulation. In: *Handbook of Counselling and Psychotherapy* (ed. C. Feltham and I. Horton), pp 102–10. London: Sage.

Merry, T. (2000). Person-centred counselling and therapy. In: *Handbook of Counselling and Psychotherapy* (ed. C. Feltham and I. Horton), pp 348–51. London: Sage.

National Institute for Health and Clinical Excellence (2007). *Drug Misuse: Psychosocial Interventions. National Clinical Practice Guideline Number 51*. London: National Collaborating Centre for Mental Health.

National Institute for Mental Health in England (2003). *Inside Outside: Improving Mental Health Services for Black and Minority Ethnic Communities in England*. London: NIMHE.

Nelson, H. (1997). *Cognitive Behavioural Therapy with Schizophrenia: A Practice Manual*. Cheltenham: Nelson Thornes.

Nelson-Jones, R. (1997). *Practical Counselling and Helping Skills*, 4th edn. London: Cassell.

Onyett, S. (1992). *Case Management in Mental Health*. London: Chapman and Hall.

Peplau, H. (1952). *Interpersonal Relations in Nursing*. New York: Putnam.

Planavsky, L. A., Mion, L. C., Litaker, D. G., Kippes, C. M., and Mehta, N. (2001). Ending a nurse practitioner–patient relationship: uncovering patients' perceptions. *Journal of the American Academy of Nurse Practitioners* 13(9), 428–35.

Quality Assurance Agency for Higher Education (2001). *Benchmark Statement: Health Care Programmes, Phase 1, Nursing*. Gloucester: QAA.

Rapp, C. A. and Goscha, R. J. (2006). *The Strengths Model: Case Management with People with Psychiatric Disabilities*, 2nd edn. Oxford: Oxford University Press.

Reddy, M. (1987). *The Manager's Guide to Counselling at Work*. London: British Psychological Society/Methuen.

Repper, J. (2002). The helping relationship. In: *Psychosocial Interventions for People with Schizophrenia* (ed. N. Harris, S. Williams, and T. Bradshaw), pp 39–52. Basingstoke: Palgrave.

Repper, J. and Perkins, R. (2003). *Social Inclusion and Recovery: A Model for Mental Health Services*. London: Baillière Tindall.

Repper, J., Ford, R., and Cooke, A. (1994). How can nurses build trusting relationships with people who have severe and long term mental health problems? Experiences of case managers and their clients. *Journal of Advanced Nursing* 19, 1096–104.

Rogers, C. R. (1951). *Client-Centred Therapy: Its Current Practice, Implications and Theory*. Boston: Houghton Mifflin.

Rogers, C. R. (1957). The necessary and sufficient conditions of therapeutic personality change. *Journal of Consulting Psychology* 21, 95–103.

Rogers, C. R. (1959). A theory of therapy, personality and interpersonal relationships as developed in the client-centred framework. In: *Psychology: A Study of Science* (ed. S. Koch), pp 184–256. New York: McGraw-Hill.

Rogers, C. R. (1961). *On Becoming a Person*. Boston: Houghton Mifflin.

Rogers, C. R. (1962). The interpersonal relationship: the core of guidance. *Harvard Educational Review* 3, 416–29.

Rogers, C. R. (1975). Empathy: an unappreciated way of being. *Counselling Psychologist* 21, 95–103.

Rogers, C. R. (1980). *A Way of Being*. Boston: Houghton Mifflin.

Sainsbury Centre for Mental Health (1998). *Keys to Engagement: Review of Care for People with Severe Mental Illness who are Hard to Engage with Services*. London: Sainsbury Centre for Mental Health.

Sainsbury Centre for Mental Health (2001). *The Capable Practitioner: A Framework and List of the Practitioner Capabilities*. London: Sainsbury Centre for Mental Health.

Shattell, M. M., Starr, S. S., and Thomas, S. P. (2007). 'Take my hand, help me out': Mental health service recipients' experience of the therapeutic relationship. *International Journal of Mental Health Nursing* 16(4), 274–84.

Stickley, T. (2002). Counselling and mental health nursing: a qualitative study. *Journal of Psychiatric and Mental Health Nursing* 9(3), 301–8.

Stiles, W. B., Shapiro, D. A., and Elliott, R. (1986). Are all psychotherapies equivalent? *American Psychologist* 41(2), 165–80.

Tilley, S. and Ryan, D. (2005). Introduction. In: *Psychiatric and Mental Health Nursing: The Field of Knowledge* (ed. S. Tilley), pp 3–14. Oxford: Blackwell.

Truax, C. B. (1966). Reinforcement and non-reinforcement in Rogerian psychotherapy. *Journal of Abnormal Psychology* 71, 1–9.

Watkins, P. (2001). *Mental Health Nursing: The Art of Compassionate Care*. Oxford: Butterworth Heinemann.

(8) Working in partnership

Alan Simpson　　　　　　　　**Geoff Brennan**

▼ Introduction

Developing and sustaining positive therapeutic relationships with service users, their families, and other carers is central to the role of the mental health nurse. This is emphasized in England with the Chief Nursing Officer's review of mental health nursing (Department of Health [DH] 2006a), in Wales within Standard 8 of *Raising the Standard* (Welsh Assembly Government 2005), in Scotland within Key Aim No. 4 (Promoting and Supporting Recovery) of the *National Programme for Improving Mental Health and Well-Being* (Scottish Executive 2003). In addition, the Northern Irish Executive commissioned an independent review of mental health and learning disability services, and the resultant strategy contains this statement from its Service User Reference Group:

> 'One element must be changed and that is the attitudes of the professionals and all those who engage with us. Essential to empowerment and recovery is a person centred approach. Understanding the person on their own terms and placing them at the centre of the process.'

Bamford Review of Mental Health and Learning Disabilities
(Northern Ireland) (2005, p.7)

In brief, all of these documents highlight that the relationship between the mental health nurse and service users needs to be positive, trusting, meaningful, and therapeutic. Modern mental health nursing requires the nurse to build on that positive therapeutic relationship and take things to another level by **working in partnership** with service users. Working in partnership is a collaborative, more empowering way of helping service users and is a key feature of the **recovery approach** (Box 8.1).

The key principles and values of the recovery approach should inform mental health nursing practice in all areas of

Box 8.1 Recovery approach and mental health nursing

'Recovery can be defined as a personal process of tackling the adverse impacts of experiencing mental health problems, despite their continuing or long-term presence. It involves personal development and change, including acceptance there are problems to face, a sense of involvement and control over one's life, the cultivation of hope and using the support from others, including direct collaboration in joint problem-solving between people using services, workers and professionals. Recovery starts with the individual and works from the inside out. For this reason it is personalised and challenges traditional service approaches.'

Frak (2005, p. 1)

care and underpin service structures, individual practice, and educational preparation (DH 2006a). Nurses need to:

- value the aims of service users
- work in partnership and offer meaningful choice
- be optimistic and offer hope about the possibilities of positive change
- value the social inclusion of people with mental health problems.

In working collaboratively, the mental health nurse recognizes the unique knowledge and expertise service users have about their own life and experiences. At the same time, the nurse offers to draw on their own skills and professional understanding to jointly develop and agree strategies aimed at helping the person move forward and regain control over their health and life.

As nurses working in partnership, we offer our expertise and knowledge to help the person recognize and understand the choices they have and to resolve problems in a way that is beneficial and acceptable to them. This can be empowering for service users as the nurse is trying to help them find their own solutions and build on their own strengths and resources, rather than disempowering and even infantilizing users by taking over and making decisions for them.

Working in partnership is not necessarily easy for either nurses or service users. We all tend to carry age-old ideas about nurses caring *for* the patient, doing things *for* the patient—and sometimes that is still exactly what is required. However, the challenge for the effective mental health nurse is to recognize and build on the numerous opportunities available within positive therapeutic relationships to encourage and enable service users to find their own ways forward. The nurse can then help service users develop and draw on these skills to deal with other challenges along their personal journey to recovery.

In this chapter, we outline some of the skills and approaches that the mental health nurse requires in order to work in partnership. Obviously, in one chapter we can provide only a limited number of examples and illustrations of the skills required, but we aim to consider these across the various life stages the nurse is likely to encounter in their work. One highly important aspect of partnership working we will not cover in this chapter is working with family members and others in caring roles. Working with families and carers requires more detailed exploration than could be done here, so we have directed you to useful information at the end of the chapter. We will, however, aim to show some of the challenges and difficulties that may be encountered in trying to work in partnership, and how these might be reframed and resolved. In particular, we will demonstrate some of the very real challenges that exist when trying to implement these skills in the 'real world' of mental health services, in which staff often face seemingly impossible demands and insufficient resources (Brennan et al. 2006).

Learning outcomes

By the end of this chapter you should be better able to:

1 Demonstrate an understanding of skills required to work in partnership with service users

2 Describe potential areas of conflict in working collaboratively with users and how to resolve them

3 Identify some of the theories and approaches that underpin these skills

4 Use a range of partnership working skills in practice.

The evidence base

Best practice in mental health nursing is underpinned by a number of frameworks that shape and inform the outcomes of mental health education and training (DH 2006b). In particular, working in partnership is contained within the very first of the Ten Essential Shared Capabilities (Box 8.2) and is then threaded throughout the rest of the core capabilities for mental health staff. Partnership working is an essential aspect in:

- respecting the user's diversity
- providing care and treatment
- challenging inequality, stigma, and discrimination
- promoting recovery
- identifying people's needs and strengths
- providing person-centred care
- promoting safety and positive risk-taking.

In other words, partnership working is an absolutely central component of mental health nursing—and arguably the cornerstone of good mental health nursing.

In most modern mental health services, mental health care is also provided within a framework of **case management** in which service users' needs are assessed and addressed by a case manager working as part of a **multidisciplinary team**. In the UK, case management is known as the Care Programme Approach (CPA) (DH 1999, 2008) and the case manager is known as a **care coordinator**, a role most often carried out by mental health nurses.

> **Box 8.2** Working in partnership: first of the Ten Essential Capabilities for Mental Health Practice
>
> *'Developing and maintaining constructive working relationships with service users, carers, families, colleagues, lay people and wider community networks. Working positively with any tensions created by conflicts of interest or aspiration that may arise between the partners in care.'*
>
> DH (2006b, p. 25)

The care coordinator is required to work in partnership with service users to assess their strengths and health and social care needs, to write a care plan in collaboration with them, and then to ensure the care plan is implemented and reviewed by members of the multidisciplinary team and other agencies. Members of users' families and other informal carers may also be consulted when appropriate and should be provided with a copy of the plan.

The CPA has often been dismissed as a bureaucratic measure that produces copious paper work but with insufficient resources to ensure care plans are fully implemented (Simpson et al. 2003). However, the care coordinator role is intended to be a genuine attempt to formalize and encourage partnership working between clinicians and service users (Simpson 2005).

However, a systematic review of the literature on service users' and carers' views on mental health nursing suggests that mental health nurses too often fail to ensure that partnership working takes place (Bee et al. 2008; also see Chapter 2). The review reported that, although service users tend to place a positive value on mental health nurses and hold their listening skills in high regard, nurses rarely provide them with sufficient information to make informed choices and tend not to provide suitable opportunities for collaborating in their own care.

When aiming to explore the evidence base for partnership working it is difficult, even impossible, simply to search for clinical trials or systematic reviews of partnership working. Working in partnership or collaboratively with someone tends to emerge or grow out of a therapeutic relationship built on empathic understanding, warmth or positive regard, and genuineness or congruence (see Chapter 7). These are the three conditions that Carl Rogers (1961) identified through research and practice as 'necessary and sufficient' in any person trying to help another achieve personal growth or therapeutic change. Consequently, it is difficult and arguably futile to tease out or unpack those aspects of such a relationship most associated with 'partnership working' and subject them to a randomized controlled trial.

It is also difficult to measure and regulate components of a partnership relationship, which necessarily involves participants' personalities, personal styles, and culture, or to control for the influences of personal histories, experiences, and current contextual factors such as age, gender, and ethnicity. Neither could you deliberately allocate groups of people to no or abusive partnership working and measure against good partnership working. This is clearly unethical.

This does not mean that there has been no analysis of partnership working, but we should be aware that 'gold standards' of research are very difficult to apply in such complex contexts

(Repper and Brooker 1997). We are, however, able to identify some of the specific skills associated with partnership working and consider the evidence base for them. In order to do this, we have to look at other knowledge streams to extend our understanding such as individual reflective analyses, case studies, and learning through experience. Often the most useful sources are key texts that deal directly with the formulation of partnership working and what it is like for the worker. These often come from practitioners with counselling and psychotherapeutic skills, as well as mental health nursing, and tend to be derived from many years of experience in working with users and supervising workers. We can also draw on studies that have collated and analysed the accounts and perspectives of the patient or service user, including studies designed and conducted by service users (Rose 2001).

There is a growing body of research into the effectiveness of various interpersonal, psychotherapeutic, or conversational approaches (Roth and Fonagy 1996). Many of these are being adapted and employed in mainstream mental health and psychiatric settings (Parry 1996). In particular, **cognitive behavioural therapy (CBT)** is considered effective for a range of conditions (Newell and Gournay 2000), with variable evidence available as to effectiveness in routine practice (Durham et al. 2000).

CBT helps people talk about how they think about themselves and the people around them, and how what they do affects their thoughts and feelings. It can help people change how they think (cognitive) and what they do (behaviour), which can help them feel better and more in control. CBT focuses on 'here and now' problems and difficulties, rather than searching for the causes of distress or symptoms in the past, and can help to make sense of overwhelming problems by breaking them down into smaller parts. **Psychosocial interventions** have been developed for people with psychosis; they take many of the principles and techniques of CBT and use them alongside family work and case management to assist the person with psychotic experiences (Healy et al. 2006). Within substance misuse services, **motivational interviewing** techniques serve a similar function in assisting service users to understand their motivation to change and taking them through the challenges of change (Rollnick and Miller 1995).

Service users can become stuck in a cycle of disempowerment and despair as they respond to life situations over which they feel they have no influence or control. Deegan (1992) has argued that this **'learned helplessness'** develops when service users, and too often mental health staff, buy into the idea that psychiatric illness or vulnerability necessarily means that service users have limited capacity for reasoned thought and even less capability to take sensible, meaningful actions.

Understandably, service users may initially feel overwhelmed and powerless in the face of mental distress and experiences that are frightening, depressing, and disorienting. Such powerlessness can then be reinforced by the stigmatizing and discriminatory attitudes frequently shown in society towards people with mental illness. Where such beliefs are then further reinforced by health care staff, perhaps influenced by a limiting, medicalized view of mental distress, nurses and others start to take responsibility *for* users—whether it is necessary or not.

Another approach that provides a very useful, collaborative, and empowering framework for working in partnership with users is Egan's (1994) Skilled Helper Model. Originally developed in psychological counselling, this person-centred, problem-solving approach to helping has been adapted by many people working in psychiatric settings. Egan argued that people are often poor at solving problems, and that mental distress develops when people try to ignore or deny problems, or get stuck repeatedly attempting the same unsuccessful solutions. The nurse's task within this approach is to help the user become more able to manage the problems they are faced with. To achieve this, Egan identifies three stages:

1 Help the person identify and clarify their difficulties, needs, and problems, but also the things that are going well.

2 Help the person identify what they would like to do and achieve—to help them construct a better future.

3 Help the person create strategies to move towards those goals.

The nurse aims to engage the user in a process that moves through the three stages, whilst acknowledging that the person brings a unique knowledge and understanding of their life story and particular situation. The nurse offers to share knowledge of the helping process so that people can become more resourceful and self-supporting (Watkins 2001). We shall look at these approaches in more detail below.

In helping the person develop better problem-solving or coping strategies, it is important to recognize that many people will already be using strategies they have found helpful themselves. Research studies conducted with people diagnosed with schizophrenia (Barrowclough and Tarrier 1997) and bipolar disorder (Lam et al. 1999) found that the majority of people employed various coping techniques, with varying levels of success.

By enquiring about and acknowledging a user's own attempts to manage distressing or challenging experiences and situations, nurses actively demonstrate a commitment to partnership working and can reinforce the person's determination to self-manage. Nurses can then draw on their knowledge and experience to discuss and suggest additional coping mechanisms to help users broaden and strengthen their repertoire of coping skills. Watkins (2001) suggests that a number of interventions drawn from solution-focused therapy can be effective in helping people find strategies to move forward in their recovery. By asking solution-focused questions the nurse can help the user identify strategies that they are already employing and encourage them to develop new ones.

However, it is also important that nurses consider how best to adapt and integrate such skills within a conversational, collaborative style of working that recognizes nurses' unique roles within practice settings (Gamble and Brennan 2006, Repper and Perkins 1996). Such an approach helps to normalize the application of these complex skills (Brandon 1996), making their use more acceptable.

Finally, we need to consider that working in partnership to provide people with more choice sometimes involves an element of risk: '*The possibility of risk is an inevitable consequence of empowered people taking decisions about their own lives*' (DH 2007, p. 8).

Although there is insufficient space in this chapter to explore these issues in detail, it is worth directing readers to recent guidance that aims to support the principle of empowerment through managing choice and risk in a responsible, considered way (DH 2007). The guidance encourages multidisciplinary teams and health and social care organizations to foster a common, agreed approach to risk and to share the responsibility for risk in a transparent and constructive way.

Step-by-step guide to partnership working

In this section we consider the following elements of partnership working:

- Why form a partnership?
- How do we form a partnership?
- Engagement
- Problem-solving
- Difficulties
- Endings.

Why form a partnership?

Why do nurses form partnerships with users? The simple answer to this question is that partnerships are formed to help users to get better. But then we must ask, 'What does "better" mean?'. Well, 'better' means helping users create a healthier future, with more chance of a good quality of life, and a higher chance of mental and physical health, combined with social opportunities in the form of meaningful relationships, housing, employment, and education. These are all aspects of what has already been referred to as the recovery approach. In essence, then, we form partnerships with users to facilitate recovery.

We are still left with questions, however, as recovery has different meanings for people with different issues. Many aspects of recovery—quality of life, health, relationships, and employment—are dependent on individual characteristics, cultural norms, and stage of life. Take a look at Table 8.1 and ask yourself whether you agree with the broad statements about recovery as applied to different user groups.

Thus, recovery needs to be defined for any given client with any given problem. This makes it virtually impossible to discuss recovery in any more than general terms, unless related to a given individual. It should also be remembered that recovery came from the user movement and that nurses 'borrow' the term when they use it (Davidson 2005). It does not belong to nurses or other professionals. In addition, within specific services such as those dealing with people with dementia, there is considerable debate as to the appropriateness of the word 'recovery' owing to concerns that the word may be read as 'cure' or a return of full function (Adams 2007). In general, therefore, although we may all agree with the principles of the personal focus and respect for personhood in the concept of recovery, we may have to find careful ways to communicate these ideals within specific services. An illustration of this is provided in the Practice Example overleaf.

Table 8.1 Recovery for different user groups

For people who are dealing with ...	Recovery allows:	Recovery should not include:
Dementia (see web materials)	• Recognition of personhood (personality, life history, choices, preferences) • Realignment of key relationships • Comfort and dignity as condition progresses • Dignity in end of life	• Denial of the progressive worsening of the condition • False hope for user and carer • Dismissal of previous biography and life choices
Psychosis	• Remission or control of psychotic symptoms • Access to same life choices as people without psychotic symptoms • Active and visual confrontation of stigma	• False hope for user and carer • Denial of the disabling effects of psychosis for many • Denial of social needs such as housing, employment
Personality disorder	• Acknowledgement of the right to access care • Supportive relationships that set boundaries and allow growth • Recognition of the difficulties in processing emotion	• Denial of right to treatment • User being blamed for difficulties • Iatrogenic problems through inappropriate treatments
Depression and suicidal urges	• Protection from self-destructive impulses • Hope for a better future	• Freedom to commit suicide • Inability to take therapeutic risks

✖ Practice Example: Life story work

Life story work is a specific intervention designed for people with dementia. It is designed to assist in retaining a sense of self and personhood in the face of memory loss (Clarke et al. 2003).

On Jasmine Ward in Prospect Park Hospital, Reading, England, the ward team offer life story work to inpatients such as Bob. In this, Bob is engaged in relating the important aspects of his life in terms of relationships, significant events, work experiences, personal preferences, and anything else

that has meaning for him. Bob's family were also asked to assist in providing information and material such as photographs and other memorabilia. This was all collated together using a book-like template designed by Central and North West London NHS Trust and the dementia charity 'For Dementia' (Thompson 2007). The end product becomes Bob's property. Staff on the ward report that the work helps them to see the person behind the condition and appreciate Bob's uniqueness.

How do we form a partnership?

There are basic behaviours that any nurse should adhere to in all interactions. These include:

- being respectful
- keeping promises
- being honest (e.g. about availability)
- paying attention to privacy and dignity.

Although covered in previous chapters, it is worth reminding ourselves that partnerships are based in the bedrock of mutual respect. Nurses signal this respect in the first instance by paying attention to the basic common courtesies. Once a respectful relationship has been established (and there are users—and indeed some nurses—who find it very difficult to build a respectful relationship), partnership working can be defined by two basic features: engagement and problem-solving.

Engagement

You may be asking, 'What is the difference between a respectful relationship and engagement?'. The difference is that you enter into a respectful relationship, but once in it you engage with each other towards a specific goal. We can have respectful relationships with anyone. Engagement means making an active commitment to do some joint work. Nurses engage with users to facilitate problem-solving. This is the work of the partnership. At first glance this statement can seem quite cold and clinical, but it is not.

Problem-solving

If users and professionals engage to achieve goals, problem-solving is the vehicle that gets them there. Problem-solving can be broken down into distinct steps (Box 8.3) and builds on

Box 8.3 Steps in problem-solving

Helping users identify and clarify needs and problems

- Helping them tell their story ('Why are you here?').
- Helping them unload.
- Avoiding assumptions, interpretations, OUR solutions.
- Establishing and agreeing shared understanding of what the situation is and what needs to change.
- Measuring the need or problem and how it affects the user.
- Identifying how we can help them.

Develop an intervention or set of interventions designed to satisfy the need or alleviate the problem

- Bring in prior knowledge or find knowledge about the evidence base for that particular problem or need.
- Negotiate areas of responsibility in carrying out the intervention.
- Describe, in terms the user can understand, who will do what within a timeframe.
- Record this, again in ways understood by the user of the service. This is the basis of good care planning under the CPA.

Box 8.3 *Continued*

Evaluate the intervention

- We do this simply by measuring the outcome against our previous measurement (quantitative, e.g. a recognized measurement of anxiety or depression) and asking the user, 'Did it work?' (qualitative).

- If it didn't achieve the required outcome, change. It is important in this that nurses avoid blaming the user or themselves. If the attempt was honest, we have learned a valuable lesson. It is important to know what does not work at a given time. It gets us nearer to what will work.

- Few interventions are completely successful in all departments right away. We learn what we can from each attempt.

Egan's (1994) model, discussed earlier. A brief case example is provided in the Practice Example below.

Difficulties

In many ways the Practice Example below is an ideal scenario in that two capable people put their expertise together and aim jointly to problem-solve a difficulty. In mental health working there may be other factors that can impact negatively on the formation of a partnership between users and nurses (Table 8.2).

For some people, being in a partnership and agreeing a plan can be extremely difficult and challenging (Box 8.4, page 89). Being able to trust another person and work with them so closely can in itself be very frightening. In good partnership working, nurses will encourage sensitive discussion of any challenging emotions aroused. Sometimes the problem-solving needs to be stopped temporarily to reassure, re-negotiate, and re-establish the partnership.

The nurse's good intentions to work respectfully and collaboratively can also be frustrated as they repeatedly encounter people that are weary, suspicious, mistrustful, ambivalent, and angry—or who appear to undermine, manipulate, or 'sabotage' genuine attempts at partnership (Bowers 2003). Compassion and emotional energy are not inexhaustible commodities, and continual stressful encounters can cause intense anxiety and lead nurses to withdraw psychologically and physically from users for self-protection (Bray 1999, Menzies 1960). We often hear complaints of nurses spending too much time in the office, rather than engaging with users. In order consistently to make use of oneself, to apply subtle interactive skills, and to work collaboratively with enthusiasm and empathy, mental health nurses need to be enabled and encouraged to make use of personal reflection, supportive colleagues, teamwork, and clinical supervision.

Endings

Partnerships between users and nurses will inevitably end. It is important for both nurses and users to recognize that ending is important. Given that partnership working involves the investment of emotional energy, the ending of the partnership

✖ Practice Example: Problem-solving erratic sleep

Jane is on an acute admission ward recovering from an acute psychotic relapse. She is well enough to undertake a mental state examination with Jack, the nurse. This reveals she has no ongoing psychotic symptoms but an erratic and distressing sleep pattern. Jane and Jack agree to work on this using a sleep diary and an anxiety scale to measure the problem.

Jane believes in the power of crystals and meditation. Jack gets some information on sleep hygiene. After looking at Jane's night-time routine, they agree to changes which include bits from Jane (using crystals and practising yoga in the evening) and bits from Jack (reduction in caffeine, advice on the use of hypnotics). Although this has limited success at first in terms of hours of sleep, Jane feels less anxious. The intervention is changed to include listening to soothing music on her MP3 player as she gets into bed. Over time the intervention is felt to be working by Jane. There is a reduction in her anxiety score and she states she is less anxious. Hours slept, however, do not improve.

Table 8.2 Difficulties encountered in working in partnership

Circumstance	Considerations
An absence of capacity in the user. Can be due to many reasons: • Confusion (as in dementia) • Acute psychosis	Be aware of the Mental Capacity Act and guidance. Work with wider network but still including and informing the user. Do not make decisions in isolation, but discuss with other colleagues and carers, and take consideration of previous life choices such as advanced directives.
User does not identify nurse as someone who can help them. Can be due to: • Difficulties in accepting condition • Perceptions of nurse by the service user	Accept where the person is, rather than force the issue. Maintain a position of open and honest working. Allow the user to choose other workers (including those outside services such as advocates) and support this partnership.
External factors that influence partnership: • Partnership working within the criminal justice system • Partnership working within forensic services • Partnership working within the Mental Health Act	Be totally honest regarding what will happen to shared information. Accept that there may be conflicts of interest, but be honest about any external demands for information outside the partnership. Allow the user to judge how much to collaborate in the partnership. Share any written or verbal feedback with others if possible and appropriate.
The nurse lacks competence or knowledge	Be honest about your weaknesses and lack of knowledge. Allow yourself to learn. Seek information and supervision. Actively seek out role models from whom you can learn. Ask service users how other nurses have helped them.

should be as healthy as possible for both parties. What we mean by this is that nurses will, inevitably, form many partnerships in the course of their career. Some of these partnerships will adhere to the positive principles outlined in this chapter. Some will be challenged by the difficulties outlined in this chapter. In order to remain optimistic and giving of oneself, all partnerships need to be reflected upon, as indicated earlier. In our experience, many nurses are able to remain optimistic and giving because they experience both positive partnerships with users and positive support from colleagues when difficulties arise.

If it is possible to end the partnership in a healthy manner, it is important for nurses and users to meet and evaluate. In this both parties can learn valuable lessons as to what helped and what hindered the partnership. This meeting should be structured to allow the exchange of experiences and, if appropriate, a reflection on difficulties. If it is not possible to meet the user, nurses should use supervision to reflect on the partnership and any feelings they are left with. While it is sometimes appropriate to communicate these reflections to the user via a letter or phone call, the nurse should always be clear that the user is able to receive these communications in the spirit they are given. In other words, nurses should ensure that their motives for communicating are not to lecture, blame, or punish, but a genuine attempt at reconciliation of the partnership. It is important to remember that many users will continue to need services and form other partnerships, and the nurse has a responsibility beyond their own interactions with users to help them to believe that services are aimed at truly assisting them in spite of any difficulties.

Box 8.4 Absconding research

Absconding is an emotive and difficult issue in many acute inpatient environments. Recent research has allowed a deeper understanding of why some clients actively run away from partnerships. Different types of client profile have been identified that indicate why people go missing or abscond (Bowers et al. 2003). Often, service users have domestic concerns they wish to attend to, or are upset or disturbed by events on the ward. The evidence-based effective interventions recommended for these clients reflect many of the qualities in this chapter. For example, nurses are advised to spend more time with patients who are actively disengaging, to elicit and respect their concerns, and be sensitive in the breaking of bad news or negotiations around leave and access to the community (Bowers et al. 2005). Working in partnership with service users, their family, and members of the multidisciplinary team is the key to implementing all of these solutions. See the online material accompanying this chapter for more details.

 www.oxfordtextbooks.co.uk/orc/callaghan

▲ Conclusion

All services are now signed up to the **principles** of recovery, even if it is difficult to use the word 'recovery' in all service areas. This commitment is enshrined in many of the policy documents of the last decade. At the core of recovery is a new focus for the relationship between service users and mental health professionals, including nurses. There has been an active shift towards collaborative work aimed at assisting users to solve the effects of mental health problems rather than prescriptive interventions that do not take into account personal preferences. This collaborative work is what partnership working is all about. Nurses need to attend actively to the principles of partnership working, in spite of the many difficulties.

w Website

You may find it helpful to work through our short online quiz and self-assessment exercise intended to help you to develop and apply the skills in this chapter. Please go to:

 www.oxfordtextbooks.co.uk/orc/callaghan

Further reading and URLs

Watkins, P. (2001). *Mental Health Nursing: The Art of Compassionate Care*. London: Butterworth-Heinemann. A very helpful, accessible book for students and qualified mental health nurses that includes several chapters on aspects of partnership or the working alliance.

Absconding
http://www.citypsych.com/

Cognitive behavioural therapy (CBT)
http://www.rcpsych.ac.uk/
    mentalhealthinformation/therapies/
    cognitivebehaviouraltherapy.aspx

Mental health of older people
http://www.scie.org.uk/publications/elearning/
    mentalhealth/index.asp

Mental Capacity Act and related issues
http://www.dh.gov.uk/en/Publicationsandstatistics/
    Publications/PublicationsPolicyAndGuidance/
    DH_074491

Motivational interviewing
http://www.motivationalinterview.org/

Psychosocial interventions (CBT for psychosis)
http://www.hearingvoices.org.uk/info_carersleaflet3.
    html
http://www.sign.ac.uk/guidelines/fulltext/30/index.
    html

Recovery, self-management, and related themes
http://www.rethink.org/living_with_mental_illness/
    recovery_and_self_management/
http://www.samh.org.uk/assets/files/113.pdf
http://www.scottishrecovery.net/content/

Service user involvement
http://www.voxscotland.org.uk/sitebuildercontent/
    sitebuilderfiles/voxguidanceongoodpracticeinservice-
    userinvolvement1.doc

The Ten Essential Capabilities and Involving users and carers (modules 2 and 3)
http://visit.lincoln.ac.uk/C6/C12/CCAWI/default.aspx

Working with families and carers
http://www.citypsych.com/docs/Carersfinal.pdf
http://www.dh.gov.uk/en/Publicationsandstatistics/
  Publications/PublicationsPolicyAndGuidance/
  DH_4009233

http://www.rethink.org/how_we_can_help/
  research/our_research/carers.html

✤ References

Adams, T. (2007). *Dementia Care Nursing: Promoting Well-being in People with Dementia and their Families*. London: Palgrave.

Bamford Review of Mental Health and Learning Disabilities (Northern Ireland) (2005). *A Strategic Framework for Adult Mental Health Services*. http://www.rmhldni.gov.uk/adult_mental_health_report.pdf [accessed 30 Mar 2008].

Barrowclough, C. and Tarrier, N. (1997). *Families of Schizophrenic Patients: Cognitive Behavioural Interventions*. London: Thornes.

Bee, P., Playle, J. F., Lovell, K., Barnes, P., Gray, R., and Keeley, P. (2008). Service user views and expectations of UK-registered mental health nurses: a systematic review of empirical research. *International Journal of Nursing Studies* 45, 442–57.

Bowers, L. (2003). Manipulation: searching for an understanding. *Journal of Psychiatric and Mental Health Nursing* 10, 329–34.

Bowers, L., Simpson, A., and Alexander, J. (2003). Patient–staff conflict: results of a survey on acute psychiatric wards. *Social Psychiatry and Psychiatric Epidemiology* 38(7), 402–8.

Bowers, L., Simpson, A., and Alexander, J. (2005). Real world application of an intervention to reduce absconding. *Journal of Psychiatric and Mental Health Nursing* 12(5), 598–602.

Brandon, D. (1996). Normalising professional skills. In: *Mental Health Matters* (ed. T. Heller, J. Reynolds, R. Gomm, R. Muston, and S. Pattison), pp 297–303. Basingstoke: McMillan/Open University Press.

Bray, J. (1999). An ethnographic study of psychiatric nursing. *Journal of Psychiatric and Mental Health Nursing* 6(4), 297–305.

Brennan, G., Flood, C., and Bowers, L. (2006). Constraints and blocks to change and improvement on acute psychiatric wards—lessons from the City Nurses project. *Journal of Psychiatric and Mental Health Nursing* 13, 475–82.

Clarke, A., Hanson, E., and Ross, H. (2003). Seeing the person behind the patient; enhancing the care of older people using a biographical approach. *Journal of Clinical Nursing* 12(5), 697–706.

Davidson, L. (2005). Recovery, self management and the expert patient–changing the culture of mental health from a UK perspective. *Journal of Mental Health* 14(1), 25–35.

Deegan, P. (1992). The independent living movement and people with psychiatric disabilities: taking back control over our own lives. *Psychosocial Rehabilitation Journal* 15(3), 4–19.

Department of Health (1999). *Effective Care Co-ordination in Mental Health Services: Modernising the Care Programme Approach. A Policy Booklet*. London: HMSO.

Department of Health (2006a). *From Values to Action: The Chief Nursing Officer's Review of Mental Health Nursing*. London: DH.

Department of Health (2006b). *Best Practice Competencies and Capabilities for Pre-registration Mental Health Nurses in England: The Chief Nursing Officer's Review of Mental Health*. London: DH.

Department of Health (2007). *Independence, Choice and Risk: A Guide to Best Practice in Supported Decision Making*. London: DH.

Department of Health (2008). *Refocusing the Care Programme Approach: Policy and Positive Practice Guidance*. London: DH.

Durham, R. C., Swan, J. S., and Fisher, P. L. (2000). Complexity and collaboration in routine practice of CBT: what doesn't work with whom and how might it work better? *Journal of Mental Health* 9(4), 429–44.

Egan, G. (1994). *The Skilled Helper: A Problem-management Approach to Helping*, 5th edn. Pacific Grove, CA: Brooks/Cole Publishing.

Frak, D. (2005). *Recovery Learning: A Report on the Work of the Recovery Learning Sites and other Recovery-orientated Activities and its Incorporation into The Rethink Plan 2004–08*. London: Rethink. http://www.rethink.org/living_with_mental_illness/recovery_and_self_management/recovery/ [accessed 16 Dec 2007].

Gamble, C. and Brennan, G. (ed.) (2006). *Working with Serious Mental Illness: A Manual for Clinical Practice*, 2nd edn. London: Elsevier.

Healy, H., Reader, D., and Midence, K. (2006). An introduction to and rationale for psychosocial interventions. In: *Working with Serious Mental Illness: A Manual for Clinical Practice*, 2nd edn (ed. C. Gamble and G. Brennan), pp 55–70. London: Elsevier.

Lam, D. H., Jones, S., Hayward, P., and Bright, J. (1999). *Cognitive Therapy for Bipolar Disorders: A Therapist's Guide to Concepts, Methods, and Practice*. Chichester: Wiley.

Menzies, I. (1960). Social systems as a structured defence against anxiety. *Human Relations* 13, 95–121.

Newell, M. and Gournay, K. (2000). *Mental Health Nursing: An Evidence-based Approach*. Edinburgh: Churchill Livingstone.

Parry, G. (1996). *NHS Psychotherapy Services in England: Review of Strategic Policy*. London: DH.

Repper, J. and Brooker, C. (1997). Difficulties in the measurement of outcome in people who have serious mental health problems. *Journal of Advanced Nursing* 27, 75–82.

Repper, J. and Perkins, R. (1996). *Working Alongside People with Long Term Mental Health Problems*. London: Chapman and Hall.

Rogers, C. (1961). *On Becoming a Person. A Therapist's View of Psychotherapy*. London: Constable.

Rollnick, S. and Miller, W. R. (1995). What is motivational interviewing? *Behavioural and Cognitive Psychotherapy* 23, 325–34. http://www.motivationalinterview.org/clinical/whatismi.html [accessed 30 Mar 2008].

Rose, D. (2001). *Users' Voices: The Perspectives of Mental Health Service Users on Community and Hospital Care*. London: Sainsbury Centre for Mental Health.

Roth, A. and Fonagy, P. (1996). *What Works for Whom? A Critical Review of Psychotherapy Research*. London: Guilford Press.

Scottish Executive (2003). *National Programme for Improving Mental Health and Well-Being: Action Plan 2003–2006*. Edinburgh: Scottish Executive.

Simpson, A. (2005). Community psychiatric nurses and the care co-ordinator role: squeezed to provide 'limited nursing'. *Journal of Advanced Nursing* 52(6), 689–99.

Simpson, A., Miller, C., and Bowers, L. (2003). The history of the care programme approach in England: Where did it go wrong? *Journal of Mental Health* 12(5), 489–504.

Thompson, R. (2007). Older people's mental health services; supporting and developing health care assistants. *Mental Health Practice* 10(10), 34–8.

Watkins, P. (2001). *Mental Health Nursing: The Art of Compassionate Care*. London: Butterworth-Heinemann.

Welsh Assembly Government (2005). *Raising the Standard: The Revised Adult Mental Health National Service Framework and an Action Plan for Wales*. Cardiff: WAG. http://wales.nhs.uk/sites3/page.cfm?orgid=438&pid=11071 [accessed 30 Mar 2008].

9 Recovery and social inclusion

Julie Repper   Rachel Perkins

▼ Introduction

In mental health services we are very used to thinking about 'the patient in our services'. We usually think about what we do in terms of the things that services provide and the professionals who provide them. We think about the people we work with in terms of their symptoms and what we need to do to reduce or get rid of their symptoms: the medication, inpatient care, community outreach services, the medical, nursing, psychological therapy, occupational therapy, and social care services that we consider might be effective. However, the UK government's *National Health Service (NHS) Plan* (Department of Health [DH] 2000) and subsequent policy documents make it clear that this is the wrong place to start. The Plan states:

> 'Patients are the most important people in the health service. It doesn't always appear that way. Too many patients feel talked at, rather than listened to. This has to change. NHS care has to be shaped around the convenience and concerns of patients. To bring this about, patients must have more say in their own treatment and more influence over the way the NHS works.'

Most recent health and social care policy in the UK, such as the *NHS Improvement Plan* (DH 2004a), *National Standards, Local Action* (DH 2004b), *Independence, Well-being and Choice* (DH 2005a), *Creating a Patient-led NHS* (DH 2005b), and *Our Health, Our Care, Our Say* (DH 2006), makes it clear that we have to move beyond care and services that focus primarily on treating illness to a **recovery**-based approach that:

- positively promotes health and well-being
- maximizes people's life chances
- enables people to take control over their lives and their own self-care
- helps people to do the things they want to do and live the lives they wish to lead.

If we are really to create services that are tailored around those whom we serve, our starting point cannot be 'the patient in our services'. Instead we must think about 'the person in their life'. We must start by understanding the challenges that people with mental health problems face in living their lives within and beyond limits imposed by the problems they face. Services and the assistance we offer need to be understood in terms of the extent to which they facilitate or hinder this process of recovery.

Learning outcomes

By the end of this chapter you should be better able to:

1 Outline the nature and focus of recovery-based approaches for people who have experienced mental health problems

2 Identify and describe the key beliefs and principles underpinning recovery-based approaches

3 Describe strategies to promote recovery and social inclusion drawing on factors identified as assisting the recovery journey

4 Reflect on your own practice and current mental health services, identifying ways in which these could be further developed to incorporate a greater focus on recovery.

What is recovery all about?

Unlike so many ideas in the mental health arena, ideas about recovery were not born of academics and professionals. Instead, they emerged from the writings of those people who have themselves faced the challenge of life with a mental health problem. Deegan (1988) defines recovery as referring to:

> '… the lived or real life experience of people as they accept and overcome the challenge of the disability … they experience themselves as recovering a new sense of self and of purpose within and beyond the limits of the disability.'

Based on a systematic analysis of personal accounts of recovery, Andresen et al. (2003) have suggested that recovery comprises four key components:

1 Finding and maintaining hope
2 Re-establishing a positive identity
3 Building a meaningful life
4 Taking responsibility and control.

Anthony (1993) expresses similar ideas:

> '… a deeply personal, unique process of changing one's attitudes, values, feelings, goals, skills, and/or roles. It is a way of living a satisfying, hopeful, and contributing life even with limitations caused by illness. Recovery involves the development of new meaning and purpose in one's life as one grows beyond the catastrophic effects of mental illness.'

The starting point is the individual's experience

It is difficult to describe what it is like to experience mental health problems in our society. Although many people work with others who have mental health problems, they cannot understand recovery until they have considered how it feels to have experienced mental health problems. For many who have experienced such problems it feels like the bottom has fallen out of their world. Sayce (2000) describes such an experience:

> 'When I was diagnosed I felt this is the end of my life. It was a thing to isolate me from other human beings. I felt I was not viable … I felt flawed, defective.'

You have to cope with strange and often frightening symptoms that may stop you being able to think properly, stop you doing the ordinary everyday things that everyone takes for granted, cause you to have experiences that no one around you believes, cause your confidence and belief in yourself to hit rock bottom. You can feel very alone, and very frightened—not only about what is happening to you but also about using mental health services. Everyone knows what it is like to go to their family doctor or go into a general hospital (either as patient or visitor), but mental health

services remain, for most people, sinister and mysterious places. Unthinkable things may happen to you like being picked up by the police, admitted to hospital against your will, or forcibly medicated—all reinforcing the stereotypical bedlam images.

In addition to all of this you experience the stigma and discrimination that go hand in hand with mental health problems in our society; all of a sudden those dreadful headlines in the newspapers, 'Dangerous Psychos', 'Mad Axe Murderer', are referring to you.

> 'All I knew were the stereotypes I had seen on television or in the movies. To me, mental illness meant Dr Jekyll and Mr Hyde, psychopathic serial killers, loony bins, morons, schizos, fruitcakes, nuts, straightjackets, and raving lunatics. They were all I knew about mental illness and what terrified me was that professionals were saying I was one of them.'
>
> Deegan (1993)

People start treating you differently—as if you are dangerous, or stupid, or both. They start talking *about you* rather than *to you*, feel that they need to tread carefully around you in case you dissolve into tears or explode into anger. As a result of the fear and ignorance surrounding mental illness, you risk losing many things that are important to you: your job, your college place, your friends, even your home.

People who experience mental health problems are among the most excluded in our society. Too many have lost everything that they valued in life and are at greater risk of losing their lives, and not just through suicide. People with serious mental health problems are more likely to suffer from the major physical diseases, more likely to get them younger, and more likely to die from them more quickly, resulting in a life expectancy some ten years less than that of the rest of the population (Disability Rights Commission 2006).

We must also remember that the stigma and discrimination that exists in the wider society also exists within mental health services. Too often mental health workers hold a pessimistic view about what people with mental health problems can achieve. If the people who are there to help you believe you will never amount to very much, what hope is there? The barriers between 'them' and 'us' remain very real. Too often people feel that they are not taken seriously and are treated as second-class citizens within mental health services. Such ideas are frequently reinforced by common dehumanizing practices that, although they may seem relatively minor to staff, exemplify the sense of separateness and segregation between users of services and staff. Common examples include having separate staff cups, staff crockery, and staff toilets.

In the face of all of this it is easy either to reject the notion that there is anything wrong with you at all, because the idea of being a 'mental patient' is just too terrible to contemplate, or to give up on yourself and your life completely. But it does not have to be like this.

Experiencing serious mental health problems is a catastrophic and life-changing experience. There is no way back to how things were before the problems started, but there is a way forward. Many people with mental health problems have demonstrated that it is possible to rebuild a meaningful, valued, and satisfying life. Recovery is possible.

As well as the many famous people who have had mental health problems—statesmen such as Parnell and Churchill, scientists such as Einstein and Babbage (who invented the first computer), scholars such as Ruskin and Wittgenstein, composers such as Ravel, artists such as Van Gogh, writers and poets such as Auden and Chesterton, businessmen such as Ted Turner who set up Cable Network News—there are also many thousands of ordinary people who have their own homes and network of family and friends, and who contribute to our communities in so many ways. Despite mental health problems and the accompanying discrimination, there are millions of people with mental health problems who are husbands, mothers, friends, and work colleagues.

Recovery is as relevant to children, older people, and those with learning disabilities as it is to working age adults with mental health problems. The UK government publication *Every Child Matters: Change for Children* (Department for Education and Skills 2003) emphasizes the importance of 'enjoying and achieving' and 'making a positive contribution', to enable all children, whether or not they have mental health or behavioural problems, to get the most out of life, develop the skills for adulthood, and be involved as valued members of the community and society.

As we get older, sources of meaning and value may increasingly lie in our past—what we have done, rather than what we will do in the future. But older people can and do remain part of their communities and continue to make valuable contributions unless they are prevented from doing so by prejudice or failure to provide the support and adjustments they need. For many, dementia may signal the end of life, but it is not immediately fatal. If people are to make the most of the lives that are left to them, then it is living with, rather than dying from, dementia that is critical. As with people of all ages who develop other terminal physical illnesses, the challenge becomes one of living as valued and meaningful a life as possible for as long as possible. The UK government report *Everybody's Business: Integrated Mental Health Service for Older Adults* (DH/Care Services Improvement Partnership [CSIP] 2005) emphasizes the importance of promoting respect and dignity, encouraging older people to be as independent as possible, providing them with the integrated support and assistive technologies they need to live independently at home as far as is possible, and the need for care in residential settings to promote **social inclusion**. Similarly, for those with learning disabilities, the essence of the UK government publication *Valuing People: A New Strategy for Learning Disability for the 21st Century* (DH 2001a) lies in promoting citizenship, inclusion, and independence, and in ensuring that everyone is valued no matter what, or how severe, their impairments. For those with addiction problems, the challenge lies in rebuilding a life that does not revolve around drugs and alcohol.

Principles of recovery

People with mental health problems may benefit from a wide range of support and treatment, and it is critical that these are available to people of all ages and to those who may experience additional discrimination and disadvantage as a consequence of physical impairments, drug and alcohol problems, forensic history, learning disabilities, progressive organic conditions, or their ethnicity, sexuality, or religion. However, the central question is whether this support and treatment helps the person to pursue their ambitions and make the most of their life. Therefore, the philosophy and principles guiding our work as mental health practitioners and the services provided are particularly important. The key principles of recovery are outlined in Box 9.1.

Recovery is about people's whole lives, not just their symptoms

There is a variety of different ways in which people may gain relief from distressing symptoms associated with mental health problems. These may include medication, psychological therapy, self-help, self-management, and a range of complementary therapies. However, it is rarely a person's ambition in life merely to get rid of distressing and disabling symptoms: people wish for this in order to be able to do the things they want to do and to live the lives they wish to lead. Recovery is about:

- enabling people to have the homes, friends, jobs, educational opportunities, or other opportunities to contribute to the communities in which we live that lend everyone's life meaning and through which we get our sense of value

- enabling people to access accommodation, material resources, employment, education, relationships, social and leisure activities

- ensuring people's safety from exploitation and abuse, at least as, if not more, important in the recovery process as reducing the mental health problems themselves.

Recovery is not a professional intervention like medication or therapy

As outlined earlier, a key focus of much current mental health provision is about offering interventions to the 'patient *in* our services'. However, recovery is about the journey of people who have mental health problems in rebuilding a meaningful, valued, and satisfying life. A recovery-based approach is therefore a very different approach to simply offering interventions; it is based on a different set of fundamental beliefs and values. Whilst mental health workers with our various treatments and supports can help facilitate recovery, we can also hinder recovery—snuffing out the embers of hope, further taking away the control that a person has over their life, and further eroding their chances of doing the things they want to do.

Box 9.1 Key principles of recovery

- Recovery is about people's whole lives, not just their symptoms.
- Recovery is not a professional intervention like medication or therapy.
- Recovery is not the same as cure.
- Recovery is about growth.
- Recovery does not refer to an end product or a result: it is a continuing journey.
- Recovery can and does occur without professional intervention.
- A recovery vision is not limited to a particular theory about the nature and causes of mental health problems.
- Recovery is about people taking back control over their life.
- Recovery is not a linear process.
- Recovery is possible for everyone.
- Carers, relatives, and friends also face the challenge of recovery.
- Everyone's recovery journey is different and deeply personal.
- Recovery is not specific to mental health problems; it is a common human condition.

Recovery is not the same as cure

Recovery does not mean that all symptoms have disappeared, that all suffering has been eliminated, or that functioning has been completely restored. Rather, it means that remaining symptoms and problems interfere less with a person's life. To take a parallel with physical impairment, someone with a severed spine may never be able to walk again, but they can rebuild a meaningful and satisfying life, doing the things they want to do, growing within and beyond the limits of their impairment. Even if a person has problems that recur, or are ever present, this does not mean they cannot rebuild a meaningful and valued life.

Recovery is about growth

Recovery is about growing within and beyond the limits imposed by ongoing symptoms and difficulties. It is about being and becoming more than a 'mental patient', taking control over your life and doing the things you want to do.

Recovery does not refer to an end product or a result: it is a continuing journey

'Recovery is a process. It is a way of life. It is an attitude and a way of approaching the day's challenges … Recovery is marked by an ever-deepening acceptance of our limitations. But now, rather than being an occasion for despair, we find our personal limitations are the ground from which springs our own unique possibilities. This is the paradox of recovery … that in accepting what we cannot do or be, we begin to discover what we can be and what we can do.'

Deegan (1992)

People cannot be 'fixed' as one might mend a television or refurbish a building. If recovery is a continuing journey, then assistance and adjustments often need to be thought of as a continuing process of supporting people in that journey. This must involve not only helping the person to move forward, but also helping them to maintain and celebrate what they have already achieved. Mental health nurses and other professionals can play a key role in facilitating such assistance, adjustments, and support. However, it is important to note that recovery can develop without, and at times in spite of, professional help.

Recovery can and does occur without professional intervention

Whilst mental health workers may play a part in facilitating recovery, they do not hold the key to recovery. It is a person's own resources and those available to them outside of traditional mental health services that are central. The expertise of experience is also important. Many people have described the enormous support they have received from others who have faced similar challenges. The vital support of others may often be realized via self-help groups, user/survivor organizations, and more informal friendships and networks within which people can share experiences and support one another's journeys. It can also be facilitated by including the expertise of personal experience of mental health problems in the staff 'skill mix' available within mental health teams.

A recovery vision is not limited to a particular theory about the nature and causes of mental health problems

A recovery vision does not commit one to a specific social, psychological, spiritual, or organic model for understanding mental health problems. Whatever understanding of their situation chosen by a person, recovery is an equally important process.

Recovery is about people taking back control over their life

Mental health problems are often presented and perceived as uncontrollable, or their control is seen as the province of 'experts'. Recovery involves people with mental health problems taking back control: control over their problems, the help and support they receive, and over their life more generally.

> 'To me, recovery means I try to stay in the driver's seat of my life. I don't let my illness run me. Over the years I have worked hard to become an expert in my own self-care … over the years I have learned different ways of helping myself. Sometimes I use medications, therapy, self-help and mutual support groups, friends, my relationship with God, work, exercise, spending time in nature— all of these measures help me remain whole and healthy, even though I have a disability.'
>
> Deegan (1993)

Recovery is not a linear process

Recovery is not a simplistic linear process; it is about trying and trying again. Deegan (1992) describes the recovery process as '…a series of small beginnings and very small steps. At times our course is erratic and we falter, slide back, re-group and start again …'. Relapse should not be considered as 'failure', but a normal part of the recovery process—an opportunity to learn what is possible and what is not, at least for now. Relapse can provide an opportunity for the person to move beyond

their limitations by identifying the additional support and adjustments that they, or those around them, may need to successfully pursue their ambitions.

Recovery is possible for everyone

Recovery is not only for those who are more able. Some people will remain profoundly disabled by mental health problems, but with the right kind of support all people can find sources of value and meaning in order to move forward in their lives. Some people deny their need for services and reject professional help, but they can still achieve the support and encouragement they need to pursue their ambitions outside of traditional mental health services—among those friends, family members, and agencies that exist to help all citizens. The critical issue then becomes not whether the individual has appropriate support from mental health practitioners or services, but whether friends, family, and community agencies receive the help they need to accommodate the person with mental health difficulties.

Carers, relatives, and friends also face the challenge of recovery

It is not only people who experience mental health problems who face the challenge of recovery. Mental health problems have a profound effect not only on the life of the person who experiences them, but also on those who are close to them— partners, relatives, and friends. These people also face the challenge of recovery. As it is not mental health services, but informal carers, who provide most of the support received by people with mental health and related problems, partners, relatives, and friends have a critical role to play in promoting recovery and facilitating social inclusion. If they are to do this, it is important that they understand the person's situation, the challenges they face, and receive the support that they need to contribute to helping the person to make the most of their life. It is too often the case that relatives, carers, and friends feel ill-informed and unsupported. Mental health workers frequently fail to recognize the significant contribution made by those in the person's wider networks of social support and the difficulties they face. Some continue to feel that professionals and services implicitly, or at times explicitly, blame them for their relative's problems.

Family and friends of the person with mental health problems also face the challenge of recovery in their own right, often having to re-evaluate their own lives, accommodating what has happened and any adjustments required. Relatives, carers, and friends must discover new sources of value and meaning for themselves, in their loved one, and in their relationship with them. Too often, informal carers find their own social networks, contacts, and opportunities diminished, and they too may experience stigma and social exclusion. It is therefore important that mental health services facilitate the recovery of carers and people who are close to the person, helping them to accommodate and make sense of what has happened, rebuild their own lives, and access those opportunities that they value.

Everyone's recovery journey is different and deeply personal

There are no rules of recovery, no single formula for success: different people choose different roads. However, the individual nature of recovery does not mean that it is impossible to support people in their recovery journey; instead it means that there is no one 'right' way to do this—the individual's wishes and preferences are paramount. Deegan (1992) argues that each person's recovery journey is unique and that each individual must find their own way, something that no one else can do for them. In light of this she warns against trying to standardize recovery:

> 'Once recovery becomes systematised, you've got it wrong. Once it is reduced to a set of principles it is wrong. It is a unique and individualised process.'

> Deegan (1989)

Recovery is not specific to mental health problems; it is a common human condition

Everyone faces the challenge of recovery at many points in their lives. All of us will at times be required to re-evaluate and rebuild our lives when we experience the loss of something we value such as a partner, a relative, a job. Other experiences such as traumas, crises, physical illness or injury—setbacks that happen to us all at intervals throughout our lives—similarly require adjustment. Perhaps the best way of understanding recovery is by considering a difficult event in our own lives. How did we feel? How did we behave? How did it change our views? What helped us to recover?

Facilitating recovery, promoting inclusion

If, as mental health practitioners, we are to help people rebuild their lives, we need to move beyond simplistic and at times inappropriate 'treatment and cure' thinking. Reducing distressing and disabling symptoms through various sorts of

treatment and therapy is important, but in itself does not provide a useful guiding vision for our work as mental health practitioners.

Moving beyond treatment and cure

A number of key principles or beliefs underpin the move from 'treatment and cure' thinking to a more person-centred, recovery-based approach. First, treatment and therapy designed to reduce distress are important only in so far as they promote recovery and social inclusion, helping people to live the lives they want to lead and do the things they want to do. Second, getting rid of a person's symptoms and problems is not essential for recovery. Many people have symptoms and problems that recur from time to time, and a few people have symptoms and problems that are ever present. However, this does not and should not preclude the possibility of that person rebuilding a meaningful, valued, and satisfying life. Deegan (1993) in her account of recovery following a diagnosis of schizophrenia describes how:

> 'One of the biggest lessons I have had to accept is that recovery is not the same thing as being cured. After 21 years of living with this thing it still hasn't gone away.'

Third, getting rid of a person's symptoms and problems does not guarantee recovery. In the time it takes for a person to get rid of their symptoms and problems, they may well have lost a great many valued roles, relationships, and activities, and will need extra help if they are to get them back. Fourth, the prejudice, discrimination, ignorance, and fear that surround mental health problems extend beyond the presence of symptoms. The commonly held public, and sadly often still professional, assumptions that 'once a schizophrenic always a schizophrenic' and 'once a mental patient always a mental patient' mean that people who have been diagnosed with mental health problems in the past may still be prevented from doing the things they want to do because of this one part of their history.

While treatments to reduce distressing and debilitating symptoms are important, they are clearly only one part of a person's recovery journey. Rebuilding a meaningful and valued life requires more than the treatment of symptoms. If we are to do this we must look to the expertise of personal experience for guidance. People recovering from mental health and related problems have identified a number of common features that seem to be important in recovery. These are outlined in Box 9.2.

Putting all of these things together, it seems that if mental health practitioners are really to support people in their recovery journey then three interrelated components are central:

1 Fostering hope and hope-inspiring relationships

2 Facilitating personal adaptation and taking back control

3 Promoting opportunity and social inclusion.

Fostering hope and hope-inspiring relationships

'For those of us who have been diagnosed with mental illness and who have lived in sometimes desolate wastelands of mental health programmes, hope is not just a nice sounding euphemism. It is a matter of life and death.'

Deegan (1993)

This means that as mental health practitioners we need to think about things such as how we make people feel welcomed and valued as individuals; how we create relationships that help them to see the possibility of a decent future for themselves; how we support people in developing and maintaining relationships with people outside the mental health system—family, friends, partners, others who may be important to the person. It also means finding ways in which we can promote peer support, enabling people with mental health problems to share their experiences and benefit from one another's expertise on the recovery journey.

Facilitating personal adaptation and taking back control

'Over the years I've worked hard to become an expert in my own self care … I've learned different ways of helping myself.'

Deegan (1993)

Of course, one part of facilitating personal adaptation and helping people to take back control of their own lives includes

> **Box 9.2** Common features identified by service users as important in the recovery process
>
> - A sense of hope
> - Relationships: having someone to believe in you when you cannot believe in yourself
> - The experience of others who have faced similar challenges
> - Coping with loss
> - Spirituality, philosophy, and understanding
> - Taking back control
> - Finding meaning and purpose in life
> - Having the opportunity to do the things that you value

trying to reduce symptoms and distress with a range of different types of treatment: medication, talking therapies, and various kinds of complementary therapy. However, as highlighted previously, whilst this is one element of the recovery journey it is not the central focus of recovery. It also means:

- Helping people to understand and accommodate what has happened to them.
- Enabling people to become experts in their own self-care, enabling and promoting self-help and self-management. This will include a number of elements, including helping people to think about what they can do to keep themselves happy and healthy, notice when things are going wrong, plan what they will do when things do start to go wrong, and work out how they are going to resume their life once a crisis has passed.
- Helping people to think about the types of help they would like both to stay well and at times of crisis; this should include help both from within the mental health system and outside.
- Helping people to think about what they would like to do with their lives and articulate their dreams and ambitions.

Promoting opportunity and social inclusion

'I don't want a CPN, I want a life.'

Rose (2001)

Promoting opportunity and social inclusion means getting the basics right: making sure that people have access to the material resources and supports they need—things such as money, food, housing, transport, physical health care, personal safety. However, it also involves going beyond mere survival and should be about enabling people to make the most of their lives, accessing those activities, roles, and relationships that they value. For many, satisfying work is central. In relation to this aspect of recovery, Rogers (1995, p. 6) argues that:

> *'It [work] offers more than a pay check; it boosts self-esteem and provides a sense of purpose and accomplishment. Work enables people to enter, or re-enter, the mainstream after hospitalisation.'*

However, it is important to remember that meaning and purpose vary from person to person, and can include a range of activities and roles: motherhood, politics, friendship, sports, environmental activism, church membership, drama, arts, voluntary work, education, etc. All of these are very different from the activities traditionally offered by mental health services to people with mental health problems, such as 'occupational therapy' and 'day centre attendance'. If people with mental health problems are to be and feel included in their communities, they must have access to the broad range of valued opportunities within them. This means supporting both the individual and at times the organization or facility they are joining. Areas where the individual may need support and where mental health practitioners may be able to assist are outlined in Box 9.3.

Organizations accessed as part of social inclusion activities may need information and support so that they understand the skills of the person joining them, the areas in which the person may require help, the sorts of adjustment to the role and the environment that might make it more accessible, and where they can access further information or advice if they need it. This is vital as traditionally the emphasis and expectations have been placed on changing the individual to fit in with the expectations of the world. A more socially inclusive approach demands a move towards changing the world so that people with mental health problems have access to all of the opportunities available.

The three components outlined above do not necessarily follow a logical sequence. They are intimately interrelated, and in helping people in their recovery we often need to think about all three at the same time. It is not necessarily the case that mental health practitioners must first develop hope-inspiring relationships and then move on in a stepwise fashion. For example, helping people with practical things such as income/benefits, housing, and purposeful activities can be important in the process of developing hope-inspiring relationships. Similarly, it may be that through beginning to do things that the person values and that value the person they begin to develop confidence and control over their life and are able to undertake practical tasks more readily. A positive feedback loop can develop whereby increased confidence and control leads to greater success in developing meaningful roles and relationships, which in turn further increases confidence and hope. This is illustrated in the model outlined in Figure 9.1.

Box 9.3 Areas where individuals may need support for social inclusion and recovery

- Identifying and maintaining the roles, relationships, and activities they already have

- Discovering new sources of interest, meaning, and value

- Finding out about, visiting, and trying out new opportunities, activities, and facilities with support

- Identifying the skills they will require to pursue new interests

- Developing, practising, and rehearsing new skills

- Reviewing progress regularly and planning accordingly

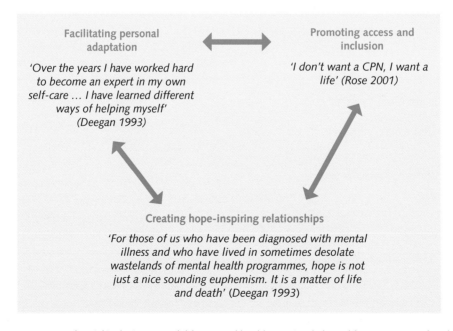

Figure 9.1 Recovery and social inclusion: a model for mental health practice (adapted from Repper and Perkins 2003).

✖ Practice Example and Tips: Recovery

Scenario

In moving towards a recovery approach, your team has decided to consider the therapeutic environment in which they work with service users (this may be an inpatient or residential area, a community team base, or a day facility). The team begins by identifying aspects of the environment that might diminish hope.

Consider therapeutic environments you have worked in. Did they inspire hope and recovery?

Go to ⊕ www.oxfordtextbooks.co.uk/orc/callaghan to consider how practices can inspire or diminish a recovery approach and see the authors' suggested answers.

'Ten top tips for recovery'

Based on Shepherd et al. (2008)

1 Help the person identify and prioritize their personal goals for recovery—*not* professional goals

2 Demonstrate a belief in the person's existing strengths in relation to the pursuit of these goals

---

3 Pay particular attention to the importance of goals which take the person out of the 'sick role' and enable them to contribute and help others

4 Identify non-mental health resources—friends, contacts, organizations—relevant to the achievement of these goals

5 Encourage self-management of mental health problems (by providing information, reinforcing existing coping strategies, etc.)

6 Listen to what the person wants in terms of therapeutic interventions, e.g. psychological treatments, alternative therapies, joint crisis planning, etc.; show that you have listened

7 Behave at all times so as to convey an attitude of respect for the person and a desire for an equal partnership in working together

8 Indicate a willingness to 'go the extra mile' to help the person achieve their goals

9 Identify examples from my own 'lived experience', or that of other service users, which inspire and validate hope

10 While accepting that the future is uncertain and setbacks will occur, continue to express support for the possibility of achieving these self-defined goals—maintaining hope and positive expectations

▲ Conclusion

At the heart of the recovery approach described here is the process of rebuilding a meaningful life despite the continuing presence of mental health problems. Recovery is based on service user-led ideas of self-determination and self-management. It emphasizes the importance of hope in sustaining motivation and supporting expectations of a rich and fulfilled life. It provides a new rationale for mental health services and has become the governing principle of mental health provision in New Zealand (Mental Health Commission 1998), Australia (National Health Plan; Australian Government 2003), the USA (Department of Health and Human Services 2003), and Ireland (Mental Health Commission 2005). In England, it has received support from the DH (2001b), and more recently from CSIP, the Royal College of Psychiatrists, and the Social Care Institute for Excellence (CSIP 2007). It has generally proved to be a dynamic, inspiring, and

creative approach that can substitute hope for despair. It circumvents sterile arguments between competing intervention models (medication vs therapy vs employment vs self-help vs complementary therapy). All or none of these may contribute to the central goal of growth and development. The highly individualized nature of the recovery process means that different people will find different approaches helpful in their journey to rebuilding a valued, meaningful, and satisfying life.

For mental health practitioners the recovery model poses a range of questions and challenges. It means that traditional power relationships must change, that we must believe in people with mental health problems having the same aspirations as those without, that we must work with non-mental health resources (friends, community facilities, and organizations) to help people achieve their goals, that we must put ourselves and our skills at the disposal of those with whom we work, and that we measure our success by the extent to which people also access other sources of support. Shepherd et al. (2008) have made a start in identifying 'Ten top tips for recovery', a list of how we can tell whether we are really 'doing' recovery in practice (in the Practice Example and Tips box). This list is embryonic, but is a useful beginning with many potential uses: as a clinical supervision tool, a list of change indicators, a charter for service users, or a poster that might serve as a reminder for staff.

However, if, as mental health practitioners, we are fully to embrace a recovery approach, we need to embrace a significant change in the culture and organization of services as well as in our own roles and relationships with the people with whom we work.

w   Website

You may find it helpful to work through our short online quiz and case study intended to help you to develop and apply the skills in this chapter. Please go to:

 www.oxfordtextbooks.co.uk/orc/callaghan

✛   References

Andresen, R., Oades, L., and Caputi, S. (2003). The experience of recovery from schizophrenia: towards an empirically validated stage model. *Australian and New Zealand Journal of Psychiatry* 37, 586–94.

Anthony, W. A. (1993). Recovery from mental illness: the guiding vision of the mental health service system in the 1990s. *Psychosocial Rehabilitation Journal* 16, 11–23.

Australian Government (2003). *Australian Health Minister's National Mental Health Plan 2003–2008.* Canberra: Australian Government: www.mentalhealth. gov.au

Care Services Improvement Partnership (2007). *National Social Inclusion Programme Capabilities for Inclusive Practice.* London: National Social Inclusion Programme/CSIP. www.socialinclusion.org.uk

Deegan, P. (1988). Recovery: the lived experience of rehabilitation. *Psychosocial Rehabilitation Journal* 11(4), 11–19.

Deegan, P. (1989). *A letter to my friend who is giving up.* Paper presented to the Connecticut Conference on Supported Employment, Connecticut Association of Rehabilitation facilities, Cromwell, CT.

Deegan, P. (1992). *Recovery, Rehabilitation and the Conspiracy of Hope: A Keynote Address.* Burlington, VT: Center for Community Change Through Housing and Support.

Deegan, P. (1993). Recovering our sense of value after being labelled. *Journal of Psychosocial Nursing* 31(4), 7–11.

Department for Education and Skills (2003). *Every Child Matters: Change for Children.* London: Department for Education and Skills.

Department of Health (2000). *The NHS Plan: A Plan for Investment, a Plan for Reform.* London: DH.

Department of Health (2001a). *Valuing People: A New Strategy for Learning Disability for the 21st Century.* London: DH.

Department of Health (2001b). *The Journey of Recovery: The Government's Vision for Mental Health Care.* London: DH.

Department of Health (2004a). *NHS Improvement Plan 2004: Putting People at the Heart of Public Services.* London: DH.

Department of Health (2004b). *National Standards, Local Action: Health and Social Care Standards and Planning Framework 2005/06–2007/08.* London: DH.

Department of Health (2005a). *Independence, Well-being and Choice: Our Vision of the Future of Social Care for Adults in England.* London: DH.

Department of Health (2005b). *Creating a Patient-led NHS: Delivering the NHS Improvement Plan.* London: DH.

Department of Health (2006). *Our Health, Our Care, Our Say: A New Direction for Community Services.* London: DH.

Department of Health/Care Services Improvement Partnership (2005). *Everybody's Business: Integrated Mental Health Service for Older Adults.* London: DH.

Department of Health and Human Services (2003). *Achieving the Promise: Transforming Mental Health Care in America.* President's New Freedom Commission on Mental Health, Publication No. SMA-03–3832. Rockville, MD: Department of Health and Human Services.

Disability Rights Commission (2006). *Equal Treatment: Closing the Gap.* London: Disability Rights Commission.

Mental Health Commission (1998). *Blueprint for Mental Health Services in New Zealand.* Wellington: Mental Health Commission.

Mental Health Commission (2005). *A Vision for a Recovery Model in Irish Mental Health Services.* Dublin: Mental Health Commission.

Repper, J. and Perkins, R. (2003). *Social Inclusion and Recovery. A Model for Mental Health Practice.* Edinburgh: Baillière Tindall.

Rogers, J. (1995). Work is key to recovery. *Psychosocial Rehabilitation Journal* 18, 5–10.

Rose, D. (2001). *Users' Voices.* London: Sainsbury Centre for Mental Health.

Sayce, L. (2000). *From Psychiatric Patient to Citizen. Overcoming Discrimination and Social Exclusion.* London: Macmillan.

Shepherd, G. Boardman, J., and Slade, M. (2008). *Making Recovery a Reality.* London: Sainsbury centre for mental Health.

10 The essence of physical health care

Helen Waldock

▼ Introduction

Physical health assessment is part of the comprehensive holistic assessment offered by mental health nurses, forming one of the core paradigms of all nursing models and theories. It has, however, been one of the most neglected areas of practice despite the known interactions between mental and physical health. This chapter addresses the central characteristics of physical health, physical health assessment, and health promotion to enable practitioners to incorporate and integrate physical health assessments and interventions into mental health care planning. The chapter has been organized so that it moves through the levels of a developing therapeutic relationship from general observations, through more intimate questioning and examination, to collaborative health care and health promotion. The central and underlying skill set relates to the establishment and development of a rapport through assessment and engaging collaboratively in enabling service users to consider and initiate changes to lifestyle. Physical health assessment has to be considered in the context of the individual and where they are in their individual health–illness continuum.

Learning outcomes

By the end of this chapter you should be better able to:

1 Outline some common physical health needs and risk factors for people with mental health problems

2 Understand the significance of and utilize a systematic approach to taking a physical health history

3 Identify the essential skills and equipment required to perform a routine physical health care assessment

4 Undertake and interpret the results from a range of routine physical health measures and investigations

5 Demonstrate an understanding of health promotion in relation to identified risk factors and courses of action to promote the physical health of individuals.

The evidence base

It is estimated that 17.5 million adults in Great Britain may be living with a chronic illness, with the highest incidence being among the most disadvantaged groups, such as those who are unemployed and those with a mental illness (Department of Health [DH] 2005). Mental health nurses need to develop physical health care assessment skills and engage actively in health promotion strategies with service users as recommended by the UK White Paper *Choosing Health: Making Healthy Choices Easier* (DH 2004), for example by encouraging physical exercise and an improved diet.

People who suffer from mental disorder, particularly of a severity requiring hospital admission, are known to be more likely to suffer physical ill health compared with the general population. Studies have shown that service users with severe mental illness (SMI) such as schizophrenia and bipolar affective disorder have a significantly higher incidence of a range of physical health problems. These include cardiovascular disease, obesity, type 2 diabetes, sexual health problems, stroke, **osteoarthritis, hyperprolactinaemia**, dental problems, HIV/AIDS, hepatitis C, respiratory problems, irritable bowel syndrome, and some cancers (Goldman 1999, Lambert and Velakoulis 2003, Östby and Correia 2000, Richardson and Faulkner 2005). On average, patients with SMI die 10–15 years earlier than people without SMI (Richardson and Faulkner 2005), and annual age-adjusted death rates are two to four times higher than in the general population. The National

Confidential Inquiry into avoidable deaths in the UK in people with mental illness (University of Manchester 2006) found that almost half the patients in the study had cardiovascular and respiratory disease. Such figures have led to an increased awareness of, and focus on, the physical health needs of this group, as indicated in the Chief Nursing Officer's review of mental health nursing (DH 2006). The mental health delivery plan for Scotland (Scottish Executive 2006) sets out targets and commitments for the development of mental health services for those with SMI by ensuring that every such patient, where possible and appropriate, has a physical health assessment at least once every 15 months.

The majority of patients with SMI in the UK are managed in the community by their family doctor and primary care services, in conjunction with community and outpatient mental health teams (secondary care services). However, there are risks in relying on primary care practitioners having performed thorough physical examinations, given the difficulties this group of service users may have in engaging with and using such services (Cohen and Hove 2001). Despite being at increased risk of developing various physical health problems, the detection rate and treatment of such illness among those with a mental illness is very poor (Phelan et al. 2001).

Previous research has suggested that the reasons for increased health risks among people with SMI are complex. They are likely to include poverty, lifestyle, access to health assessments and treatments, and side effects of antipsychotic and mood-stabilizing medication (Phelan et al. 2001). The evident inequalities cannot be explained by mental health problems alone (Samele 2004). Further reasons for such increased incidence may include a lack of awareness and/or late recognition of symptoms, low expectations of health care services, difficulties in attending doctor's surgeries, and potentially long waiting times. Difficulties in communicating with health care professionals and stigma and discrimination, as well as problems with registering with a family doctor, have also been found. Research indicates that staff and carers often believe that mental health service users are uninterested in their physical health, although service users do not share this view (Dean et al. 2001, Meddings and Perkins 2002).

There is sufficient evidence to demonstrate that those with mental health problems are less likely to have their physical health needs recognized and, even when they are, such needs tend to be managed poorly. A number of studies suggest that people who use mental health services are much less likely than the general population to be offered routine blood pressure, cholesterol, urine, or weight checks, or to receive opportunistic advice on smoking cessation, alcohol use, exercise, or diet (Sherr 1998).

Secondary care mental health services should undertake regular and full assessments of the mental and physical health of service users, addressing all issues relevant to the individual's quality of life and well-being. Physical health checks should pay particular attention to potential endocrine disorders such as diabetes and hyperprolactinaemia, cardiovascular risk factors such as blood pressure and lipids, side effects of medication, and lifestyle factors such as smoking and diet (National Institute for Clinical Excellence 2002).

A physical examination and assessment at the point of admission to hospital or entry into mental health services will, for many service users, be the only such physical assessments they receive. It is therefore vital that these assessments are of a sufficient standard to pick up significant abnormalities in order to enable appropriate management. In addition, a competent and comprehensive physical assessment may help to tailor medication prescribing and provide a baseline for comparison should there be emerging medication side effects or other changes in the individual's physical condition (Garden 2005).

Specific factors leading to poor physical health amongst those with mental health problems include:

- **Lifestyle:** smoking, poor diet, lack of exercise, alcohol consumption, substance abuse, sexual behaviours/activities, living conditions/homelessness.

- **Self-neglect:** people with SMI generally do not tend to look after themselves well due to the negative symptoms associated with their illness. Often those with SMI lack the social skills to communicate a medical problem effectively.

- **Psychotropic medication:** movement disorders, weight gain, toxicity issues.

Health variations and ethnicity

The 1999 Health Survey for England found that Pakistani and Bangladeshi people generally reported worse health than the general population, with men in these groups having higher rates of cardiovascular disease. Asians and Black Caribbeans were more likely to suffer from diabetes than the general population. In all minority ethnic groups in England, except the Irish, people were less likely to drink alcohol or at least consumed less than the general population. Bangladeshi and Irish men were more likely than the general population to smoke, and both Bangladeshi men and women were more likely to chew tobacco than other Asian groups. These factors are relevant in that members of the Black Caribbean male population in the UK are more likely to be admitted to psychiatric units, to be locked in wards, or to experience compulsory detention under the Mental Health Act 1983. This is despite the rate of psychosis among Black Caribbean men being the same as for white men. They are therefore more likely to be presenting with higher than average health risks.

Physical health assessment

To prepare you to support the physical health needs of service users, we will look at the following:

- General observation
- Current health state review
- History
- Baseline observations
- Further physical assessment
- Recommended equipment for physical examination on psychiatric wards
- Chaperones.

Assessment is focused on the collection of various types of information about the person being assessed. Such information may be reported subjectively by the individual (e.g. pain or feelings of worthlessness) or observed or measured objectively by the professional (e.g. vomiting or posture). Objective information can be assessed at any time, and such assessment should form a basic component of any mental health professional's core competencies. The core skill of observation can be applied to physical health care as part of the overall physical health assessment. Key factors relevant to physical assessment are described below.

General observation

- **Age:** the person appears to be their stated age
- **Development:** is appropriate for age and sex
- **Consciousness:** alertness, orientation, ability to attend to questions
- **Skin colour:** tone is even, skin is intact, no obvious lesions
- **Facial features:** symmetrical with movement
- **Stature:** height appears within the normal range for age and sex
- **Nutrition:** weight appears within the normal range for height and body build; body fat distribution appears even
- **Symmetry:** body parts look equal bilaterally and in relative proportion to one another

- **Gait:** walk is smooth, even, well balanced; associated movements such as arm swings are present
- **Range of motion:** movement is deliberate, accurate, smooth, and coordinated; no involuntary movement is present
- **Speech:** articulation (the ability to form words) is clear, fluent, and evenly paced
- **Personal hygiene:** appears clean and well groomed
- **Obvious physical deformities:** note any congenital or acquired defects.

Current health state review

The purpose of a current health state review is to enable the service user to report any current changes that they may not recognize as significant, or that had changed gradually and so had gone unnoticed, and to give an opportunity to discuss any physical concerns they may not have had the opportunity to discuss before. The structure of the review can be needs led in that the client can discuss what is important to them. However, the practitioner is advised to have a framework in mind to ensure that no bodily system is omitted in the review. Sensitivity and diplomacy need to be employed when discussing bodily functions, taking into account the culture, age, and religion of both the individual and the professional, to avoid embarrassment. The systems headings outlined in Box 10.1 are suggested as a guide.

History

Where possible a history should provide a record of what has happened since birth, giving clues to current predisposing or potential risk factors. History-taking is a collaborative effort within the multidisciplinary team, and often occurs as a natural disclosure when building a relationship with the service user. Some important elements of history-taking include:

- **Family:** composition, ages, health, and causes of death of blood relatives, specifically any family history of heart disease, high blood pressure, stroke, diabetes, cancer, sickle cell anaemia, allergies, obesity, alcoholism, mental illness, or seizures
- **Past health:** client's perception of level of current health, childhood illnesses, allergies, serious accidents/injuries, adult illnesses, surgical procedures, other hospitalizations, immunizations (especially hepatitis for intravenous drug users), smoking
- **Prescribed medication:** types, dose, and frequency; whether the individual is currently taking it, what this is for, any borrowed medication, concordance, side effects, dose, and frequency

Box 10.1   Example of a physical health review

Skin: any skin ailments (eczema, psoriasis); pigment or colour change; change in moles; excessive dryness; pruritus (itching); bruising; rash or lesion

Hair: recent loss or change in texture

Nails: change in shape, colour, or brittleness

Head: unusually frequent or severe headache; any head injury; syncope (dizziness) or vertigo

Eyes: difficulty with vision (acuity, blurring, blind spots, eye pain, diplopia [double vision]); redness; swelling; watering or discharge

Ears: earaches or infections; discharge; tinnitus or vertigo

Nose and sinuses: unusually severe or frequent colds; sinus pain; nasal obstruction; nose bleeds; change in sense of smell

Mouth and throat: pain; frequent sore throat; bleeding gums; toothache; dysphagia (problems swallowing); voice change; altered taste

Neck: pain; limitation of movement; lumps or swellings

Breast: pain; lump; nipple discharge; rash; symmetrical; change in appearance or sensation

Breathing: pain with breathing; wheezy or noisy breathing; shortness of breath (SOB); how much activity produces SOB; cough; sputum (colour and amount)

Cardiac: chest pain; palpitations; dyspnoea (difficulty breathing); orthopnoea (inability to breathe easily unless sitting up straight or standing erect); paroxysmal nocturnal dyspnoea (difficulty breathing after lying flat); hypertension; coronary artery disease

Peripheral vascular: coldness, numbness, tingling, discoloration, or swelling of extremities (hands and feet); varicose veins; aching, crampy, tired, and sometimes burning pain in the legs that comes and goes usually with exercise (intermittent claudication); leg ulcers

Gastrointestinal: appetite; food intolerance; dysphagia; heartburn; reflux; indigestion; pain associated with eating; nausea and/or vomiting (characteristics, e.g. before or after eating); vomiting blood; previous ulcer, gall bladder, jaundice, appendicitis, colitis, irritable

bowel; recent change in bowel movements (constipation, diarrhoea, black stools, rectal bleeding)

Urinary: frequency or urgency; nocturia (excessive urinating at night); dysuria (pain); oliguria (less than usual); hesitancy or straining; urine colour; incontinence; previous kidney stones; urinary tract infections (UTIs); prostate problems (men); pain in flank, groin, suprapubic region, or lower back

Male genital: penile or testicular pain, sores, lesions; penile discharge; lumps

Female genital: menstrual history (age at menarche, last period, cycle length, duration); amenorrhagia (lack of periods); menorrhagia (excessive bleeding); premenstrual syndrome; dysmenorrhagia (pain); intermenstrual spotting; vaginal itching or discharge; age at menopause, menopause symptoms, postmenopausal bleeding

Sexual health: current sexual activity; dyspareunia (painful intercourse in females); changes in erection or ejaculation (male); contraception; previous or suspected sexually transmitted disease (gonorrhoea, herpes, chlamydia, warts, HIV/AIDS, syphilis)

Musculoskeletal: joint pain, stiffness, swelling, deformity, limitation of movement or noise with joint motion; muscle pain, cramps, weakness, gait, or coordination problems

Neurological: history of seizure, stroke, fainting or blackouts; any weaknesses, tics, tremors, paralysis, or coordination problems; sensory function; numbness or tingling; cognitive function; memory (long and short term) changes

Haematological: bleeding of skin or mucous membrane; excessive bruising; blood transfusions or reactions; anaemia

Endocrine: history of diabetes or diabetic symptoms; polyuria (frequent micturition); polydipsia (thirst); polyphagia (eating large amounts of food); history of thyroid disease; intolerance to heat and cold; changes in skin pigmentation or texture; excessive sweating; relationship between appetite and weight; abnormal hair distribution; nervousness or tremors

- **Over-the-counter medication:** as for prescribed medication; include any use of alternative and complementary substances, vitamins, etc.
- **Drugs and alcohol:** frequency and quantity.

Baseline observations

Routine baseline observations provide a relative norm for an individual against which change can be measured over time. The practical procedures of taking such routine observations provide an ideal opportunity for further observation and communication about physical health concerns with a logic and fluency that is relevant to the moment, thereby putting the individual at ease. For example, raised blood pressure is often a side effect of some high-dose antidepressants; respiration and pulse monitoring can be used as a means of directly giving feedback to an individual who is anxious or having a panic attack. It is important that such procedures are always explained to the client and that their consent and cooperation is gained. Key factors to remember include: ensuring clean hands by washing or use of alcohol gel to prevent cross-infection; protecting clients' privacy to reduce anxiety; helping clients into a suitable position for the procedure, either sitting or lying.

Temperature

Normal body temperature range in a resting person is 35.8–37.3°C. Infants have a wider normal range, and older adults tend generally to have a lower temperature. High temperature may be indicative of viral or bacterial infection, inflammatory disorders, or dehydration. Low temperature may be indicative of exposure to cold or an underlying problem or condition such as hypothyroidism, diabetes, liver failure, kidney failure, excessive use of alcohol or illicit drugs, or side effects of medications such as phenothiazines, barbiturates, opiates, clonidine, lithium, and benzodiazepines.

There are several devices for taking temperatures and these will vary across clinical areas (Box 10.2). Note that use of electronic ear thermometers is the most common way to measure temperature (Figure 10.1). Some common devices are listed in Box 10.2; manufacturer's instructions must be followed for any device used.

Pulse

In a resting adult, the normal heart rate range is 60–100 beats per minute. The rate varies with age, being more rapid in infancy. Females after puberty have a slightly higher rate than males. Pulses are found where arteries pass close to or above bones and can therefore be easily palpated. The most

Box 10.2 Devices for taking a temperature

- **Digital thermometers:** can be used in the mouth, **axilla**, or rectum
- **Electronic ear thermometers:** measure the temperature inside the ear canal (most commonly used)
- **Plastic strip thermometers:** small plastic strips pressed on the forehead
- **Glass mercury thermometers:** although previously common, should no longer be used

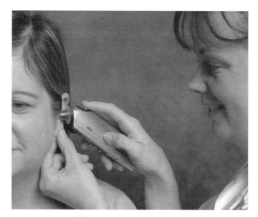

Figure 10.1 Taking temperature using an electronic ear thermometer.

common and least intrusive site for measuring the pulse rate is at the wrist (radial pulse). A fast heart rate may be caused by activity or exercise, anaemia, decongestants, fever, hyperthyroidism, medication for the treatment of asthma, and stimulants such as caffeine and stress. A slow heart rate may be caused by heart disease, heart medication, high levels of fitness, or hypothyroidism. The procedure for taking and recording a radial pulse rate is outlined in Box 10.3.

Respiration

A person's breathing when resting is normally relaxed, regular, automatic, and silent. Resting respiration rates for most adults are usually between 10–20 breaths per minute. Increased respirations could indicate chest infection, fever, pain, recent exercise, or anaemia. Decreased respirations could indicate hypothermia, opium-based drugs, or sedation. When recording respirations you should count the breaths for a full minute, and assess the depth, rhythm,

Box 10.3 Taking a radial pulse

- Place the pads of the first three fingers at the flexor aspect (below the thumb) of the wrist.

- Increase the pressure gently until the strongest pulsation is felt.

- Count the number of beats for a full minute.

- Record the pulse rate in beats per minute, noting any irregularities in the rhythm and strength (is it fast and full **[bounding]**, or is it weak and feeble **[thready]**).

Box 10.4 How to record blood pressure

- Familiarize yourself with the type of sphygmomanometer equipment available (increasingly electronic rather than manual) and follow the manufacturer's directions for use.

- Remove restrictive clothing from arm.

- Apply the cuff 3–5 cm above the point at which the brachial artery (inner aspect of the crook of the arm) can be palpated (Figure 10.2). The cuff should be applied smoothly and firmly, covering 80% of arm circumference.

- Ask the client to rest their arm on a suitable firm surface.

- Inflate and deflate the cuff to the point where you can achieve a clear recording of the systolic and diastolic.

- Completely deflate the cuff and remove from client.

- Document findings, comparing with available past readings. Note any differences, detect trends, and report abnormal findings immediately.

and any use of accessory muscles (shoulder movements). You should record respiration as breaths per minute.

Blood pressure (BP)

Blood pressure is the force of the blood pushing against the side of the vessel wall. The **systolic** force is the maximum pressure felt on the artery wall during left ventricular heart contraction. The **diastolic** pressure is the elastic recoil or resting pressure between each ventricular contraction. Average BP in a healthy adult is normally 100–130 systolic over 60–85 diastolic

in millimetres of mercury (mmHg). BP can be influenced by sex (postpubescent females have a lower BP than males), weight (higher in obesity), and exercise/exertion; increased BP due to increased activity should return to normal within five minutes. Instructions for recording a BP are outlined in Box 10.4.

Remember that pulse, respirations, and BP are affected by anxiety and distress, and therefore it is essential that the client is as relaxed as possible when such baseline observations are recorded.

Further physical assessment

The introduction of annual physical health checks for people with SMI in England (every 15 months in Scotland), either through primary care services or as part of an enhanced care programme, necessitates the need to move beyond baseline observations. Not all mental health practitioners will routinely be involved with further physical assessment, but some discussion of it is important as an admission episode may provide the opportunity to undertake such assessments. Some of the skills involved are also applicable for use with those who already have a confirmed diagnosis such as diabetes, asthma, or an eating disorder. Such assessments can also be used as part of the feedback or evaluation for a package of care with a health promotion component.

Urinalysis

Urinalysis can reveal health problems and diseases such as diabetes mellitus, various forms of kidney disease, and UTIs that may have gone unnoticed due to a lack of external signs or symptoms. The first part of conducting a urinalysis is direct visual observation of a urine sample. Normal, fresh urine should be pale to dark yellow or amber in colour, clear, and free of sediment. Normal urine volume output is 750–2000 mL per 24 hours. A readily available microchemistry system, often referred to as 'dipstick analysis', is frequently used as a first-line investigation. Box 10.5 outlines the procedure for obtaining and testing a urine specimen using this method. Box 10.6 outlines what the readings produced by the dipstick are and what positive (+ve) results might mean.

Peak flow

A peak flow meter is a small device that is blown into to measure airflow expiration. It records airflow in litres per minute (L/min). There are no normative values for peak flow as they vary depending on age, size, and sex (charts are often available in clinical areas). However, the chart in Figure 10.3 can be used as a rough guide.

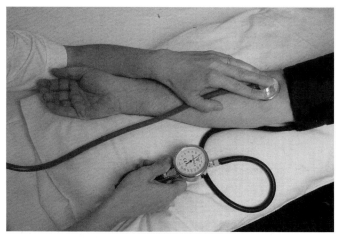

Figure 10.2 Position of cuff and stethoscope when taking blood pressure.

Box 10.5 How to obtain and test a urine specimen using dipstick analysis

- Read instructions on bottle as there are time differences for each reading.

- Explain the reason for a routine urinalysis to the client; provide a suitable, clean specimen container; ask them to provide a 'clean catch' of mid-stream urine.

- Immerse the dipstick completely in the sample of fresh urine and withdraw immediately, drawing the edge along rim of container to remove excess.

- Hold the dipstick horizontally before reading each measure.

- Clearly record observations, even if there are no abnormalities. Where any abnormalities exist, report these immediately.

Height (cm)	120	130	140	150	160	170	180+
Peak flow (L/min)	215	260	300	350	400	450	500

Figure 10.3 Chart of peak flow values.

One limitation of peak flow readings is that they measure the condition only of the large airways. If there are problems in the smaller airways, a person can be symptomatic but still have good peak flow readings. Instructions for taking a peak flow reading are outlined in Box 10.7.

Box 10.6 Urinalysis readings and interpretations

pH: the acidity of the urine—helpful for identifying body acid–base imbalances. Normal range is 4.6–8. High pH can indicate UTI, vomiting, or renal failure. Low pH can indicate chronic obstructive pulmonary disease, diabetic ketoacidosis, or diarrhoea.

The following readings should not be present in a normal urine sample. Positive results could indicate:

+ve glucose (glycosuria): diabetes mellitus

+ve ketones: calorie deprivation (starvation, poor self-care), diabetic ketosis, high alcohol consumption

+ve protein (proteinuria): UTI, kidney disease, heavy metal poisoning

+ve bilirubin: liver problems

+ve haemoglobin (haematuria): UTI, menstruation in women, cystitis, other kidney problems

+ve leukocytes: pyuria associated with UTI, chlamydia, viral infections, and foreign bodies

+ve nitrites: significant numbers of bacteria, UTI

Body mass index (BMI)

Also known as the 'Quetelet Index', BMI is a statistical measure of the weight of a person scaled according to height. It provides a simple numeric measure of a person's 'fatness' or 'thinness', allowing health professionals to make a more objective judgement about an individual's health status in relation to weight. However, BMI categories do not take into account many factors such as frame size and muscularity. The categories also fail to account for varying proportions of fat, bone, cartilage, and water weight. Nevertheless BMI is a useful general indicator of potential health problems and risk of disease. It is also important to remember that BMI is only one factor related to risk of disease. In order to assess more accurately an individual's likelihood of developing obesity-related diseases, the UK National Heart, Lung, and Blood Institute guidelines recommend looking at two other predictors:

- The individual's waist circumference (because abdominal fat is a good predictor of risk for obesity-related diseases)

- Other individual risk factors for diseases and conditions associated with obesity (e.g. high BP due to physical inactivity).

The means of calculating BMI are outlined in Table 10.1, and you can find useful online BMI calculators such as this one at: www.nhsdirect.nhs.uk/magazine/interactive/bmi/index.aspx.

The World Health Organization (WHO 1995) BMI classification is as follows:

$<18.5\,kg/m^2$	Underweight, Thin
$18.6–24.9\,kg/m^2$	Healthy weight, Healthy
$25.0–29.9\,kg/m^2$	Grade 1 obesity, Overweight
$30.0–39.9\,kg/m^2$	Grade 2 obesity, Obesity
$>40.0\,kg/m^2$	Grade 3 obesity, Morbid Obesity

Box 10.7 How to take a peak flow reading

- Explain the procedure to the client and familiarize yourself with the equipment available.

- Check that the pointer is at zero.

- Preferably stand or sit the client in a comfortable, upright position.

- Hold the peak flow meter level (horizontally) to the mouth of the client, keeping your fingers away from the pointer to enable free movement.

- Ask the client to take a deep breath and, closing their lips firmly around the mouthpiece, blow as hard as they can into the meter (as if they were blowing out candles on a birthday cake).

- Look at the pointer and note the reading.

- Reset the pointer back to zero.

- Do this three times and record the highest reading.

- Compare with the readings in Figure 10.3.

Table 10.1 How to calculate BMI

Measurement units	Formula and calculation
Kilograms and metres (or centimetres)	**Formula: weight (kg) / height² (m²)** With the metric system, the formula for BMI is weight in kilograms divided by height squared in metres. As height is commonly measured in centimetres, divide height in centimetres by 100 to obtain height in metres. Example: weight = 68 kg, height = 165 cm (1.65 m) Calculation: $68 / 1.65^2 = 24.98$
Pounds and inches	**Formula: weight (lbs) / height² (in²) × 703** Calculate BMI by dividing weight in pounds (lbs) by height squared in inches (in) and multiplying by a conversion factor of 703. Example: weight = 150 lbs, height = 5′ 5″ (65″) Calculation: $(150 / 65^2) \times 703 = 24.96$

Waist circumference

As identified earlier, waist circumference, which reflects abdominal fat, is a predictor of risk for cardiac disease (Rexrode et al. 1998). Individuals who carry fat mainly around the waist are more likely to develop health problems than those who carry fat mainly in the hips and thighs (Mitka 2005). Although there are no universally accepted norms for this measurement (Yusuf et al. 2005), the following can be used as a guide:

- **Males:** If the circumference is 94–102 cm, cardiovascular risk is increased 1.5–2-fold. If the circumference is more than 102 cm, cardiovascular risk is increased 4.6-fold.
- **Females:** If the circumference is 80–88 cm, cardiovascular risk is increased 1.5–2-fold. If the circumference is more than 88 cm, cardiovascular risk is increased 2.6-fold.

The circumference of waist size can be measured as follows using a flexible tape measure. Ask the client to stand up straight with relaxed abdominal muscles. Place the tape measure around the stomach at the level of the belly button (navel); measure and record the circumference.

Lipid profile

The lipid profile is a group of blood tests that are undertaken together to determine risk of coronary heart disease (CHD) and to help determine preventive treatment. The well established tests that make up a lipid profile are useful to determine whether someone is likely to have a heart attack or stroke caused by atheroma or arteriosclerosis (Anderson et al. 1987, McBride 2007). A lipid profile includes: total cholesterol; HDL (high density lipoprotein) cholesterol (often called 'good cholesterol', which carries cholesterol to the liver where it is removed from the body); LDL (low density lipoprotein) cholesterol (often called 'bad cholesterol' as it can build up in the blood and increase the risk of heart

disease); and triglycerides, which store energy (a high level of triglycerides can block blood vessels and cause other health problems such as abdominal pain and pancreatitis).

Sometimes the laboratory report will include additional calculated values such as HDL : cholesterol ratio, or a risk score based on lipid profile results, age, sex, and other factors. Key ranges for a lipid profile report are outlined in Figure 10.4.

Pain assessment

Pain is a highly complex and subjective experience that originates from the central and/or peripheral nervous systems. The subjective report of pain is the most reliable indicator of pain. Information needs to be gathered from clients about the site of the pain; description of the pain (aching, throbbing, sharp, burning, crushing, shooting, etc.); and comparison with any previous experiences. The speed of onset, duration, frequency, and influences such as movement, heat, and cold all need to be considered in conjunction with any associated symptoms such as swelling, numbness, or 'pins and needles' when assessing pain. Pain is usually indicative of underlying pathology or injury and should not be considered as something to be tolerated (see Further reading and Useful websites).

Recommended equipment for physical examination on psychiatric wards

To complete a thorough physical examination and assessment the equipment outlined in Box 10.8 is recommended as a minimum.

If patients decline a physical assessment and examination, this must be documented clearly in the multidisciplinary records and on any physical health assessment form. Practitioners are encouraged to record basic observable physical signs such as

---

Total Cholesterol (lower ↓ is better)

Best = <200 mg/dL
Borderline high = 200–239 mg/dL
High = 240 mg/dL or higher

Triglycerides (lower ↓ is better)

Best = <150 mg/dL
Borderline high = 150–199 mg/dL
High = 200–499 mg/dL
Very high = 500 mg/dL or higher

LDL Cholesterol (lower ↓ is better)

Best = <100 mg/dL
Good = 100–129 mg/dL
Borderline high = 130–159 mg/dL
High = 160–189 mg/dL
Very high = 190 mg/dL or higher

HDL Cholesterol (higher ↑ is better)

Low = <40 mg/dL
Best = 60 mg/dL or higher

Figure 10.4 Key ranges for a lipid profile report.

Box 10.8 Minimum equipment required for physical examination and assessment

- Examination couch or bed
- Stethoscope—used to detect heart, lung, stomach, and other sounds in humans, e.g. normal and abnormal respiratory, cardiac, pleural, arterial, venous, uterine, and intestinal sounds
- Sphygmomanometer (non-mercury)—device used to measure arterial blood pressure
- Thermometer (non-mercury)
- Small torch (for checking pupil reactions)
- Reflex hammer—to test deep tendon reflexes to detect abnormalities in the central or peripheral nervous system
- Diagnostic set—containing ophthalmoscope for examining the eyes; auroscope (also called otoscope) for examining the external ear
- Weighing scales
- Height measure
- Flexible tape measure
- Tuning fork (256 Hz)—used to detect conductive hearing loss
- Urinalysis sticks
- Alcometer—digital breathalyser for alcohol detection
- Neurological testing—stimulation of the skin
- Snellen chart—eye chart used to measure visual acuity
- Disposable gloves

levels of consciousness or current motor functioning. Further attempts to undertake a physical assessment should be made at a later time, possibly when the patient is more settled.

Chaperones

Any physical health assessment that involves a patient undressing and/or intimate examinations should be undertaken in the presence of a chaperone. This protects service users and staff from inappropriate actions or allegations of inappropriate behaviours or actions. This is particularly, but not exclusively, important in the case of physical examinations or procedures involving the opposite sex. Gender, religious, and cultural sensitivities regarding physical assessments, intimate examinations, and undressing should always be considered.

Adequate information and explanation as to why the examination or procedure is required should be provided and, where necessary, easily understood literature and diagrams can support verbal information. In addition, careful and sympathetic explanation of the examination techniques to be used should be given throughout the procedure. It is unwise to assume that the patient understands why certain examinations are being conducted or why they are done in a certain manner. For example, patients need to be told why both breasts are examined when they may complain of a lump in only one, or why a vaginal examination may be necessary if a woman complains of abdominal pain (Gerada and Warner 2005).

Physical health risk management and health promotion

There is overwhelming evidence to demonstrate that having a mental health problem is associated with both deteriorations in physical health and poorer access to appropriate physical health care services. As a consequence, people with mental health problems, particularly those with SMI, require a holistic

Table 10.2 Physical health risks, health screening, and health promotion opportunities for people with mental illness

Issue	Risk factors	Associated risk	Health screen (look for)	Health promotion
Antipsychotic medication (APM)	Movement disorders First-episode SMI Female stigma	**Dyskinesia** **Dystonia** Tremors **Hypokinesia** Sedation **Akathisia**	Is either taking APM or it is being considered First episode of schizophrenia Female sex	Educate the client and carer(s) about recognizing side effects Consider possible use of vitamins E and B6 Consider one dose at night or larger dose at night

Issue	Risk factors	Associated risk	Health screen (look for)	Health promotion
			Changes to bodily movements Changes in sleep pattern Assess for side effects using a validated rating scale Take medication history	Avoid intermittent use of APM and only one APM at a time Where sedation is an issue, advise against driving and/or operating machinery Liaise with GP
Respiratory disease	Smoking Family history Asthma Bronchitis Emphysema	Wheeziness, SOB, chest tightness, cough Worse at night and provoked by triggers, e.g. pollen, animals, exercise	Family history Age 35 years Smoker or ex-smoker Breathlessness on mild exertion Persistent cough/sputum production Frequent winter colds Asthma Peak flow rate	Inhaler technique education Personal asthma action plans Smoking cessation Self-management Education Consider annual influenza vaccination Consider pneumococcal vaccination Refer to specialist Liaise with GP
Diabetes	Family history Unbalanced diet Obesity Black and minority ethnic groups APM	**Hyperglycaemia** **Dyslipidaemia** Hypertension **Retinopathy** Renal disease **Neuropathy** Heart disease Depression	Tiredness, lethargy, thirst, weight loss, and blurred vision Glucometer levels <4–7 mmol/L and >9 mmol/L Urinalysis: presence of ketones and protein BMI Unbalanced diet Pregnancy APM (olanzapine, respiridone, quetiapine)	Patient information Balanced diet Smoking cessation Physical exercise Referral to specialist Liaise with GP
Weight gain (obesity)	APM Neuroleptic medication Lack of exercise Poor diet	Hypertension Diabetes mellitus CHD Stroke Osteoarthritis	APM (olanzapine, zotepine, risperidone, amisulpride) Recent smoking cessation Possible pregnancy	Dietary advice Lifestyle changes Regular weight monitoring Exercise on prescription

Issue	Risk factors	Associated risk	Health screen (look for)	Health promotion
			Other medicines (e.g. mood stabilizers, anti-hypertensives) Lack of activity Poor diet BMI Waist circumference **FPS**	Consider referral to dietician Consider thyroid function tests Liaise with GP
Cardiovascular disease	Family history Lifestyle issues Smoking Diet Lack of exercise Alcohol Neuroleptic medication	Hypertension **Hyperlipidaemia**	BP >140/90 mmHg Age: males >45 years; females >55 years Postmenopausal (women only) Family history Smoking Physically inactive Medication types Alcohol Two or more risk factors Consider FPS Lipid profile ECG	Smoking cessation Dietary advice Exercise on prescription Medication review If >20% on FPS, consider cholesterol-lowering or antihypertensive medication, or aspirin/clopidogrel Possible referral to dietician Liaise with GP
Sexual health	Family history Postmenopausal women Unprotected sex Multiple sexual partners Intravenous drug use Bipolar disorder Childhood sexual abuse Neuroleptic medication	Breast, cervical, and testicular cancer STIs Chlamydia Hyperprolactinaemia HIV/AIDS Pregnancy Infertility Hepatitis B and C	Family history Postmenopause Age: females: 50–65 years; males: 15–45 years Caucasian men Previous testicular tumour Sexual dysfunction Smear test >3 years ago Amenorrhoea Gynaecomastia Sexual history Contraceptive history Check prolactin levels	Self-examination techniques Self-help groups Family planning/contraceptive advice Healthy living advice Counselling Screening: mammography; smear; STI/HIV testing Consider hepatitis B vaccination

lifestyle management approach in order to combat the clear physical health risks that exist for them. The notable risk areas, what to look for when health screening, further actions to be taken, and potential opportunities for health promotion are highlighted in Table 10.2.

Health promotion plays a key role in the physical health assessment and management of people with SMI, although health promotion information is rarely targeted as particularly relevant and important to this group (Nocon 2004, Sherr 1998). The mental health practitioner needs to be aware of the potential risks in making suggestions and should seek to empower clients to ask for further assistance from appropriate professionals as well as enabling them to do this. Mental health practitioners also need to be in a good position to liaise with other agencies to ensure equality of access and reduce discrimination.

It is well known that lifestyle changes such as increasing exercise levels, losing weight, and eating a better diet can help to decrease the risks of cardiovascular disease and diabetes. There is a plethora of advice and information leaflets available, although it needs to be acknowledged that the evidence base for effectiveness of some interventions is limited.

What is known is that effective interventions to encourage increases in general levels of physical activity work best when they focus on empowering people to make their own choices about strategies to increase physical activity levels, counselling from an exercise specialist, and participation in walking programmes. Such interventions are more effective than attendance at a facility like a gym (Thorogood et al. 2003). Family doctor-based lifestyle interventions such as advice on smoking, diet, exercise, and alcohol have been shown to produce small behavioural changes (Ashenden et al. 1997). Effective interventions to promote weight loss include contact with a therapist and family support programmes that are weight focused (Thorogood et al. 2003) and combined diet and exercise supported by behavioural therapy (Mulvihill and Quigley 2003). Group-based approaches have also been shown to be effective in helping patients with schizophrenia to stop smoking (Addington et al. 1998).

Mass media campaigns or classroom-based health education and educational packages and seminars to promote physical activity have not demonstrated any major change (Kahn et al. 2002, Mulvihill and Quigley 2003). Furthermore a systematic review of the nursing literature on health behaviour found that motivation did not appear to be a significant factor in more than one-third of the studies, although it was concluded that either overall motivation is not being measured effectively, or motivation is not an essential determinant of health behaviour (Carter and Kulbok 2002). The difficulties and ethics surrounding health promotion have been much discussed and further reading is recommended. However, physical health promotion needs to form an integrated component of the individualized user-focused package of care offered to all those with mental health problems.

▲ Conclusion

Physical health needs, based on a thorough physical health assessment, should always be considered as part of a holistic care plan including discharge planning. The assessment of physical health needs should include awareness of physical complications associated with common psychiatric conditions and treatments, especially medications such as antipsychotics. Assessment and management of physical health needs will require the mental health practitioner to liaise and cooperate with a range of health care agencies (e.g. primary care, dietician services, smoking cessation services, acute medical or surgical care services).

Complex physical health needs often require specialist input, and consideration needs to be given to the most appropriate setting for care. This will require consideration of specific staff competencies and the care environment. Specialist referral and input should be documented as part of the ongoing care review process and, although it is not always possible for medical specialists to attend such reviews, their input and advice should form a key part of care planning and intervention. The involvement of specialist health care staff or services in a service user's care must be judged according to the patient's needs and the skills and competencies of the mental health team.

w Useful websites

Information for health and well-being: www.rethink.org/living_with_mental_illness/everyday_living/physical_health_and_wellbeing/

Patient-focused information on all aspects of health and illness, screening and health promotion, including sleep, anxiety, depression, diet, and exercise: www.patient.co.uk

National guidelines for monitoring and treating high blood pressure and cholesterol: www.nhlbi.nih.gov/guidelines/index.htm

Leaflets and information sheets that can be printed off the website around overdose prevention and safer drug use: www.nta.nhs.uk

Smoking cessation website: www.ash.org.uk

Partners Against Pain is an alliance of patients, caregivers, and health care providers working together to alleviate unnecessary suffering by leading efforts to advance standards of pain care through education and advocacy: www.partnersagainstpain.com

➤ Further reading

Barkauskas, V., Baumann, L., and Darling-Fisher, C. (2002). *Health and Physical Assessment*, 3rd edn. London: Mosby.
Holistic health assessment in a unique narrative format that is practical and easy to understand. Introductory chapters reinforce basic skills, from interviewing techniques, to assessment of health beliefs and behaviours. Subsequent assessment chapters are organized by body system, and consistently explore anatomy and physiology, examination, and variations from health.

Robson, D. and Gray, R. (2006). Serious mental illness and physical health problems: a discussion paper. *International Journal of Nursing Studies* 44(3), 457–66.

Turk, D. C. and Melzack, R. (ed.) (2001). *Handbook of Pain Assessment*, 2nd edn. New York: Guilford Press.
A comprehensive text discussing all kinds of pain, including useful pain measurement instruments for assessing and understanding the pain patients may be experiencing. It includes the assessment in different kinds of people such as children, the elderly, persons with limited communication, and couples and families.

Vagnini, F. J. and Yeager, S. (2007). *30 Minutes a Day to a Healthy Heart: One Simple Plan to Conquer All Six Major Threats to Your Heart.* Reader's Digest Association.
Practical guide to looking after your heart, includes diet and exercise.

✦ References

Addington, J., el-Guebaly, N., Campbell, W., Hodgins, D. C., and Addington, D. (1998). Smoking cessation treatment for patients with schizophrenia. *American Journal of Psychiatry* 155, 974–6.

Anderson, K. M., Castelli, W. P., and Levy, D. (1987). Cholesterol and mortality: 30 years of follow-up from the Framingham Study. *Journal of the American Medical Association* 257, 2176–80.

Ashenden, R., Silagy, C., and Weller, D. (1997). A systematic review of the effectiveness of promoting lifestyle change in general practice. *Family Practice* 14, 160–76.

Carter, K. F. and Kulbok, P. A. (2002). Motivation for health behaviours: a systematic review of the nursing literature. *Journal of Advanced Nursing* 40, 316–30.

Cohen, A. and Hove, M. (2001). *Physical Health of the Severe and Enduring Mentally Ill*. London: Sainsbury Centre for Mental Health.

Dean, J., Todd, G., Morrow, H., and Sheldon, K. (2001). Mum, I used to be good looking…Look at me now: the physical health needs of adults with mental health problems: the perspectives of users, carers and front-line staff. *International Journal of Mental Health Promotion* 3(4), 16–24.

Department of Health (2004). *Choosing Health: Making Healthy Choices Easier*. London: DH.

Department of Health (2005). *Supporting People with Long Term Conditions*. London: DH.

Department of Health (2006). *From Values to Action: The Chief Nursing Officer's Review of Mental Health Nursing*. London: DH.

Garden, G. (2005). Physical examination in psychiatric practice. *Advances in Psychiatric Treatment* 11, 142–9.

Gerada, C. and Warner, L. (2005). *Model Chaperone Framework: Guidance on the Role and Effective Use of Chaperones in Primary and Community Care Settings.* Leicester: NHS Clinical Governance Support Team.

Goldman, L. S. (1999). Medical illness in patients with schizophrenia. *British Journal of Clinical Psychiatry* 60(suppl 21), 10–15.

Kahn, E. B., Ramsey, L. T., Brownson, R. C., et al. (2002). The effectiveness of interventions to increase physical activity. A systematic review. *American Journal of Preventative Medicine* 22, 73–107.

Lambert, T. J. R. and Velakoulis, D. (2003). Medical co-morbidity in schizophrenia. *Medical Journal of Australia* 178, 67–70.

McBride, P. E. (2007). Triglycerides and risk for coronary heart disease. *Journal of the American Medical Association* 298, 336–8.

Meddings, S. and Perkins, R. (2002). What 'getting better' means to staff and users of a rehabilitation service: an exploratory study. *Journal of Mental Health* 11(3), 319–25.

Mitka, M. (2005). Obesity's role in heart disease requires apples and pears comparison. *Journal of the American Medical Association* 294, 3071–2.

Mulvihill, C. and Quigley, R. (2003). *The management of obesity and overweight. An analysis of reviews of diet, physical activity and behavioural approaches. Evidence briefing.* London: Health Development Agency.

National Institute for Clinical Excellence (2002). *Clinical Guideline 1: Core Interventions in the Treatment and Management of Schizophrenia in Primary and Secondary Care.* London: NICE.

Nocon, A. (2004). *Background Evidence for the DRC's Formal Investigation into Health Inequalities Experienced by People with Learning Difficulties or Mental Health Problems.* London: Disability Rights Commission.

Ösby, U. and Correia, N. (2000). Mortality and causes of death in schizophrenia in Stockholm County, Sweden. *Schizophrenia Research* 45, 21–8.

Phelan, M., Stradins, L., and Morrison, S. (2001). Physical health of people with severe mental illness. *British Medical Journal* 322, 443–4.

Rexrode, K. M., Carey, V. J., Hennekens, C. H., et al. (1998). Abdominal adiposity and coronary heart disease in women. *Journal of the American Medical Association* 280, 1843–8.

Richardson, C. R. and Faulkner, G. (2005). Integrating physical activity into mental health services for persons with serious mental illness. *Psychiatric Services* 56(3), 324–31.

Samele, C. (2004). Factors leading to poor physical health in people with psychosis. *Epidemiologia Psichiatria Sociale* 13, 141–5.

Scottish Executive, Health Department (2006). *Delivering for Mental Health.* Edinburgh: Scottish Executive.

Sherr, L. (1998). Health promotion and mental illness—an overview. *Psychology, Health and Medicine* 3(1), 5–18.

Thorogood, M., Hillsdon, M., and Summerbell, C. (2003). Cardiovascular disorders. Changing behaviour. *Clinical Evidence* Dec (10), 95–117.

University of Manchester (2006). *Five Year Report by the National Confidential Inquiry into Suicide and Homicide by People with Mental Illness.* Manchester: University of Manchester.

World Health Organization (1995). *Physical Status: The Use and Interpretation of Anthropometry. Report of a WHO Expert Committee.* WHO Technical Report Series 854. Geneva: WHO.

Yusuf, S., Hawken, S., Ôunpuu, S., et al. (2005). Obesity and the risk of myocardial infarction in 270 000 participants from 52 countries: a case–control study. *Lancet* 366, 1640–9.

(11) Fostering guided self-help

Judith Gellatly　　　　**Karina Lovell**

▼ Introduction

At the point of registration mental health nursing students should be confident in providing evidence-based clinical interventions that optimize health, well-being, and quality of life for patients using a range of communication skills. Central to such interventions is the establishment of a relationship with individuals with mental health problems and the provision of feedback that is constructive and facilitates positive change.

Whilst in the past UK health policies have focused primarily on severe mental health problems such as schizophrenia, more recently there has been a growing acknowledgement of the need to address more common mental health problems (CMHPs). CMHPs such as anxiety and depression cause significant personal distress and social disability, and have economic consequences for patients, families, and wider society. CMHPs account for a large proportion of consultation time within primary care settings (Jenkins et al. 2002). Based on evidence of clinical effectiveness, cognitive behavioural therapy (CBT) is the psychological treatment of choice for both anxiety and depression (National Collaborating Centre for Mental Health [NCCMH] 2004). Although such psychological treatment is provided within primary care, a huge disparity exists between need and provision within current services, with many people not receiving effective treatment (Kessler et al. 1999). Service provision is often characterized by long waiting lists (Lovell et al. 2003), with many patients waiting months or even years to receive psychological treatment (Anderson et al. 2005, Lovell and Richards 2000). A large UK survey of around 25 000 patients by the Healthcare Commission indicated that over a period of ten months only 40% of patients had been offered access to talking therapies (Commission for Healthcare Audit and Inspection 2005).

The adoption of a **stepped care** system has been proposed to overcome these problems (Scogin et al. 2003). Stepped care attempts to enhance the efficiency and effectiveness of service delivery, and can be described as a sequence of treatment options offering simpler and less expensive interventions, such as low-intensity 'minimal interventions', in the first instance and more complex and expensive options if the patient does not benefit. A stepped care model, in a general sense, involves four qualitatively different steps starting with pure self-help, moving to **guided self-help (GSH)**/group therapy, then to brief individual therapy, and finally to longer-term individual therapy (Bower and Gilbody 2005).

The UK National Institute for Clinical Excellence (NICE) in their guidelines for depression and anxiety propose such an approach for the effective and efficient management of such problems (NCCMH 2004). The most appropriate 'minimal interventions' are those that are less dependent on the availability of therapists, and focus on patient-initiated use of evidence-based CBT techniques. Such interventions are generally described under the broad label of 'guided self-help', where CBT techniques are used by patients and facilitated by a 'health technology'. Health technologies in this case may include the use of books, video and audiotapes, computer programs, and internet sites. The NICE guidelines for depression propose the use of GSH at step two, between 'watchful waiting' and brief psychological therapy, and define GSH as involving a CBT-based self-help resource *and* limited support from a health care professional.

Current policy initiatives have thus focused on changing and improving mental health services, with particular emphasis on the incorporation of more brief evidence-based psychological therapies to overcome the problems in delivery and access. As a result there has been growing interest in developing the roles of mental health nurses in the delivery of such approaches. With the increased emphasis on patient empowerment, mental health nurses need to widen their skills in assessment, health promotion, and psychological therapies.

Self-help forms the basis of these therapies, and GSH interventions that require minimal therapist contact are increasingly being adopted in primary care services.

This chapter provides an overview of GSH, including its rationale, evidence base, and application in practice. In particular it highlights the use of GSH in primary care mental health for people suffering from anxiety and depression.

Learning outcomes

By the end of this chapter you should be better able to:

1 Demonstrate an understanding of the nature of GSH for anxiety and depression

2 Be familiar with the evidence base for GSH

3 Identify the key skills involved in the delivery of GSH

4 Apply knowledge and skills of GSH to your nursing practice with patients.

What is guided self-help?

GSH refers to self-help interventions that require minimal therapist contact and aim to provide the optimal balance between efficiency and effectiveness (Gellatly et al. 2007). NICE, in its guidelines for the treatment of depression, define GSH as: '*A self-administered intervention designed to treat depression, which makes use of a range of books or a self-help manual that is based on an evidence-based intervention, mainly CBT, and is designed specifically for the purpose*' (NCCMH 2007, p. 61). CBT is a 'talking therapy' that is based on the belief that thoughts (cognitions), physical sensations (feelings), and actions (behaviour) are all interlinked; for example,

---

Box 11.1 Underlying principles of guided self-help

- Based on CBT principles
- Usually mediated through a health technology, e.g. **bibliotherapy**, video/audiotapes, computer administered/web-based packages
- Intervention is focused on enhancing patient self-management
- Limited support from a health care professional (or paraprofessional)—main role is facilitative: supporting, monitoring, and reviewing patient's progress
- Should involve no more than three hours of total contact with the health professional

---

negative thoughts often lead to distressing feelings, which can then affect mood and behaviour. Using a set of structured techniques such as exposure therapy and behavioural activation over a time-limited period, CBT helps people to identify unhelpful thoughts and behaviours in order to reduce distress and improve functioning. The evidence base for CBT is established for treating a wide variety of mental health problems (Butler et al. 2006).

GSH is aimed at patients experiencing mild to moderate symptoms of depression and anxiety, with minimal or no risk factors. There are a number of underlying principles associated with GSH (Box 11.1).

The evidence base

There is an increasing body of evidence indicating that GSH can be successful for a range of mental health problems. However, this chapter focuses on the evidence base for the application of GSH for people experiencing depression or anxiety, and more commonly those with coexisting depression and anxiety.

There is a wealth of evidence for the effectiveness of GSH in treating depression alone including a number of **systematic reviews** (Anderson et al. 2005, Bower et al. 2001). Gellatly and colleagues (2007) undertook a systematic review to examine the factors that determine the effectiveness of GSH with patients with depression. Findings indicated that a range of different delivery methods, professionals, and content can be employed successfully when delivering GSH and that the health technology used is less critical. Further analysis of a range of studies of self-help for depression demonstrated better outcomes for GSH than unguided self-help.

A recent **randomized controlled trial** (RCT) by Anderson et al. (2005) additionally indicated that GSH delivered via the internet with minimal therapist contact led to greater reductions in depressive symptoms and increased benefits to quality of life than a waiting-list control group, with improvements being maintained at six-month follow-up.

Anxiety often coexists alongside depression, and most studies in primary care have examined both of these conditions together. However, one study by van Boeijen et al. (2005) focused specifically on the effectiveness and feasibility of GSH for people who were suffering from anxiety disorders alone. This RCT compared GSH delivered by family doctors in primary care with CBT delivered by CBT therapists in specialist mental health services (secondary care). The findings demonstrated that the outcomes of both treatments were comparable, with significant symptom improvements at the 12- and 52-week follow-up for both groups.

The majority of studies of GSH have focused on its effectiveness with coexisting depression and anxiety. Evidence from a large number of such studies generally supports the use and effectiveness of GSH with such conditions. Increased technological sophistication and greater access to the internet by the general population has seen a growing interest amongst researchers in the design and evaluation of internet-based GSH interventions for CMHPs. Proudfoot et al. (2004) conducted a RCT to examine the effectiveness of an interactive web-based package designed for people presenting in primary care with mild, moderate, and severe depression or mixed anxiety and depression (Beating the Blues™, Ultrasis plc; www.ultrasis.com). The package comprised eight computer-based sessions with 'homework' projects between each session. The package was evaluated positively by patients in terms of overall satisfaction, and results demonstrated reduction in clinical symptoms and accompanying improvements in work and social functioning. These changes were sustained at six-month follow-up, with the outcomes being comparable to those of traditional face to face therapy.

Gega et al. (2004) examined a number of computer-aided self-help programs for anxiety and depression, including Fearfighter™ (Kenwright et al. 2001), Cope™ (Osgood-Hynes et al. 1998), and BTSteps™ (Greist et al. 2002). They found that all the programs resulted in symptom improvement and positive patient outcomes, with patients reporting high levels of satisfaction with the treatment and the guidance received from clinicians. In addition to positive patient outcomes, the use of these technologies enabled clinicians to treat more patients in the same period of time than face to face approaches, and reduced treatment costs overall.

The studies outlined above indicate that there is encouraging evidence for the use of GSH in terms of its effectiveness in treating anxiety and depression. GSH is demonstrably more effective than no treatment or waiting-list control, and can prove more acceptable and cost effective when compared to other more traditional approaches to psychological treatments. GSH as an intervention of choice is increasingly becoming a central component of stepped care models of depression care, in both the USA and the UK (NCCMH 2004, Scogin et al. 2003).

In contrast, however, a number of recent studies have indicated that these findings are not fully conclusive. Mead et al. (2005) conducted a RCT that compared patients with anxiety and depression receiving GSH (using a manual) with waiting-list controls. They found that, whilst GSH patients reported high levels of satisfaction with the relationship with the deliverer and positively evaluated the manual overall, no significant benefits in terms of depression and anxiety symptoms were demonstrated. Although there was some evidence of significant benefit to social functioning, this finding was difficult to interpret and thus these authors concluded that, on the basis of their findings, there is no clear evidence for GSH as a beneficial treatment for people waiting for psychological therapy. Richards et al. (2003) conducted a RCT comparing GSH for people suffering from anxiety and depression facilitated by a general practice nurse to usual care by a family doctor over a three-month period. Although they found that the GSH group had achieved much better clinical outcomes than the usual care group at one month, these differences had disappeared at three-month follow-up. Whilst this study failed to demonstrate effectiveness of GSH in the longer term, GSH patients remained more satisfied with their treatment than those in the usual care group.

In a meta-analysis evaluating the effectiveness of self-help books for mild to moderate depression, Anderson et al. (2005) suggested that a number of the studies comparing GSH and delayed treatment are small, of poor quality, and contain some aspects of bias. They did recognize that with additional facilitated guidance the use of self-help books can be of benefit, but argued that the evidence for use of self-help books alone for depression is weak and cautioned against generalization to primary care without further investigation.

In summary, there is growing evidence indicating that GSH is an effective treatment for the management of depression and anxiety. Although evidence of effectiveness is not uniformly positive, this is perhaps due to the need for more definitive trials. However, the incorporation of GSH into stepped care models has highlighted its value, particularly for people who would otherwise receive little in terms of psychological help when on waiting lists for psychological therapy.

Application of GSH in clinical practice

Although the concept of GSH is relatively simple, implementing it as part of routine clinical practice requires application and skill. The role of the mental health nurse, and other mental health workers, in using GSH is to work in partnership with patients to support, guide, and monitor the use of GSH using a health technology (such as a book, computer program, internet site, etc.).

The key roles of the mental health nurse or other mental health worker in facilitating GSH are listed in Box 11.2.

Conducting a patient-focused assessment

A prerequisite for any intervention is a thorough assessment. The mental health nurse should conduct a patient-centred assessment using a semi-structured interview schedule to elicit information focusing on the patient's needs rather than on diagnosis (Mead and Bower 2000, Newell 2000). An outline for a semi-structured, patient-centred interview is shown in Box 11.3.

The assessment should focus on gaining an understanding of patients' main problems using general open questions, specific open questions, and closed questioning, thus ensuring that the patient is able to 'tell their story'. The four 'W' questions in Box 11.3 provide a useful starting point, followed by identifying the autonomic, behavioural, and cognitive aspects of the problem. Other areas highlighted in Box 11.3 are also important. A thorough assessment is an essential starting point in assisting the mental health nurse to develop an in-depth and specific understanding of the problem, gaining sufficient information to help them work with the patient to select an appropriate GSH intervention.

On completion of the assessment, a problem statement should be derived between the mental health nurse and the patient, ensuring that there is a 'shared understanding' of the current difficulties. A problem statement is a brief statement about the problem (drawing on the patient's own words) that includes the triggers to and impact of the difficulty. In addition to the problem statement, the nurse should work with the patient to set some specific patient-centred goals for achievement. It is

also useful to use a standardized outcome measure. There is a wealth of standardized outcome measures available, including CORE-OM (Evans et al. 2000), the Beck Depression Inventory (Beck et al. 1961, 1996), and the Hospital Anxiety and Depression Scale (HADS) (Zigmond and Snaith 1983). Selection should be dependent on the patient's difficulties and which measures are used in local services. The PHQ-9 (Kroenke et al. 2001) is a relatively simple and quick measure that has been shown to be acceptable to both patients and professionals to monitor depression. Importantly it has been found to be acceptable whether

---

Box 11.2 Key roles of the mental health worker in facilitating GSH

- Conduct a patient-centred assessment
- 'Selling' the rationale for GSH—based on information regarding nature, roles, and evidence
- Selecting the appropriate health technology
- Guiding and supporting patients to use the health technology
- Monitoring and reviewing progress
- Relapse prevention

Box 11.3 Format for a patient-centred semi-structured assessment

4 Ws

- **What** is the problem?
- **Where** does the problem occur?
- **When** does the problem happen?
- **With whom** is the problem better or worse?

ABC

- **A**utonomic—physical feelings
- **B**ehavioural—behaviour (e.g. avoidance)
- **C**ognitive—thoughts

Current triggers

- Is there anything that particularly triggers the problem, such as time of day, specific events, etc.

Impact

- Specific effects of the problem on various aspects of life—work, home, social, private leisure, family/relationship functioning

Risk assessment

Other important information

- Modifying factors—things that make the problem worse or better
- Onset and course of the problem
- Client expectations and goals
- Past treatment
- Drug and alcohol use
- Any other relevant information the client wishes to discuss

Problem statement and goal-setting

used face to face or on the telephone (Richards et al. 2006). A baseline standardized measure can be used at the first interview and at subsequent points during treatment. It is useful to enable the nurse and the patient to monitor and review progress in a measurable way, as well as for service evaluation and/or audit.

Delivering the rationale for GSH

Delivering a coherent rationale for any intervention is an essential clinical skill which requires providing sufficient information and explanation to enable patients to make an informed choice. The key elements in delivering a rationale for GSH are detailed in Box 11.4. Patients' understandings of self-help are often based on their previous experience of mental health services and/or their awareness of the concept of self-help as an approach to change (Khan et al. 2007, Rogers et al. 2004). The structure and concept of self-help should be discussed explicitly with the user. The roles of the patient and nurse should also be explained, emphasizing the nurse's role in support, guidance, monitoring, and review, and the active, central role of the patient. One useful way to explain this is to use the analogy of the personal fitness trainer, explaining that a personal fitness trainer does not do the actual physical work of getting an individual fit, but helps the individual to devise, plan, and monitor their own fitness programme. This helps to emphasize aspects of partnership and that the patient is in control of their own programme of care. The structure of planned sessions should be explained: that they are brief, usually between 15 and 30 minutes in duration, and that they can be delivered either face to face, by telephone, or by email.

Selecting the GSH health technology

The health technology is an essential feature of GSH and there are a number of key issues that should be considered in selecting which one to use from the range of self-help technologies described earlier. Although some promising research is available for some computerized CBT (CCBT) and web-based programmes (for instance, *Beating the Blues*™ and *Fearfighter*™ have been recommended for the management of mild to moderate depression and panic and phobias respectively [Kaltenthaler et al. 2006]), a more rigorous evaluation of these, and in particular self-help books, is required. Whichever health technology is to be used, it should be based on the principles of CBT where evidence for effectiveness is strongest (Gellatly et al. 2007, NCCMH 2004). Such evidence-based interventions that may form part of a GSH programme include behavioural activation, **problem solving, exposure therapy, cognitive**

restructuring, and **relaxation techniques** (Bond and Dryden 2002). In addition, further consideration should be given to the characteristics of the health technology, including the type of health technology used, presentation, etc.

A recent systematic review suggests that the actual type of health technology used in GSH may not be critical to effectiveness (Gellatly et al. 2007). This suggests that the health technology selected should be based on patient preference in conjunction with the specific types of technology available. The experience of the authors of this chapter suggests that inclusion of a choice of evidence-based interventions within

Box 11.4 Rationale for guided self-help

What is GSH?

* Explain emphasis on patient self-management
* Nature, frequency, and length of contact sessions—between 15 and 30 minutes
* Format of sessions—can be face to face, by telephone, or by email (offer choice)

Role of the user

* Explain emphasis on active role of patient in self-management
* They are the expert in their experience of low mood and anxiety

Role of the nurse

* To facilitate, support, and guide the patient with the use of the health technology
* Use analogy of nurse likened to a personal fitness trainer
* Nurses are the experts in evidence-based interventions

Role of the health technology

* Explanation of the health technology to be used (offer choice and check literacy)
* Explain the structure of the technology (e.g. contents, how to navigate, etc.)

Role of family and friends

* Explain how family and friends can help—being supportive, encouraging
* If the user wishes, the nurse would be happy to discuss any aspects of the GSH programme with family or friends

the materials is what is important, enabling patients to make informed choices as to the intervention that they feel will help them best. In addition, the layout of the materials should be considered. Whether web based or printed, many people find it difficult to read dense and difficult text. For people with literacy difficulties this is essential, and for many people with depression or anxiety concentration is already impaired. Thus, the material should be selected with care, paying particular attention to ease of readability and how user friendly the technology generally is. If materials are being designed, readability scores can easily be checked in most word processing packages using the Flesch readability scale (Flesch 1948). Text is rated on a 100-point scale: the higher the rating, the easier the text is to understand. Most written material should aim for a score of approximately 60–70 on this scale, which equates to the national average reading age. Simple but accurate explanations and guidance are essential, and together with clear illustrations and case histories can enhance understanding. With all GSH materials it is essential that the nurse facilitating the GSH knows and understands it to assist the patient.

Guiding and supporting people to use the health technology

Following the assessment and selection of the appropriate health technology, treatment sessions, whether face to face, by telephone, or by email, should focus on guiding and supporting the patient in its use. Owing to the relative brevity of contact sessions in this approach, it is important that they are structured well to maximize potential.

Sessions should begin with a collaboratively set agenda identifying shared aims for the session. These usually include a general review of the previous week, risk, and mood. Following on from this, review how the technology is being used, including exercises contained in the material. Most health technologies contain specific interventions based on CBT and include various self-monitoring diaries to obtain a baseline and measure of progress related to thoughts (in the case of cognitive restructuring) or activity (in the case of behavioural activation). Examples are often given of how to change, evaluating and challenging thoughts in cognitive restructuring, or how to increase activity gradually in behavioural activation. The role of the nurse as facilitator is to discuss the diaries completed by the patient and to work in partnership with the patient to problem-solve any difficulties arising. One common obstacle that arises is that patients are unable to complete an exercise. Careful and sensitive

questioning about what the specific difficulties are should be sought and relevant solutions advised.

When patients are working well with the material, the focus should move to the next steps of the intervention. For example, if a patient has selected behavioural activation through the use of a book, the nurse would ask them to go through the diaries and collaboratively set specific achievable activity tasks for the next session. If cognitive restructuring is being used, the nurse might focus on how the patient has identified or challenged unhelpful thinking. Sometimes, to enhance understanding, it may be necessary to complete an exercise within the contact session. For example, patients often find it difficult to evaluate their thoughts, however good the health technology is, and working through one example of a particular thought in the session can be helpful. Towards the end of contact sessions the nurse should summarize the salient points that have arisen, ensure that the patient understands the next steps, and provide opportunities for any final questions.

Monitoring progress

Monitoring progress is an important part of GSH, providing regular feedback to the patient and nurse, helping to review progress, and aiding clinical decision-making. There is a range of ways of doing this, but it should involve discussion with the patient and the use of both **process** (i.e. patient diaries) and **outcome** (i.e. standardized measures—see Patient-focused assessment on page 124) measures. Monitoring should always be a collaborative process using all the information available and, although an ongoing process, it is useful to plan a formal review every 3–4 weeks.

Relapse prevention

Towards the end of the intervention, and as the patient begins to improve, it is important that the nurse discusses the issue of relapse prevention. A discussion about 'staying well' can help highlight some of the triggers that have precipitated previous bouts of depression, enabling the patient to identify early warning signs. The nurse should help devise a plan of action with the patient (including teaching people to monitor their own mood and/or anxiety using some of the outcome measures described above). This should also include identifying actions that the patient found helpful during the intervention and restarting them as necessary. Once again, this process emphasizes a central feature of GSH in that it focuses on what the patient can do for themselves.

✖ Practice Example

Paul is 35 and experiencing moderate depression. His family doctor has referred him to see a mental health nurse in the primary care mental health team. During the initial interview Paul describes regularly waking at about 4.30 a.m. and not being able to get back to sleep, and general loss of interest and pleasure in many previously enjoyed activities (such as socializing with his friends, running, and films). He feels he has made a 'mess' of his life and has achieved nothing. He spends most of his day sitting around doing nothing, and recently has taken to sleeping on the sofa instead of in bed.

His depression began six months ago after his third business failed and a difficult separation from his girlfriend. He has a 3-year-old child whom he sees on a weekly basis. Paul has been taking antidepressants for three months and feels that they have made a slight improvement. Paul was not a risk to himself or others.

After the assessment Paul wrote the following goals: 'To go to the cinema once each week with friends' and 'To run two miles twice a week' and 'To negotiate with my ex-girlfriend to have my son overnight once a week'. The nurse offered GSH and gave a detailed rationale of how this could help to lift his mood and reduce the impact his depression was having on his life. The self-help book used had a range of evidence-based interventions that were accompanied by stories of people who had recovered from depression using these techniques. The nurse suggested that Paul read the stories and choose the intervention that he felt would benefit him the most. At the second session a week later, Paul had read the 'stories' and decided that he felt that behavioural activation (see Chapter 12) was the intervention he could work with. The nurse ensured that Paul understood the rationale for behavioural activation and provided him with a baseline diary to complete, outlining his current levels of activity (see Chapter 12). In the following session Paul and the nurse discussed the diary and collaboratively set some tasks that aimed gradually to increase his activity levels. These consisted of (a) going to bed at 11.30 p.m. at night, (b) walking for about 15 minutes a day, and (c) cooking a meal every day. Paul wrote these in his diary and a further telephone appointment was agreed for a week later.

Over the next six phone contact sessions Paul gradually increased his activity levels each week and his mood started to improve. The nurse supported and encouraged him to continue his programme and discussed with Paul how best to approach his ex-partner about having his son to stay one night. They agreed that the best way forward was to write to her. The nurse also spent some time problem-solving other difficulties with Paul. For example, one week Paul identified particular difficulty completing his activity schedule. The nurse reiterated the rationale for scheduling and, after agreeing some modifications of the tasks, this difficulty was overcome. By session ten Paul had managed to come to a mutual agreement with his ex-partner for his son to sleep over every two weeks, was socializing more, and continued running. His mood had lifted and he was enjoying life once again. Relapse prevention was discussed with Paul, and together with the nurse he drew up an individual plan for staying well. This included maintaining his socializing and exercise, and finding a running partner to enhance his motivation. The nurse also taught him how to rate and interpret the PHQ-9 (the nine-item depression scale of the Patient Health Questionnaire) so that he could self-monitor over the coming months.

The online resource centre for this chapter has another practice example that you can work through yourself.

 www.oxfordtextbooks.co.uk/orc/callaghan

▲ Conclusion

In conclusion, GSH is firmly established as a patient-focused approach to intervention that fits well with a stepped care model for CMHPs. The evidence base is promising, but further research is essential. The key role of the mental health nurse (and other mental health workers) in using GSH is to work in partnership with patients to support, guide, and monitor them using an evidence-based health technology.

w   Website

You may find it helpful to work through our short online quiz and scenario intended to help you to develop and apply the skills in this chapter. Please go to:

 www.oxfordtextbooks.co.uk/orc/callaghan

✚   References

Anderson, L., Lewis, G., Araya, R., et al. (2005). Self-help books for depression: how can practitioners and patients make the right choice? *British Journal of General Practice* 55, 387–92.

Beck, A. T., Steer, R. A., and Brown, G. K. (1996). *Beck Depression Inventory*, 2nd edn. San Antonio, TX: The Psychological Corporation.

Beck, A. T., Ward, C. H., Mendelson, M., Mock, J., and Erbaugh, J. (1961). An inventory for measuring depression. *Archives of General Psychiatry* 4, 561–71.

Bond, F. W. and Dryden, W. (ed.) (2002). *Handbook of Brief Cognitive Behaviour Therapy*. Chichester: John Wiley.

Bower, P. and Gilbody, S. (2005). Stepped care in psychological therapies: access, effectiveness and efficiency. *British Journal of Psychiatry* 186, 11–17.

Bower, P., Richards, D., and Lovell, K. (2001). The clinical and cost effectiveness of self-help treatments for anxiety and depressive disorders in primary care: a systematic review. *British Journal of General Practice* 51, 838–45.

Butler, A. C., Chapman, J. E., Forman, E. M., and Beck, A. T. (2006). The empirical status of cognitive-behavioral therapy: a review of meta-analyses. *Clinical Psychology Review* 26, 17–31.

Commission for Healthcare Audit and Inspection (2005). *Survey of Users 2005: Mental Health Services*. London: Commission for Healthcare Audit and Inspection.

Evans, C., Mellor-Clark, J., Margison, F., et al. (2000). Clinical Outcomes in Routine Evaluation: the CORE-OM. *Journal of Mental Health* 9, 247–55.

Flesch, R. (1948). A new readability yardstick. *Journal of Abnormal Psychology* 32, 221–33.

Gega, L., Marks, I., and Mataix-Cols, D. (2004). Computer-aided CBT self help for anxiety and depressive disorders: experience of a London clinic and future directions. *Journal of Clinical Psychology* 60, 147–57.

Gellatly, J., Bower, P., Hennessy, S., Richards, D., Gilbody, S., and Lovell, K. (2007). What makes self-help interventions effective in the management of depressive symptoms? Meta-analysis and meta-regression. *Psychological Medicine* 37, 1217–28.

Greist, J. H., Marks, I. M., Baer, L., et al. (2002). Behaviour therapy for obsessive compulsive disorder guided by a computer or by a clinician compared with relaxation as a control. *Journal of Clinical Psychiatry* 63, 138–45.

Jenkins R., McCulloch A., Friedli L., and Parker C. (2002). *Developing a National Mental Health Policy*. Maudsley Monograph 43. Hove: Psychology Press.

Kaltenthaler, E., Brazier, J., De Nigris, E., et al. (2006). Computerised cognitive behaviour therapy for depression and anxiety update: a systematic review and economic evaluation. *Health Technology Assessment* 10(33), 1–168.

Kenwright, M., Liness, S., and Marks, I. M. (2001). Reducing demands on clinicians by offering computer-aided self-help for phobia/panic. Feasibility study. *British Journal of Psychiatry* 179, 456–9.

Kessler, D., Lloyd, K., Lewis, G., et al. (1999). Cross sectional study of symptom attribution and recognition of depression and anxiety in primary care. *British Medical Journal* 318, 436–40.

Khan, N., Bower, P., and Rogers, A. (2007). Guided self-help in primary care mental health: meta-synthesis of qualitative studies of patient experience. *British Journal of Psychiatry* 191, 206–11.

Kroenke, K., Spitzer, R. L., and Williams, J. B. (2001). The PHQ-9: validity of a brief depression severity measure. *Journal of General Internal Medicine* 16, 606–13.

Lovell, K. and Richards, D. (2000). Multiple access points and levels of entry (MAPLE): ensuring choice, accessibility and equity of CBT services. *Behavioural and Cognitive Psychotherapy* 28, 379–91.

Lovell, K., Richards, D. A., and Bower, P. (2003). Improving access to primary mental health care: uncontrolled evaluation of a pilot self-help clinic. *British Journal of General Practice* 53, 133–5.

Mead, N. and Bower, P. (2000). Patient centredness: a conceptual framework and review of the empirical literature. *Social Science and Medicine* 51, 1087–110.

Mead, N., MacDonald, W., Bower, P., et al. (2005). The clinical effectiveness of guided self-help versus waiting-list control in the management of anxiety and depression: a randomized controlled trial. *Psychological Medicine* 35(11), 1633–43.

National Collaborating Centre for Mental Health (2004). *Management of Depression in Primary and Secondary Care*. National Clinical Practice Guideline 23. London: National Institute for Clinical Excellence.

National Collaborating Centre for Mental Health (2007). *Management of Depression in Primary and Secondary Care*. National Clinical Practice Guideline 23 (amended). London: National Institute for Clinical Excellence.

Newell, R. (2000). General consultation skills. In: *Mental Health Nursing: An Evidence Based Approach* (ed. R. Newell and K. Gournay), pp 79–102. Edinburgh: Churchill Livingstone.

Osgood-Hynes, D. J., Greist, J. H., Marks, I. M., et al. (1998). Self-administered psychotherapy for depression using a telephone-accessed computer system plus booklets: An open US–UK study. *Journal of Clinical Psychiatry* 58, 358–65.

Proudfoot, J., Ryden, C., Everitt, B., et al. (2004). Clinical efficacy of computerised cognitive-behavioural therapy for anxiety and depression in primary care: a randomised controlled trial. *British Journal of Psychiatry* 185, 46–54.

Richards, A., Barkham, M., Cahill, J., Richards, D., Williams, C., and Heywood, P. (2003). PHASE: a randomised, controlled trial of supervised self-help cognitive behavioural therapy in primary care. *British Journal of General Practice* 53, 764–70.

Richards, D. A., Lankshear, A. J., Fletcher, J., et al. (2006). Developing a UK protocol for collaborative care: a qualitative study. *General Hospital Psychiatry* 28(4), 296–305.

Rogers, A., Oliver, D., Bower, P., Lovell, K., and Richards, D. (2004). People's understanding of primary care based mental health self-help clinic. *Patient Education and Counseling* 53, 41–6.

Scogin, F., Hanson, A., and Welsh, D. (2003). Self-administered treatment in stepped-care models of depression treatment. *Journal of Clinical Psychology* 59, 341–9.

van Boeijen, C. A., van Oppen, P., van Balkom, A. J. L. M., et al. (2005). Treatment of anxiety disorders in primary care practice: a randomised controlled trial. *British Journal of General Practice* 55, 763–9.

Zigmond, A. S. and Snaith, R. P. (1983). The Hospital Anxiety and Depression Scale. *Acta Psychiatrica Scandinavica* 67, 361–70.

(12) **Behavioural activation**

Dave Richards

▼ Introduction

This chapter will describe the skill known as **behavioural activation (BA)**. BA is one of the most effective psychotherapeutic techniques for patients experiencing depression and is relatively simple to apply. It forms a major part of recent developments in **low-intensity psychological treatment** such as guided self-help and other therapeutic work involving only brief contact between mental health workers and patients, as well as being used as a more traditional **high-intensity psychological treatment**, in which therapists and patients work together for longer and have more numerous sessions. It has shown to be equally as effective as both **cognitive therapy** and **antidepressants** (Dimidjian et al. 2006). Competence in applying BA will equip any nurse with a highly effective and acceptable psychological technique to assist people with depression.

This chapter outlines the theory, history, and evidence base for BA and describes a seven-step BA protocol (Richards et al. 2008) illustrated by practice examples. Details of how BA can be used in **relapse prevention strategies** are also described, followed by key references and further reading.

Learning outcomes

By the end of this chapter you should be better able to:

1 Understand the theoretical basis for BA and the links between behaviour and mood

2 Describe the evidence base for BA as an effective, patient-centred treatment for depression

3 Outline a seven-step protocol for implementing BA collaboratively with patients, including its role in relapse prevention and health promotion

4 Apply your understanding and the BA protocol to your nursing practice with patients.

Theoretical underpinning and evidence base

Theory

BA has a distinct theoretical base drawn from **contextual** understandings of human psychopathology. For a full description of how these theories underpin treatments based on the principles of behavioural psychology, see Richards (2007). In brief, however, these theories maintain that how we feel, what we think, and what we do are direct results of interactions we have with our physical and social environment. If we do something and our experiences of doing it are positive, we are more likely to do it again. If we avoid something because we do not like it and the experience of avoidance is relieving—we feel better because we have avoided something unpleasant—we will probably repeat this avoidance behaviour again.

The first example is called **positive reinforcement**. Reinforcement always increases the behaviour in question. Positive reinforcement does so because we like the thing we did, so we do it some more. The second example is called **negative reinforcement**. As with positive reinforcement, negative reinforcement increases a particular behaviour. In this case, however, the behaviour is avoidance of something we do not like, and the resulting relief of avoidance means that when we think about doing the same thing we are more likely to avoid it again.

Both types of reinforcement are vital to understanding depression and BA. People who are depressed generally reduce the frequency and types of behaviour they usually engage in (American Psychiatric Association 1994, World Health Organization 1992). They commonly stop going out with others, reduce interactions with friends, work colleagues, and family, and make little effort to do things they may have enjoyed previously. Essentially, people who are depressed tend to avoid things. Part of the reason for this is that the activities highlighted earlier require effort. This expenditure of effort can be tiresome. By avoiding effort, people who are feeling depressed feel less burdened and this acts as negative reinforcement.

At the same time, however, people who get into this pattern of avoidance reduce social and personal activities that bring pleasure, thus reducing their opportunity for positive reinforcement and the benefits this brings. The increased frequency of negatively reinforced avoidance means people do not have the same opportunities for pleasure or achievement. Indeed, depression is characterized by an absence of the ability to feel pleasure—**anhedonia**. People who are depressed often get stuck in a vicious circle of negatively reinforcing avoidance and reduced opportunity for pleasurable activity.

This is problematic because behaviour has a significant impact on emotion. As well as behaviours, emotion can be seen to consist of a physical element and thoughts (Lang 1979). This **three systems theory** has been very influential in understanding emotion. Increased behavioural avoidance and reductions in pleasurable activities influence and are influenced by physical symptoms of depression such as sleep difficulties, appetite changes, and poor concentration. Equally, behavioural changes can increase and follow on from negative thinking. Physical feelings and thoughts are similarly linked. Negative behaviours, thoughts, and physical feelings act as a vicious circle of depression.

Evidence for behavioural activation as a treatment

In the 1970s researchers developed a treatment based on positive reinforcement alone (e.g. Lewinsohn 1974). The treatment was designed to encourage people with depression to increase their exposure to pleasurable and constructive experiences. This was in order to increase the opportunity for positive reinforcement. **'Activity scheduling'** became very popular, so much so that it was incorporated into cognitive therapy, the new psychotherapy that swept the English-speaking Western world from 1979 onwards (Beck et al. 1979). With the development of cognitive therapy, interest in behavioural treatments declined for a number of years.

However, during the 1990s, researchers in the USA re-examined behavioural theories of depression, concluding that cognitive therapists had actually misunderstood the role of behaviour in depression, concentrating erroneously on positive reinforcement alone and on behaviour change as an initial route to cognitive change, rather than a treatment in its own

right. Jacobson and colleagues (1996, 2001) and Hopko and his team (Hopko et al. 2003a,b) outlined the central role of behavioural avoidance in the maintenance of depression, enabling a more theoretically coherent treatment to be developed. Whereas activity scheduling can be conceptualized as just one positively reinforcing strategy within a cognitive treatment paradigm, behavioural activation is a stand-alone treatment drawn from a theoretically distinct contextual paradigm that asserts the additional importance of reducing negative reinforcement as well as providing opportunities for positive reinforcement. In a large and important clinical trial, Jacobson et al. (1996, 2001) demonstrated that BA was as effective in treating depression as pure cognitive therapy or the combination of cognitive and behavioural techniques termed **cognitive behavioural therapy (CBT)**. A further trial by Dimidjian et al. (2006) demonstrated that BA was as effective as cognitive therapy or antidepressants. There was even some evidence that BA was more effective than either cognitive therapy or antidepressants for people who were suffering from severe depression.

These trials prompted a re-examination of the evidence for behavioural treatments of depression in general. Two research groups have now conducted and published systematic reviews of behavioural treatments of depression (Cuijpers et al. 2007, Ekers et al. 2007) and discovered that the evidence base for such treatments is in fact quite substantive, including 20 published randomized controlled trials. The meta-analysis by Ekers et al. (2007) included 1109 patients and showed that the effects of BA for depression were superior to no treatment, **usual care, brief psychotherapy** or **supportive therapy,** and equal to CBT. It has become clear, therefore, that BA has been inappropriately neglected; for example, it is not recommended as a standalone treatment in current guidelines (National Institute for Health and Clinical Excellence 2004). However, the recency of these new evidence reviews (Cuijpers et al. 2007, Ekers et al. 2007) means that BA is certainly being included as a treatment option in revisions of these guidelines, and is likely to be recommended in future editions. Our new understanding of the evidence base strongly suggests that BA should be offered to patients as a routine choice in care.

Step-by-step description

The following protocol for BA is drawn from a clinical trial of depression management in the UK (Richards et al. 2008). It was developed from the clinical methods described by Martell et al. (2001) and Hopko et al. (2003a).

Step 1: Explaining BA

It is essential that patients receive a full and comprehensive rationale for any proposed intervention. Such strategies are central to patient-centred practice (Mead and Bower 2000) and have been shown to improve the chances that patients will undertake therapeutic activities. The rationale should go something like this:

'When we are depressed we often feel physically unwell, have negative thoughts, and change the way we behave. These feelings, thoughts, and behaviours are all linked. We end up in a vicious circle where the worse we feel physically the more we think depressed thoughts, and the more we think depressed thoughts the more we withdraw from doing the normal things we used to do. The more we withdraw the more we feel physically unwell and the more depressed our thoughts become.

Some of the things we avoid are routine activities such as cleaning the house, doing the ironing, washing up. Other routines are disrupted such as the time we go to bed or get up, when we eat, and how we cook for ourselves. These are important life routines that help make us comfortable in our surroundings. Other activities that get disrupted are things we do for pleasure such as seeing our friends, enjoying a day out with family, or playing games with our children—things that often make us feel well. A third area where we avoid activities is in doing essential things such as paying bills or dealing with difficult situations at work.

Many people who are depressed think they need to feel completely physically well before starting to do things again. However, research evidence suggests that gradually starting to do more of the things we have been avoiding again can be a very effective form of self-help for depression. Setting goals for things we want to do can help to "act our way out" of depression rather than waiting until we are ready to "think our way out". Behavioural activation is a structured, active way of doing this. It focuses on re-establishing daily routines, increasing pleasurable activities, and addressing necessary issues. This helps us to regain important functions that have been lost or reduced during depression.'

Step 2: Understanding current activity

Although patients may verbally tell us what they are doing, having them keep a diary of a week's activity provides a more accurate baseline to measure current activity and, as treatment progresses, to evaluate changes. The second step in BA is therefore to encourage patients to complete such a diary. Table 12.1 provides an example of a blank BA diary. Each day is divided into sections and patients are asked to complete each section in terms of **four Ws; what** they did, **where** the activity took place, **when** they did it, and **who,** if anybody, they did it with. If no activities were undertaken—for example, the patient may be staying in bed until midday—then the section can be left blank or filled in with this information. Even if people think they are doing nothing, this is very helpful information. Such diaries have been used in clinical trials incorporating behavioural activation (Richards et al. 2008) and the ability to use them clinically is seen as a vital cognitive behaviour therapy competence (Roth and Pilling 2007).

Often, initially completing such a diary can be quite upsetting for patients as they may realize just how little they are doing. Alternatively, some patients find that the diary shows nothing but routine activity and reveals how few pleasurable activities figure in their schedule. Some patients find such a diary aversive and cannot complete it. This is in itself a significant piece of information. As ever, the results of the diary-keeping exercise should be treated with respect and sensitivity.

Step 3: Identifying routine, pleasurable, and necessary activities

The next key step is to help patients identify things that they would like to do. Often, though not exclusively, these are activities that they have stopped doing since they became depressed. Some of the activities may be routine ones, such as housework or cooking. Some may be pleasurable activities, such as going out and meeting people. Others may be activities that are necessary to enable people to move on in their lives, such as paying bills or dealing with conflict.

Box 12.1 shows BA Worksheet I, which can be used to list all these activities. Patients should be advised to make a list in any order they like, but to group their desired activities into three lists: **routine, pleasurable,** and **necessary.** You can print off a copy of this box from the online resource centre:

 www.oxfordtextbooks.co.uk/orc/callaghan

Step 4: Making a hierarchy of routine, pleasurable, and necessary activities

In order to plan the BA programme it is important to begin by asking the patient to order the activities identified in Step 3 into a hierarchy of difficulty: **most difficult, medium difficulty, easiest**. Box 12.2 outlines a second worksheet, Worksheet II, which can help patients organize their list—this is also available from the online resource centre:

It is important to advise patients to include some of each type of activity—routine, pleasurable, and necessary—in each category of difficulty in the hierarchy. This may be quite hard, as necessary activities are often highly aversive and the ones most ardently avoided. These activities may cluster at the top of the hierarchy but paradoxically be just the ones that are most pressing.

Step 5: Planning some routine, pleasurable, and necessary activities

This is the stage when BA actually gets 'active', with patients planning to implement some of their identified activities. Using a blank diary sheet (as in Table 12.1), patients should be encouraged to plan a programme of currently avoided activities. The key is to take examples of routine, pleasurable, and necessary activities from near the bottom of their list and plan to do them. It is not sufficient to have a vague idea of what will be attempted. Each chosen activity should be written in the diary to be undertaken at specific times, including the steps needed to undertake each activity.

Activities should be spelled out exactly and precisely using the four Ws outlined in Step 2 (**what, where, when, and who** with). Patients should be encouraged to schedule at least one activity each day—more if they wish—but it is important not to plan so many activities that achievement is unlikely. The idea is to start with small and regular activities, and gradually to increase the number and difficulty.

Table 12.1 A blank behavioural activation diary

		Monday	Tuesday	Wednesday	Thursday	Friday	Saturday	Sunday
Morning	What Where When Who							
	What Where When Who							
Afternoon	What Where When Who							
	What Where When Who							
Evening	What Where When Who							
	What Where When Who							

Box 12.1 Behavioural Activation Worksheet I

Write down your *routine* activities here (e.g. cleaning, cooking, shopping, etc.):

....
....
....
....
....
....

Write down your *pleasurable* activities here (e.g. going out/visiting friends or family):

....
....
....
....
....
....

Write down your *necessary* activities here (e.g. paying bills, etc.):

....
....
....
....
....
....

Box 12.2 Behavioural Activation Worksheet II

Now try to put your lists in order of difficulty.

Most difficult

....
....
....
....
....

Medium difficulty

....
....
....
....
....

Easiest

....
....
....
....
....

Step 6: Reviewing BA diaries

This final stage of jointly reviewing the patient's achievements in relation to planned routine, pleasurable, and necessary activities is absolutely crucial. It enables patients to reflect on their BA programme, receive feedback on progress, and problem-solve any difficulties experienced in implementation. Diaries are the essential data for collaboration between nurses and patients implementing BA programmes. Diaries should be examined together and each planned activity reviewed to see whether it went ahead, what happened when the patient tried it, and how they felt once it had been done. Some BA programmes ask people to rate 'achievement and pleasure' for each activity, often using a 0–10 scale. This is not necessary and can be burdensome for the patient. As highlighted earlier, a core symptom of depression is anhedonia, and patients are unlikely to feel pleasure, at least initially. Therefore, focusing on this aspect too much may be discouraging for patients in the early stages.

Patients often activate less than they had planned—a good reason for not scheduling too many activities, at least in the early stages. Skill is required to enable the patient not to become too discouraged. A flexible approach should be taken so that they can feel they are still making progress, even if some activities did not go as planned or were omitted. Strategies include making sure that patients know it is perfectly reasonable to reschedule activities to another day if not achieved when originally planned, problem-solving the reasons for non-completion, and choosing activities lower down the hierarchy of difficulty from Worksheet II (Box 12.2).

The most important thing about the review stage is that it is a joint and careful examination of the diary sheets. Every time the BA programme is reviewed, the diary records should be regarded respectfully. Shared decisions between nurses and patients implementing the BA programme should be based on this review. If progress is being made then this is the time to add additional planned activities. A balance needs to be struck between going too quickly, potentially resulting in failure and discouragement, and ensuring that momentum is maintained and progress made. Once again, this can only be done collaboratively.

As the BA programme is implemented, patients should begin to see that their mood is often related to their activity levels. This connection usually becomes established early on in the process. 'Bad' days are often those where planned activities were not achieved. Rather than focusing on failure, these occasions can be used to reiterate this vital connection, reinforce the power of the technique, and aid motivation. Engaging patients in discussing the relationship between their activity levels and their mood using examples of both success and failure is an important therapeutic conversation.

As the programme moves on, diary-keeping remains important but the selection and planning of activities becomes more patient directed. Nurses and other helpers should begin to step back as patients take more responsibility and initiative for scheduling and increasing activity levels. People are the best managers of their own mental health and should always take the lead after the early stages.

Step 7: Preventing relapse

Reminding patients of the connection between their recovery and the methods they used to get there is essential to maintain future health. The ideal situation is for patients to identify and be sensitive to early warning signs, using these as a cue to start the activity planning process again. If the connection between activity and mood has been established in a patient's mind, should mood begin to drop again they can go back to examining their activity levels and think about the balance of routine, pleasurable, and necessary activities. This combination of detecting warning signs (or 'triggers') and reinitiating previously successful strategies is often called 'relapse prevention' and is an important final stage in any treatment. Nurses should devote some time in a final contact session with patients implementing a BA programme to discuss the patient's future plans for managing relapse. Making the possibility of future depressive episodes explicit must be handled sensitively of course, but formally listing triggers and writing a plan for starting the programme again are extremely good ideas. The key message is that self-activation has delivered improved mood and the focus should be on the success of this programme and its likely future use to limit any subsequent episode of low mood.

✖ Practice Examples

Ken

Ken was a single, 36-year-old man who was feeling 'down'. He was tearful, felt an overwhelming sense of sadness, had great difficulty in concentrating, and his sleep was disturbed. He had lost a lot of interest in previously enjoyed activities: stopping cycling, going to the gym, and socializing with friends. He was lethargic and unmotivated to do much except go to work. As a result he spent most weekends resting or just sitting doing nothing. He had low self-esteem, thinking that he did nothing well and that he had not achieved as much as he would have liked to by this point in his life. He occasionally had suicidal thoughts, but these were only fleeting and he had no plans to take his own life.

Ken's depression was affecting his work, home, and social life. The problem had started two months previously when he learned that he was to be made redundant. He had been offered another job with the company but it involved moving 100 miles away and he did not wish to move. He had had three previous episodes of depression, all precipitated by a major life event (episode one when aged 18 and his father died; episode two when aged 27 after an accident; episode three when aged 30 following the break-up of a long-term relationship). In the past antidepressants had helped. A week ago Ken was prescribed fluoxetine (Prozac) 20 mg a day and his family doctor had made an appointment for Ken to see a mental health nurse.

In discussing his options with the nurse Ken was happy to continue with the medication but felt that he also needed some active skills to assist his recovery. He liked the sound of BA and, although he understood that it might be useful to complete a baseline activity diary, he preferred to move on to Step 3 immediately.

He started to draw up a list of activities using Worksheet I, finding it easy to identify routine and pleasurable activities but more difficult to identify necessary activities.

»

» The nurse helped him realize that taking steps towards gaining new employment was something he had been avoiding and was a necessary series of activities to undertake. He went away to think about what these steps might be and to complete Worksheet I before seeing the nurse again. At the next session he showed the nurse his completed worksheet (Box 12.3).

Ken and the nurse then worked together to combine these activities into a hierarchy of difficulty using Worksheet II (Box 12.4). As can be seen, the necessary activities tended to cluster at the top of the worksheet in the '**most difficult**' area.

As Ken moved on to Step 5 (**planning stage**), he was helped to select a range of activities from his Worksheet II and enter them into his first diary (Table 12.2). Most planned activities were routine as Ken felt his priority was getting back on top of his daily life. However, the nurse ensured that he also planned in at least one pleasurable activity and gently suggested making a move on his need to find a new job by breaking down his statement 'Look for a new job' into some preparatory steps. As can be seen, because Ken was still at work, most of his days were occupied by working and he needed to identify time at the weekends and in the evenings to undertake new activities. Ken did not start too ambitiously. This is important, as if too much is attempted this could result in failure and a sense of despondency.

The following week Ken reported that he had managed to do most of the things he had planned. He was most pleased with having cooked a proper meal, something he had not done for a while. However, although he had managed to buy a newspaper with a jobs section, there were no jobs that suited his circumstances. He was very pleased with the phone call to his friend, who had been worried about him and was glad to hear from him. After a discussion with the nurse, Ken decided that he needed more assistance with job finding. The nurse suggested that he might contact some recruitment agencies and Ken decided to schedule this into his lunchtimes (Table 12.3). He also increased the frequency of his cooking and decided to complete his cleaning. The most important thing for Ken was that he appreciated his new sense of purpose and felt that he was actually doing something positive rather than letting his mood dictate his life.

At the next contact with the nurse, Ken reported considerable satisfaction in his achievements during the previous week. He had done most of the planned cleaning and felt better about his flat. Things had not gone completely smoothly, but, although he had missed cooking one evening because he was so tired after work, he had made a meal the following night and felt that this was an acceptable compromise. He had also contacted two recruitment agencies who asked him to present his CV. This caused him some anxiety and he felt a bit

---

Box 12.3 Ken: BA Worksheet I

Write down your *routine* activities here (e.g. cleaning, cooking, shopping, etc.):

- Cleaning my flat
- Shopping (for food)
- Cooking meals using fresh ingredients
- Doing the washing
- Ironing work shirts

Write down your *pleasurable* activities here (e.g. going out/visiting friends or family):

- Going for a drink/out with my friends
- Cycling
- Gym
- Reading the paper

Write down your *necessary* activities here (e.g. paying bills, etc.):

- Look for a new job

Box 12.4 Ken: BA Worksheet II

Now try to put your lists in order of difficulty

- Gym **(most difficult)**
- Look for a new job
- Reading the paper **(medium difficulty)**
- Cooking meals using fresh ingredients
- Ironing work shirts
- Going for a drink/out with my friends
- Cycling
- Cleaning my flat **(easiest)**
- Shopping (for food)
- Doing the washing

»

» **Table 12.2** Ken's first diary

	What Where When Who	Monday	Tuesday	Wednesday	Thursday	Friday	Saturday	Sunday
Morning	What Where When Who	Work	Work	Work	Work	Work		Buy a trade paper and look for job adverts
	What Where When Who	Work	Work	Work	Work	Work		
Afternoon	What Where When Who	Work	Work	Work	Work	Work	Do some washing	
	What Where When Who	Work	Work	Work	Work	Work		Clean up living room
Evening	What Where When Who		Plan meal and shopping	Go shopping for fresh food	Cook a proper meal			
	What Where When Who					Ring up a mate		

despondent as he had never had to prepare one before. Ken and the nurse worked on this problem and together decided that an example of a CV to copy might help. Ken decided to ask a friend at work for some advice on CV layout. He also decided to plan to go for a cycle ride the following Sunday.

From then on, Ken's programme proceeded reasonably smoothly. He gradually increased both his pleasurable and necessary activities whilst maintaining his routine ones. Talking to his friend at work led to him going out for a drink one evening, something he had not done for a while, and this gave him some very positive reinforcement, particularly as the friend was concerned about, rather than dismissive of, his problems. In fact, his friend helped him compile his CV and Ken sent it to a number of recruitment agencies. Although cycling was hard at first, he began to realize how much he had missed this. He enjoyed it and so gradually increased his distances. After a further three sessions with the nurse Ken felt that he could manage on his own as he had a good understanding of the principles of BA. His depression was gradually lifting and he could clearly see the connection between increased activity and his improved mood. The nurse advised Ken to note down early warning signs of depression and to keep the BA programme instructions and diaries in a place where he could find them should he need to use them again.

»

» **Table 12.3** Ken's second diary

		Monday	Tuesday	Wednesday	Thursday	Friday	Saturday	Sunday
Morning	What Where When Who	Work	Work	Work	Work	Work		
	What Where When Who	Work	Work Contact agencies	Work Contact agencies	Work	Work		Buy and read the paper
Afternoon	What Where When Who	Work	Work	Work	Work	Work	Do some washing	
	What Where When Who	Work	Work	Work	Work	Work		Clean up bedroom
Evening	What Where When Who		Plan meal and shopping	Go shopping for fresh food	Cook a proper meal		Cook a proper meal	
	What Where When Who		Clean Kitchen	Make a list of agencies from Yellow Pages	Clean bathroom	Ring up a mate		

Jan

This case example concerns Jan, a 44-year-old woman suffering from her second episode of depression preceded by six months of feeling 'not right' prior to seeing her doctor. She had not received any treatment for a previous episode 15 years ago during a difficult divorce. Her main problems were disturbed sleep and general lack of interest in family activities. Jan lived with her husband and two children aged 9 and 13. She had become irritable and tired with thoughts that life was getting on top of her but had no suicidal thoughts or intentions. These symptoms had led Jan to disengage from family life and she was aware that she was not performing well at work.

Although Jan's family doctor had prescribed fluoxetine (Prozac) 20 mg daily one week ago, she had not taken the tablets as she was very unsure about medication. She believed that she should be able to 'pull herself together' like she did last time she was depressed. The doctor made an appointment for her to see the nurse.

The nurse enabled Jan to exercise personal choice about treatment options. After a detailed conversation with the nurse about her medication, she remained certain that she did not want to take it. The nurse and Jan agreed that they would review this decision in four weeks after giving other approaches a try. This led on to a discussion about BA. Jan took some information materials away with her to read and think about.

»

Box 12.5 Jan: BA Worksheet I

Write down your routine activities here (e.g. cleaning, cooking, shopping, etc.):

- Washing up
- Cleaning the house
- Cooking meals
- Washing clothes
- Ironing
- Food shopping

Write down your pleasurable activities here (e.g. going out/visiting friends or family):

- Reading stories to younger child
- Having a meal out with husband
- Jewellery party with work colleagues
- Watching favourite TV programmes like history programmes
- Going to the cinema

Write down your necessary activities here (e.g. paying bills, etc.):

- Paying bills
- Reorganizing work deadlines
- Doing tax return

Next time they met, Jan had already started to draw up her lists. BA fitted with her personal view that she had to tackle her mood problems herself. Box 12.5 shows Jan's routine, pleasurable, and necessary activity lists.

As can be seen, the main difference between Ken and Jan is that Jan's pleasurable activities included a range of family and social activities. These were the very activities that she reported having withdrawn from. Simply listing her activities helped her identify that she was avoiding activities she enjoyed and helped her realize the impact of her depression, confirming her view that she should make plans to try to reintegrate these activities into her life.

Thereafter, Jan's BA programme proceeded quickly and smoothly. Unlike Ken, who needed quite a lot of support initially, Jan used the connections she made between activity and mood to design and implement her own programme. When the nurse and Jan spoke on the telephone after four weeks, Jan reported that she liked the programme and was able to design it herself. She did not feel she needed to fill in diaries; for Jan, understanding the principles was enough. She told the nurse that she did not feel she needed to have further contact and that she most certainly did not think medication was an alternative now that she had taken charge of her own recovery programme.

Hema

The final case example is of a woman called Hema. When Hema asked to see someone, she was complaining of sadness, difficulty in concentrating, poor sleep, and no time for activities other than work. Her days consisted not of inactivity, but of endlessly trying to fit everything in. She was very house-proud and made sure her rooms were particularly clean. However, because of poor concentration she spent many hours at work, staying late and missing lunchtimes to complete her work and to avoid making mistakes. Occasionally, she found it almost impossible to get up in the morning and so had started to feign colds in order to take days off sick. Although she had no plans to commit suicide, she had had some thoughts that things needed to get better or she would begin to question her purpose in life.

Her depression was clearly affecting her work, home, and social life. It had started about three months previously when her relationship with her partner had ended. She had had no previous episodes of depression. Her family doctor had prescribed fluoxetine (Prozac) 20 mg, which she had taken for three weeks with some slight improvement before she saw the nurse.

Her social networks were good and she wanted advice on how to improve her mood. Table 12.4 outlines the key steps in Hema's BA programme.

Hema's baseline diary (Table 12.5) was full of activities, almost none of which provided her with any positive reinforcement. Unlike Ken and Jan, Hema was very active but her activities were universally necessary and routine. Using Hema's baseline diary, the nurse helped Hema to see she had an unbalanced activity regime and Hema appreciated for the first time just how she was structuring her life.

At first Hema believed that she could not possibly fit anything else into her time and this created some initial

»

» **Table 12.4** Key steps in Hema's behavioural activation programme

Step 1	Step 2	Step 3	Step 4	Step 5	Step 6	Step 7
Explaining behavioural activation	Understanding current activity	Identifying routine, pleasurable, and necessary activities	Making a hierarchy of routine, pleasurable, and necessary activities	Planning some routine, pleasurable, and necessary activities	Reviewing behavioural activation diaries	Preventing relapse
Basic explanation adapted to Hema's problem-specific presentation	Baseline diary to understand current activity levels and balance of activity	Review of baseline diary and reflection of amount of activity and balance between activities Identification of activities either avoided or underrepresented in baseline diary Completion of Worksheet I	Ordering of avoided and underrepresented activities from baseline diary and Worksheet I Completion of Worksheet II	Precise timetabling of underrepresented and avoided activities from Worksheet II into first behavioural activation diary	Scrutiny of first behavioural activation diary at next contact with Hema Problem-solving of completed or non-completed planned activities Making connection between behaviour and mood Planning of new activities for subsequent weeks Continuation of review contacts	Review of overall progress Recognition of triggers and warning signs Planning for the future

anxiety. However, with the nurse's help she was able to identify where she could make some space to plan pleasurable activities. After a few weeks she began to experience the value of scheduling simple, pleasurable activities, identified using Worksheet I, such as having a relaxing bath, telephoning a friend, and reading a book. For Hema, the key learning was that her mood was responsive to a change in her behaviour. Although she would always be a busy person and something of a perfectionist, through the BA programme she learned the value of activity balance and positive rewards from pleasurable activities. Step 7 involved her setting up a personal monthly 'reality check' to review the balance of her life, particularly the number of times she had done things for herself, rather than others.

»

>> **Table 12.5** Hema's first diary

		Monday	Tuesday	Wednesday	Thursday	Friday	Saturday	Sunday
Morning	What Where When Who	Office	Travel to London	Office	Office	Travel to Bristol	Shopping	Read financial pages
	What Where When Who	Office	Meetings	Office	Office	Meetings	Clean bathrooms	Church
Afternoon	What Where When Who	Office	Meetings	Office	Office	Meetings	Clean downstairs	Catch up on paper-work
	What Where When Who	Office	Meetings	Office	Office	Meetings	Wash windows	Catch up on paper-work
Evening	What Where When Who	Office	Travel back	Office	Office	Travel back	Visit elderly neighbour Cook	Cook
	What Where When Who	Cook meal	Cook	Shopping and cook	Cook	Cook	Early to bed	Prepare for office next day

Health promotion

BA is an active, skills-based, patient-centred approach to mental health intervention, where the main techniques are undertaken by patients themselves. It teaches an understanding of the connection between depression and behaviour, and how changes in behaviour can improve the thinking and physical components of mood. In particular, Step 7 sets up a self-activated relapse prevention strategy that can be implemented by patients if they detect warning signs and triggers for lowered mood. As such, the concept of health promotion is central to the BA approach.

▲ Conclusion

BA is a powerful, relatively simple, low-intensity psychological treatment for depression. It is evidence based, as effective as more complex psychological therapies (Ekers et al. 2007) and highly acceptable to people suffering from depression. The main evidence for BA comes from studies conducted in outpatient or community environments where most people with depression are treated. However, one trial did apply BA in an inpatient setting (Hopko et al. 2003b). Readers working in such environments should consider how the principles of BA might be adapted for these settings. Nurses can use BA to help large numbers of patients with depression by supporting them as they use the step-by-step techniques to learn the vital connection between mood and behaviour, and how altering behaviour can improve all components of low mood. The use of patient-centred tools such as the worksheets and diaries described here enables nurses and patients to work collaboratively using accurate feedback to problem-solve and develop a tailored individual treatment programme. Although BA requires sensitivity and skill to implement, it can be learned quickly by both nurses and patients, and studies clearly show that it can provide a viable alternative to cognitive therapy and antidepressant drugs, even for patients with 'severe' depression.

w Website

You may find it helpful to work through our short online quiz and scenario intended to help you to develop and apply the skills in this chapter. Please go to:

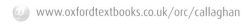

www.oxfordtextbooks.co.uk/orc/callaghan

➤ Further reading

Khan, K., ter Riet, G., Galanville, J., Sowden, A., and Kleijnen, J. (2002). *Undertaking Systematic Reviews of Research on Effectiveness: CRD's Guidance for Those Carrying Out or Commissioning Reviews. Report 4,* 2nd edn. York: University of York, Centre for Reviews and Dissemination.

Lewinsohn, P. and Graf, M. (1973). Pleasant activities and depression. *Journal of Consulting and Clinical Psychology* 41, 261–95.

Mowrer, O. H. (1950). *Learning Theory and Personality Dynamics.* New York: Arnold.

Skinner, B. F. (1953). *Science and Human Behaviour.* New York: Macmillan.

http://www.christophermartell.com/resources.php

http://www.clarku.edu/academiccatalog/facultybio. cfm?id=92

http://psychology.utk.edu/people/hopko.html

✚ References

American Psychiatric Association (1994). *Diagnostic and Statistical Manual of Mental Disorders,* 4th edn. (DSM-IV). Washington, DC: APA.

Beck, A. T., Rush, A. J., Shaw, B. J., and Emery, G. (1979). *Cognitive Therapy of Depression.* New York: Guilford Press.

Cuijpers, P., Van Stratena, A., and Warmerdama, L. (2007). Behavioral activation treatments of depression: a meta-analysis. *Clinical Psychology Review* 27(3), 318–26.

Dimidjian, S., Hollon, S., Dobson, K., et al. (2006). Randomized trial of behavioural activation, cognitive therapy, and antidepressant medication in the acute treatment of adults with major depression. *Journal of Consulting and Clinical Psychology* 74(4), 658–70.

Ekers, D., Richards, D., and Gilbody, S. (2007). A meta-analysis of randomized trials of behavioural treatment of depression. *Psychological Medicine* 35(5), 611–23.

Hopko, D. R., Lejuez, C. W., Ruggiero, K. J., and Eifert, G. H. (2003a). Contemporary behavioral activation treatments for depression: procedures, principles and progress. *Clinical Psychology Review* 23, 699–717.

Hopko, D. R., Lejuez, C. W., LePage, J. P., Hopko, S. D., and McNeil, D. W. (2003b). A brief behavioral activation treatment for depression: a randomized trial within an inpatient psychiatric hospital. *Behavior Modification* 27, 458–69.

Jacobson, N., Dobson, K., Traux, P., et al. (1996). A component analysis of cognitive-behavioural treatment of depression. *Journal of Consulting and Clinical Psychology* 64, 295–304.

Jacobson, N., Martell, C., and Dimijan, S. (2001). Behavioural activation treatment for depression: returning to contextual roots. *Clinical Psychology: Science and Practice* 8(3), 255–70.

Lang, P. (1979). A bioinformational theory of emotional imagery. *Psychophysiology* 16, 495–512.

Lewinsohn, P. M. (1974). A behavioural approach to depression. In: *Psychology of Depression: Contemporary Theory and Research* (ed. R. M. Friedman and M. M. Katz), pp 157–85. New York: Wiley.

Martell, C., Addis, M., and Jacobson, N. (2001). *Depression in Context. Strategies for Guided Action.* New York: Norton.

Mead, N. and Bower, P. (2000). Patient centredness: a conceptual framework and review of the empirical literature. *Social Science and Medicine* 51, 1087–110.

National Institute for Health and Clinical Excellence (2004). *Depression: Management of Depression in Primary and Secondary Care—NICE Guidance.* London: NICE.

Richards, D. A. (2007). Behaviour therapy. In: *Dryden's Handbook of Individual Therapy,* 5th edn. (ed. W. Dryden), pp 327–51. London: Sage.

Richards, D. A., Lovell, K., Gilbody, S., et al. (2008). Collaborative care for depression in UK primary care: a randomised controlled trial. *Psychological Medicine* 38, 279–88.

Roth, A. D. and Pilling, S. (2007). *The Competences Required to Deliver Effective Cognitive and Behavioural Therapy for People with Depression and with Anxiety Disorders.* London: Department of Health.

World Health Organization (1992). *The ICD-10 Classification of Mental and Behavioural Disorders: Clinical Descriptions and Diagnostic Guidelines.* Geneva: WHO.

(13) Medication management

Dan Bressington   Mark Wilbourn

▼ Introduction

Mental health nurses have an important role in administering and monitoring the effects of medication in addition to helping service users to maximize the benefits of treatment and minimize associated adverse effects. Medication is a very effective treatment for mental health problems, but large numbers of service users either stop taking it or take it reluctantly (World Health Organization [WHO] 2003).

Whilst we acknowledge that a good understanding of neurotransmission mechanisms, pharmacology, psychopharmacology, and drug types and actions is essential to good medication management, these aspects are not covered in this chapter. We would encourage you to access specific texts that explore these areas in more detail, and references to such texts are provided in the Further reading list at the end of the chapter. This chapter focuses on influences on medication adherence, the evidence base for a range of interventions to enhance adherence, and guidance on how to engage service users in a collaborative manner to enable effective medication management. The behaviour of taking medication should be viewed similarly to that of any other health-related behaviour, such as exercise, healthy eating, etc.

Learning outcomes

By the end of this chapter you should be better able to:

1 Outline the nature of and influences on non-adherence with medication amongst service users

2 Describe a range of evidence-based interventions for collaborative approaches to medication management

3 Outline general principles and skills for communication with service users and carers about medication that encourage service user and carer involvement in shared decision-making

4 Use a structured approach to assessment and a range of specific interventions in routine nursing practice to enhance medication management for service users.

Medication management

Mental health nurses play an essential role in the administration and management of medicines and the UK Department of Health's (DH) *Best Practice Competencies and Capabilities for Pre-registration Mental Health Nurses in England* identifies medication management as a core competency (DH 2006). In terms of monitoring medication effectively, there are four key areas that mental health nurses need to focus on: safety, symptoms, side effects, and service user satisfaction. The management of medication should be facilitated by effective communication with service users and carers that encourages a collaborative working relationship.

The UK Nursing and Midwifery Council (NMC) provide excellent guidelines about the safe storage and administration of medicines, and you are advised to be aware of these at all times (NMC 2002). In addition, you should be aware that individual National Health Service (NHS) Trusts and hospital authorities have local policies that govern the administration of medicines that need to be adhered to.

Patient safety is paramount at all times, and errors in the administration or monitoring of medicines should be reported immediately to appropriately senior members of staff so that appropriate action can be taken. The UK NHS National Patient Safety Agency (NPSA) is a useful resource that provides appropriate information about maximizing patient safety in terms of medications.

When service users require assistance in adhering to medication regimens, the NMC (2002) suggests, where appropriate, the use of **compliance aids**. These aids (i.e. weekly dosing boxes) should ideally be dispensed and sealed by a pharmacist. Where a pharmacist is unable to dispense the medications in a compliance aid, a nurse may do so, but should be aware that there is a risk of error and that they are accountable for use (NMC 2002). Compliance aids are intended for use by individuals who recognize the need for treatment but have problems in remembering to take their medication.

Where more complex reasons for non-adherence exist, a variety of psychosocial approaches may be necessary; the remainder of this chapter focuses on managing non-adherence with long-term medicines and maintaining a collaborative approach during discussions with service users and carers about treatment.

Non-adherence with long-term treatment

Not taking or ceasing to take medication is usually referred to as non-compliance or non-adherence. Definitions of non-compliance vary from total refusal to missing an occasional dose. Non-compliance is not only related to the actual taking of medication; for example, failure to attend scheduled appointments is also classed as non-compliance. Service users often feel that the words compliance or adherence are terms that imply that service uses should do as they are told by professionals and are not able to make choices themselves (Playle and Keeley 1998). These terms should therefore be avoided when discussing treatment with service users. A service user's adherence to a treatment regimen is not at a fixed point and can vary on a day-by-day basis. Osterberg and Blaschke (2005) identify a pattern of adherence in people taking long-term medicines: in one-sixth virtually all doses are taken, in one-sixth almost all doses are taken, in one-sixth there is infrequent non-adherence, in one-sixth there is frequent non-adherence, and in two-sixths few or no doses are taken.

'Concordance' is an alternative term used increasingly in the literature, and suggests a joint process between service user and service provider in terms of discussing and managing treatment; even if a service user does not take medication the process can still be concordant.

Stopping medicines in recurrent or enduring conditions places service users at a higher risk of relapse than those who continue taking treatment as prescribed. Gray et al. (2004) identified that amongst people with a psychotic illness the one-year relapse risk for service users taking medication as prescribed is about 20–30%, whereas relapse rate without medication is around 70%. Similarly, service users who respond to antidepressants and continue taking them for up to 36 months have relapse rates of around 18%, whereas those who are switched to placebo have relapse rates of more than 40% (Geddes et al. 2003). Stopping medication is not confined to users of mental health services; reviews of literature on adherence with long-term therapies have highlighted the widespread problem of non-adherence with a range of treatments (Playle and Keeley 1998, WHO 2003). The average rate of adherence in service users with chronic health conditions is 50% and varies slightly between disorders, for example 30–60% for antidepressants, 43% for asthma, and 37–83% for HIV medicines. It is important that service users and professionals recognize that it is a normal behaviour to stop taking medication against advice, and professionals should avoid directly or indirectly blaming or judging service users for making a decision to refuse medicines.

Influences on non-adherence

The WHO (2003) report on adherence states that non-adherence to long-term treatment is a worldwide problem and identifies important influencing factors. The relationship with professionals and other service-related factors has a strong influence on medication-taking behaviour. Condition-related factors, patient-related factors, and treatment effects were also highlighted as determining adherence to treatment.

The influences on adherence to treatment are complex and involve many factors. These influencing factors can be grouped under five main categories (Gray et al. 2007):

1 Illness-related factors (insight, symptom severity)

2 Treatment-related factors (side effects, treatment efficacy, and methods of administration)

3 Clinician-related factors (lack of collaborative working, authoritarian attitudes, and access to clinicians)

4 Patient-related factors (including age, sex, culture, beliefs about treatment, and beliefs around severity of illness)

5 Environmental factors (including peer pressure).

Service users' satisfaction with drug treatments have a direct influence on adherence, and higher levels of treatment satisfaction improve adherence (DH 1999).

Interventions to enhance adherence/concordance

A number of different interventions have been tested to try to help services users follow treatment advice; some of these have shown promising results. However, research into medication adherence can be complicated, as service users who agree to take part in studies may be likely to be generally more adherent than those who do not participate; a consequence of this is that the participants in trials may not represent service users seen in everyday clinical practice. A great deal of research into medication non-adherence has examined service users with psychosis, although similar approaches to manage non-adherence with medicines in other enduring conditions, for example depression (Vergouwen et al. 2003), have shown promise. A detailed systematic review of the literature on interventions to improve the taking of prescribed medication can be found in the Cochrane Library (Haynes et al. 2005). Interventions can broadly be divided into three areas: educational, behavioural, and cognitive behavioural.

Educational interventions aim to provide information to service users about both their illness and medication. Group and individual service user education has been evaluated using a variety of research approaches, with results indicating that giving information improves service users' understanding of their illness and medication but does not necessarily improve adherence rates (Macpherson et al. 1996, Gray 2000, Vergouwen et al. 2003). However, family interventions involving **psycho-education** have been shown to improve rates of adherence and can reduce the occurrence of relapse (Pekkala and Merinder 2002, Aguglia et al. 2007,).

Behavioural interventions try to help service users tailor their treatment to suit their daily routines. For example, encouraging service uses to take medication before they go to bed to minimize sedation or similarly taking medication with other routine behaviour (e.g. when leaving the house in the morning). There is some evidence that this approach can be helpful (Boczkowski et al. 1985).

Recently research to enhance adherence has examined cognitive behavioural approaches and interventions. These interventions focus on enabling the practitioner to work collaboratively with service users to explore their beliefs about illness and treatment. Lecompte and Pelc (1996) tested a cognitive behavioural programme in a randomized controlled trial and found that service users who received the intervention spent less time in hospital than those in the control group. The approach was based on five strategies: engagement, psycho-education, identifying early symptoms and developing coping strategies, behavioural strategies for reinforcing adherence, and addressing false beliefs about medication.

Kemp et al. (1998) tested 'compliance therapy', which is based on motivational interviewing and cognitive behavioural techniques. The intervention was divided into three phases. Phase 1 dealt with service users' experiences of treatment by helping them to review their illness history; phase 2 focused on discussing common worries about treatment and exploring the good and the bad things about treatment; phase 3 dealt with long-term management and strategies for avoiding relapse. The study found that treatment adherence was better in the compliance therapy group, with patients taking longer to relapse than those who received non-specific counselling.

Gray et al. (2004) combined a variety of promising interventions to produce a medication management training package for community nurses in the UK. This **cluster randomized controlled trial** demonstrated that medication management training was effective in improving clinical outcomes for people with schizophrenia.

The Cochrane Library systematic review of interventions to improve adherence (Haynes et al. 2005) confirms that interventions to improve adherence are relatively effective in the short term; however, interventions to improve adherence in long-term conditions are more complex and should incorporate a variety of approaches. The search further to establish the effectiveness of interventions to enhance adherence remains an important focus of research and one that can have far-reaching benefits.

Implications for clinical practice

Medication management approaches should try to help people to maximize the effectiveness of their medication. The aim is not to force people to take medication, but to work collaboratively with service users to enable them to make informed choices that maximize health. When clinicians work in this way, service users are more involved in the process, more satisfied with treatment, and therefore less likely to stop taking medication.

The suggested approaches aimed at maintaining concordance would be appropriate in both community and inpatient settings. It is acknowledged that it can be difficult to maintain collaboration when service users refuse treatment and are compelled to take medication under the mental health legislation. In these situations the health care professional has a duty of care to enforce treatment to maintain the health and safety of the service user and others. This duty of care at times takes priority over individual rights to autonomy and choice, and health care professionals should focus on maintaining engagement with the service user and encouraging shared decision-making where possible. **Advance patient directives** can help to maintain a client-centred approach where a service user is treated against their will under the Mental Health Act; if a service user is able to express their wishes about medicines and treatment whilst well, these views can be incorporated into future care plans.

General principles and interpersonal skills

The general principles of establishing and maintaining therapeutic relationships and working in partnership with service users (described in Chapters 7 and 8) should form the foundations of any clinical intervention. When discussing medication with service users, certain principles that underpin an effective and collaborative approach should be adhered to. Jarboe (2002) makes the following suggestions for creating and maintaining a collaborative relationship:

- Use language that reinforces a partnership, i.e. 'we' not 'you'.
- Encourage **self-efficacy** and avoid threats/coercion.
- Provide simple, accurate, and understandable information.
- Convey that services are intended to help service users, not control them.
- Answer questions honestly and give examples to explain.

Gray et al. (2003) outline the essential elements of good medication management that should be used in conjunction with other approaches to maximize collaboration:

- A client-centred approach
- An assessment of the service user's experiences with treatment, response to medication, and side effects
- Regular medication review to ensure that the prescription is appropriate and up to date
- Open exchange of information about the illness and treatment with the service user
- Working with the service user to help to integrate taking medication into the daily routine
- Use of **problem solving**, motivational interviewing, and cognitive behavioural strategies.

Structuring the clinical session

Following an interview structure can help to guide clinical sessions and enhance service user engagement and collaboration. A general guide to structuring collaborative medication management sessions is provided in Table 13.1 (🌐 you can also print this off from the online resource centre to bring along to placement or insert in your portfolio). The step-by-step instructions assume that the aforementioned general

principles are being used and are based on a cognitive therapy checklist modified by Haddock et al. (2001) and the Concordance Skills and Adherence Therapy Competency Scale (Gray and Robson 2005).

Assessment

As with all interventions, a period of assessment is required to identify medication management needs; during this process the nurse needs to be consciously aware of engagement issues. If service users are unwilling to discuss medication issues on a particular day, the nurse should respect the service user's views and address issues that the service user perceives as meaningful. The medication management assessment should focus on the service user's experiences of taking medication. Each area of assessment can be repeated at points to measure the outcomes of interventions. The assessment should be non-judgemental, conversational in nature, and cover the key areas outlined in Box 13.1.

The adherence therapy assessment devised by Gray and Robson (2005) can be a very useful collaborative assessment tool. This tool is available online at: www.adherencetherapy.com.

Suggested interventions

The range of interventions discussed in this section is based on the work of Gray et al. (2004, 2006), Kemp et al. (1998), and Lecompte and Pelc (1996). Before attempting any of the suggested medication management interventions, the nurse should have built a therapeutic alliance with the service user and collaboratively assessed the service user's need. Exchanging information about medication with service users/carers is a core task that will repeat itself throughout the medication management process. Finding out what service users know about medication and providing knowledge that the service user wants will enhance the transparent nature of the approach. If the nurse is unable to answer a question, honesty is essential, and the question should be addressed at the next opportunity. Lack of understanding and common misconceptions should be identified and addressed. Education alone is unlikely to improve adherence, but as part of a treatment package it can maintain concordance and enhance the individual's feeling of wellbeing. Psycho-educational interventions that involve family and carers have been shown to improve understanding of treatment and treatment adherence rates (Pekkala and Merinder 2002).

Table 13.1 Structuring collaborative medication management sessions

Before the session	Beginning session	During session	Ending the session
Explain that the aim is to: • Work together • Share responsibility • Give the service user choices • Help the service user achieve their goals **Be flexible around:** • Where and when to meet • The length of the session (dependent on service user's feelings and concentration) **Do not:** • Tell the service user what they must talk about in sessions • Insist on meeting if the service user is not keen or has more pressing issues **Always:** • Maintain professionalism by ensuring that you are on time for agreed meetings	**Establish a collaborative agenda for the session:** • Ask how the client has been since the last meeting • Establish client's current emotional state • Ask for how long the client would like to meet and ensure that they are aware that they can stop or take a break at any point • Ask for feedback around homework tasks (if any) • Establish the main issues that the client would like to discuss and prioritize needs • Jointly agree the content of discussion (ensure it is appropriate and achievable within the timeframe) **Do not:** Exclusively set your own agenda or be inflexible if the client wants to change the topic of conversation	**Convey understanding and use reflection:** • Regularly summarize what is being discussed to allow the service user to correct misunderstandings • Respond appropriately to non-verbal communication • Reflect back to the client your understanding of what the client has said • Reflect back to the client the subtle communication and empathic content of the discussion **Maintain collaboration:** • Encourage the client to express their viewpoints throughout the session • Offer choices where appropriate • Maintain the focus of the session towards a need/concern that was identified jointly • Be transparent and honest in approach and in response to questions • If the client has problems generating spontaneous thought, make some general suggestions, e.g. 'Have you thought about ...?'	**Winding up the session:** • Avoid abrupt endings by reminding the client that the session is coming to an end • Ask the client if there is anything that has been missed • Summarize your understanding of the session and ask the client to correct misconceptions **Eliciting feedback:** (should also be carried out during the session as appropriate) • Find out if the service user's goals have been met in the session • Directly ask the client for feedback about their thoughts and feelings about the session—ask about what was 'good' and 'not-so-good' **Recheck service user's emotional state:** • Directly ask how the client feels at the end of the session to elicit emotional responses **Homework tasks:** • If any work outside the session needs to be carried out (e.g. completing an assessment/intervention or seeking knowledge), ensure that all parties understand what is required and why

»

Table 13.1 *Continued*

Before the session	Beginning session	During session	Ending the session
		Manage resistance (signs of resistance include arguing, ignoring, interrupting, etc.): • Do not pressure the reluctant client to talk about a specific issue—back off • Emphasize that the client has personal choice and control • Do not lecture, argue, or debate **Do not:** • Tell the client what they should or must do	**Link to the following session:** • Ask for suggestions about how the next session could be improved • Obtain a rough idea about what the client would like to address in the next session

Box 13.1 Key areas for discussion in a medication management assessment

Practical issues

Does the service user know the names, doses, and purpose of treatments? Are there any practical problems (forgetting, paying for, or collecting prescriptions)? Does the service user use street drugs or alcohol (and how much)? How many doses of medication (if any) does the service user tend to miss? What makes it easier/more difficult for the service user to take medication?

Motivation

How important does the service user feel it is to take medication (score 1–10)? How confident is the service user that they can take medication (score 1–10)? How satisfied is the service user with treatment (or ready to take if considering taking medication) (score 1–10)? Why have they given themselves a particular rating? What would need to be different for the ratings to change? The assessment of motivation should be repeated after each intervention and at other appropriate points.

Beliefs about treatment

What does the service user think about their medication? What concerns does the service user have about treatment? A standardized rating scale such as the 'Drug Attitude Inventory' (Hogan and Awad 1983) or 'Adherence therapy assessment' (Gray and Robson 2005) can help to explore common concerns about treatment. In particular, issues related to perceived addiction potential, the need to take treatment in the long term, or notions that medicines cannot help with psychiatric disorders need to be addressed.

Side effects

It is essential that the adverse effects of medication are identified and managed collaboratively to reduce discomfort or distress. A service user may volunteer information or report side effects if directly asked; however, any side effects experienced may not always be attributed to treatment by the service user. In order to obtain a comprehensive assessment of adverse effects, standardized rating scales can be used, for example the

Box 13.1 *Continued*

Liverpool University Side Effect Rating Scale (Day et al. 1995). Any side effects identified should be recorded and addressed collaboratively as a practical problem by the service user and treating team. A review of the prescription may be required to address side-effect concerns. The nurse should explore the distress associated with each side effect as discomfort will vary from individual to individual and recent evidence suggests that the impact of side effects can be environmentally bound (Gray et al. 2007).

Collaborative problem solving

This approach can help service users and carers to develop problem-solving skills, which may be used to help find solutions to any problem (not just medication issues).

Service users or others may identify side effects or specific practical problems with accessing and taking medication. A structured problem-solving approach can be used to identify solutions and behavioural strategies that can be integrated into solutions to make taking medication easier for service users. From the assessment, the service user and nurse may have identified practical problems. It is recommended that the nurse ascertains which of these is causing the service user most concern and prioritizes in terms of what the service user thinks will be the easiest to solve. It may be more effective to work on a problem that seems easier to solve as this will help to maintain engagement.

A suggested problem-solving structure is detailed in Box 13.2 ( ) you can also print this off from the online

Box 13.2 Problem solving (based on the work of Falloon 2000)

What is the problem statement?

- What is the problem? (use the service user's own words)
- Where/when does it occur?
- What makes it worse or better?
- What are the consequences of the problem?

Setting a goal

- Ask the service user what they would like to achieve.
- Devise a SMART goal:

  Specific

  Measurable

  Achievable

  Realistic

  Time limited.

Thinking of solutions

- Encourage the service user to think about as many solutions as possible (these may not all be appropriate).
- If required the nurse can help to make suggestions.
- Evaluate/choose solution.
- Explore what would be good and not-so-good about each solution.
- In light of this information, ask the client to choose the solution that they think is most likely to be effective.

Action plan (needs to be detailed)

- List the steps needed to put their plan into action.
- What do they need to do?
- Who else may be able to help them?
- Might anything get in the way?
- How might they get round potential obstacles?

Implement solution

- Follow the action plan over the agreed period.
- Ask the service user to make a mental or physical note about progress.

Evaluation

- Ask the service user to score how successful the solution was—score out of ten (this encourages recognition of partial success).
- If not solved, explore why.
- If solved, what has been learned?
- Does the client want to tackle another problem on the list?

resource centre to take along placement or insert in your portfolio). The intervention should be carried out within the framework for structuring sessions outlined in Table 13.1.

A fictitious case example of the clinical application of this approach is outlined in the Practice Example box.

Looking back and using an illness timeline

This intervention aims to maximize engagement and to allow service users to tell their personal story of their experiences over time. The service user identifies when they or a significant other first recognized the start of mental health problems, and the positive and negative effects of treatment to date are plotted chronologically over time. According to Miller and Rollnick (2002) and Gray et al. (2003), this exercise has numerous benefits including: helping service users identify what was helpful and not-so-helpful in terms of mental health, highlighting any relationship between stopping medication and relapse, and allowing discussion about past negative treatment experiences. The purpose is not to identify what the service user had done 'wrong', but to identify strengths and what has worked in terms of achieving their goals. The exercise may help service users to understand that there can be a time lag between stopping taking medicines and a recurrence of symptoms.

✖ Practice Example: Collaborative problem solving

Steve

Steve is a 25-year-old man who has had a diagnosis of schizophrenia since he was 18 years old. He is currently prescribed clozapine 200 mg in the morning and 600 mg at night. Steve lives in his own rented flat and works part-time in a car showroom. He has a good relationship with his family and has a girlfriend. A medication management assessment reveals that Steve is satisfied with his treatment (score 8/10) despite experiencing some side effects, and he recognizes that it is important for him to take his medication (score 9/10). Steve reports that he forgets to take around three morning doses of clozapine weekly; as a result he scores his confidence to take medication as 4/10. When he forgets to take the morning dose he takes it at the same time as his night dose, resulting in him feeling very sedated and finding it difficult to get up the next morning. The problem was explored using the approach detailed in Box 13.2.

The problem (in Steve's words) was identified as: 'When I leave the house in the morning I sometimes forget to take my medication'. His goal was to 'remember to take my morning medication every day over the next two weeks'. Steve initially identified a number of potential solutions and evaluated the potential of each:

- To ask my mum to phone me to remind me (I would remember to take it, but don't like relying on mum and sometimes she may forget to remind me).

- To set a reminder on my mobile phone (I would remember, but I often forget to turn my phone on and don't check reminders until I get home from work).

- To ask the CPN to remind me (the CPN wouldn't forget but may not have time to do this every day).

- To put a reminder notice on the back of my front door (I would see the notice when I leave and would have time to return to my room to take my medication).

After weighing up the pros and cons of each solution, Steve decided to put a notice on the back of his front door (next to his keys) that would remind him to take his medication. The detailed plan was as follows:

'Tonight I will put a note on my front door stating: "MORNING MEDS". Each morning when I get my keys I will be reminded to take my medication before I leave the house. I will record how many doses I miss and discuss how things went with my CPN in two weeks' time.'

Steve implemented the solution over a two-week period; he reported that he had initially been reminded by the notice, but on one occasion he had put his coat over the notice and forgot his medication. As a result of this Steve moved the notice next to the kettle and has been reminded to take his medication consistently since. He scored his confidence to take medication as 7/10, indicating that the problem solving had enhanced his perception of self-efficacy.

Exploring ambivalence or uncertainty about treatment

Many people find themselves doubting the need for long-term medication and treatment. The aim of this intervention is to help the client explore these doubts and convey that it is normal and acceptable to be unsure about taking medication. Service users are helped to explore their inherent uncertainty about whether or not to take medication by using a balance sheet that lists the 'good' and 'not-so-good' things about taking and/or stopping medication as a basis for further exploration. Emphasis should be placed on the less obvious benefits of medication such as getting on better with friends or being able to go to work. Identifying the 'not-so-good' and 'good' things can reinforce the impact of the benefits of medication and give service users and clinicians ideas about the negative aspects of treatment that can be addressed. Asking service users to then re-rate their 'importance', 'confidence', and 'satisfaction' scores after the exercise will provide a measure of any changes in the client's motivation to take treatment (Kemp et al. 1998, Miller and Rollnick 2002, Gray et al. 2003).

Looking forward and making long-term plans

This intervention is designed to help service users focus on the future, looking beyond current and previous difficulties, and enhancing service users' perceptions of self-efficacy.

Service users should be encouraged to identify a realistic goal 6–12 months in the future. The goal should adhere to the SMART principles outlined in Box 13.2. If the service user identifies a long-term or end-treatment goal (e.g. 'I want a full-time job'), a shorter-term SMART goal that progresses towards the end goal can be agreed upon (e.g. 'I will go to the Job Centre this Wednesday morning and ask if any part-time jobs are available'). Potential barriers to achieving the goal are identified and strategies to overcome them are jointly constructed. Service users should be asked: 'How does medication fit into your plans?'. A problem-solving strategy is then used to identify a detailed plan of how to achieve the goal, together with contingency plans in case the initial plan does not work. Revisiting the 'looking back' exercise described previously can provide useful information about past helpful and not-so-helpful strategies (Gray et al. 2003, Miller and Rollnick 2002). The 'looking forward' exercise is an ideal intervention for health promotion and maximizing recovery. Strategies that were previously found useful by the service user can be incorporated into future plans to achieve their goals, and the collaborative and client-centred approach is often useful in engendering hope and realistic optimism.

A fictitious case example is included in the web-based material accompanying this book www.oxfordtextbooks. co.uk/orc/callaghan. We would encourage you to examine the findings of assessment and answer the short-answer questions based on what has been learned from this chapter.

▲ Conclusion

People who are prescribed long-term medication frequently find that taking medication regularly can be difficult; these issues are not confined to people with mental health problems. Uncertainty about whether or not to take medication, especially in the longer term, is a common phenomenon. A number of interventions to try to help people to enhance concordance with medication have been tested and the most promising approaches come from a combination of cognitive, behavioural, motivational interviewing, and problem-solving approaches. Sound clinical interpersonal skills should underpin collaborative approaches that aim to engage service users in talking about and self-managing their treatment.

w Website

You may find it helpful to work through our short online quiz and scenario intended to help you to develop and apply the skills in this chapter. Please go to:

www.oxfordtextbooks.co.uk/orc/callaghan

➤ Further reading

Andrews, G. and Jenkins, R. (1999). *Management of Mental Disorders*. London: World Health Organisation Collaborating Centres. [*See Chapter 2.*]

Gray, R. and Bressington, D. (2004). Pharmacological interventions and ECT. In: *The Art and Science of Mental Health Nursing. A Textbook of Principles and Practice* (ed. I. Norman and I. Ryrie), pp 306–28. Maidenhead: Open University Press.

Stahl, S. M. (2000). *Essential Psychopharmacology. Neuroscientific Basis and Practical Applications*, 2nd edn. Cambridge: Cambridge University Press.

Wilbourn, M. and Prosser, S. (2003). *The Pathology and Pharmacology of Mental Illness*. Cheltenham: Nelson Thornes.

✛ References

Aguglia, E., Pascolo-Fabrici, E., Bertossi, F., and Bassi, M. (2007). Psychoeducational intervention and prevention of relapse among schizophrenic disorders in the Italian community psychiatric network. *Clinical Practice and Epidemiology in Mental Health* 3, 7.

Boczkowski, J., Zeichner, A., and DeSanto, N. (1985). Neuroleptic compliance among chronic schizophrenic outpatients: an intervention outcome report. *Journal of Consulting and Clinical Psychology* 53, 666–71.

Day, J. C., Wood, G., Dewey, M., and Bentall, R. (1995). A self rating scale for measuring neuroleptic side effects. Validation in a group of schizophrenic patients. *British Journal of Psychiatry* 166, 650–3.

Department of Health (1999). *The National Health Service Plan: A Plan for Investment. A Plan for Reform*. London: Stationery Office.

Department of Health (2006). *Best Practice Competencies and Capabilities for Pre-registration Mental Health Nurses in England: the CNO's Review of Mental Health Nursing*. London: DH.

Falloon, I. (2000). Problem solving as a core strategy in the prevention of schizophrenia and other mental disorders. *Australian and New Zealand Journal of Psychiatry* 34(suppl 2), S185–90.

Geddes, J. R., Carney, S. M., Davies, C., et al. (2003). Relapse prevention with antidepressant drug treatment in depressive disorders: a systematic review. *Lancet* 361, 653–61.

Gray, R. (2000). Does patient education enhance compliance with clozapine? A preliminary investigation. *Journal of Psychiatric and Mental Health Nursing* 7, 285–6.

Gray, R., Brewin, E., and Bressington, D. (2003). Psychopharmacology and medication management. In: *The Handbook of Community Mental Health Nursing* (ed. B. Hannigan and M. Coffey), pp 274–86. London: Routledge.

Gray, R., Wykes, T., Edmonds, M., Leese, M., and Gournay, K. (2004). Effect of a medication management training package for nurses on clinical outcomes for patients with schizophrenia: cluster randomised controlled trial. *British Journal of Psychiatry* 185(2), 157–62.

Gray, R. and Robson, D. (2005). *Adherence Therapy/ Medication Management Treatment Manual*. London: Institute of Psychiatry. www.adherencetherapy.com

Gray, R., Leese, M., Bindman, J., et al. (2006). Adherence therapy for people with schizophrenia: European multicentre randomised controlled trial. *British Journal of Psychiatry* 189, 508–14.

Gray, R., Lathlean, J., Bressington, D., and Mills, A. (2007). *Observational Cross Sectional Pilot Study of Adherence with Antipsychotic Medication in People* with *Schizophrenia or Schizoaffective Disorders in Prisons. Report to the NHS National R & D Programme on Forensic Mental Health*. www.phrn.nhs.uk/Prison/MentalHealthDemoReport.pdf

Haddock, G., Devane, S., Bradshaw, T., et al. (2001). An investigation into the psychometric properties of the cognitive therapy scale for psychosis (CTS). *Behavioural and Cognitive Psychotherapy* 29, 221–33.

Haynes, R. B., Yao, X., Degani, A., Kripalani, S., Garg, A., and McDonald, H. P. (2005). Interventions to enhance medication adherence. *Cochrane Database of Systematic Reviews* (4)CD000011.

Hogan, T. P. and Awad, A. G. (1983). Subjective response to neuroleptics and outcome in schizophrenia: a re-examination comparing two measures. *Psychological Medicine* 22, 347–52.

Jarboe, K. (2002). Treatment nonadherence: causes and potential solutions. *Journal of the American Psychiatric Nurses Association* 8(4), S18–25.

Kemp, R., Kirov, G., Everitt, B., Hayward, P., and David, A. (1998). Randomised controlled trial of compliance therapy: 18-month follow-up. *British Journal of Psychiatry* 172, 413–19.

Lecompte, D. and Pelc, I. (1996). A cognitive-behavioural programme to improve compliance with medication in patients with schizophrenia. *International Journal of Mental Health* 25, 51–6.

Macpherson, R., Jerrom, B., and Hughes, A. (1996). A controlled study of education about drug treatment in schizophrenia. *British Journal of Psychiatry* 168, 709–17.

Miller, W. R. and Rollnick, S. (2002). *Motivational Interviewing: Preparing People for Change*. New York: Guilford Press.

Nursing and Midwifery Council (2002). *Guidelines for the Administration of Medicines*. London: NMC.

Osterberg, L. and Blaschke, T. (2005). Adherence to medication. *New England Journal of Medicine* 353, 487–97.

Pekkala, E. and Merinder, L. (2002). Psychoeducation for schizophrenia. *Cochrane Database of Systematic Reviews* (4)CD02831.

Playle, J. F. and Keeley, P. (1998). Non-compliance and professional power. *Journal of Advanced Nursing* 27, 304–11.

Vergouwen, A., Bakker, A., Katon, W., et al. (2003). Improving adherence to antidepressants: a systematic review of interventions. *Journal Clinical Psychiatry* 64(12), 1415–20.

World Health Organization (2003). *Adherence to Long-Term Therapies: Evidence for Action*. Geneva: WHO.

(14) Legal, professional, and ethical issues

Richard Griffith

▼ Introduction

A chapter on the legal and ethical issues informing mental health nursing practice may seem unusual in a book that focuses on skills. However, all the mental health nursing skills described in this book are underpinned by a requirement to deliver them ethically and in accordance with the law. The UK Nursing and Midwifery Council's code of professional conduct (NMC 2008) states that you are personally accountable for your practice. This means that you are answerable for your actions and omissions, regardless of advice or directions from another professional.

We appreciate that readers of this book will be in a variety of international locations that are governed by their own mental health laws. However, the **principles** apply to every reader, who should familiarize themselves with the legal implications for their own area of practice. The Mental Health Act (MHA) 1983 for England and Wales concerns the circumstances in which a person in these countries with a mental disorder can be detained for assessment and treatment of that disorder, and sets out processes to be followed to ensure that they are not inappropriately detained or treated. The 1983 Act emphasizes the rights of people subject to its provisions, and when introduced was seen as reining in the discretionary powers that doctors had to detain and treat patients under previous legislation. The main purpose of the legislation is to ensure that people with mental disorders that threaten their health or safety, or the safety of the public, can be treated, irrespective of their consent, where it is necessary to prevent them from harming themselves or others.

The position of the patient with mental health problems in England and Wales is now more legalized than ever before. A strong body of case law has developed that deals with fundamental issues of liberty, autonomy, and respect. It is essential that as a mental health nurse you not only apply the requirements of the legislation accurately but you do so ethically with due regard for patients' rights.

To assist you, the legislation is accompanied by codes of practice that offer guidance on the application of the law (Department for Constitutional Affairs 2007, Department of Health 2008). The codes, if followed, will allow you to demonstrate clearly that you have discharged your duties by applying the law in a transparent, ethical, and respectful way.

Learning outcomes

By the end of this chapter you should be better able to:

1 State the principles of the MHA 1983

2 Describe the requirements for compulsory admission and **detention**

3 Evaluate the safeguards designed to protect patients treated for a mental disorder

4 Discuss the principles of the Mental Capacity Act 2005

5 Describe the statutory framework for assessing decision-making capacity and determining best interests under the Mental Capacity Act 2005.

The Mental Health Act 1983

Background to the Act

In England and Wales, mental health care is regulated through the provisions of the MHA 1983 as amended by the MHA 2007, which came into force in October 2008. The development of mental health law in England and Wales, and the key principles of current legislation, are outlined in Box 14.1.

Despite a longstanding policy of community-focused service delivery and support, the legislation continues to centre on entry into, care in, and discharge from *institutions*. However, the fundamental aim of the 1983 Act was to strengthen the rights of patients made subject to its compulsory powers. This is achieved through five key principles that have a liberal thrust.

Box 14.1 Development of modern mental health law in England and Wales

MHA 1959

This legislation came at a time of great optimism in psychiatry with novel techniques and new medicines being developed. It gave doctors a lot of discretion when treating patients for their mental disorder but also sought to avoid stigma by:

- Using compulsory detention and treatment as a last resort

- Removing the need for certification by a Justice of the Peace before detention

- Taking up the mantle of community care and encouraging a range of community services.

MHA 1983

This replaced the MHA 1959 and, although using a similar framework, placed much greater emphasis on patients' rights—described as new legalism in mental health care. It gave greater protection to those with mental health problems, subject to the provisions of the MHA 1983 as opposed to protecting the 'sane'. It achieved this by:

- Reining in the discretionary powers of doctors

- Giving more authority to mental health review tribunals

- Increasing the role of approved social workers and hospital managers.

MHA 1983: 2007 amendments

These amended the MHA 1983 by:

- Changing the way the Act defines mental disorder so that a single definition applies throughout the Act

- Introducing an appropriate medical treatment test requiring medical treatment appropriate to the patient's mental disorder and all other circumstances of the case to be available to that patient before they can be detained or have their detention renewed

- Broadening the group of practitioners who can take on the functions that used to be performed by the approved social worker and responsible medical officer

- Giving patients the right to make an application to displace their nearest relative and enabling county courts to displace a nearest relative

- Introducing supervised community treatment for patients following a period of detention in hospital

- Requiring hospital managers to ensure that patients aged under 18 years admitted to hospital for mental disorder are accommodated in an environment that is suitable for their age

- Placing a duty on the appropriate national authority to make arrangements for help to be provided by independent mental health advocates

- Introducing new safeguards for patients when electroconvulsive therapy (ECT) is the proposed treatment

- Introducing deprivation of liberty safeguards through the Mental Capacity Act 2005.

1. Increased recourse to review of detention

Detention in hospital has always been limited by time since the Lunacy Act 1890, but a right of appeal for those detained for assessment was introduced for the first time by the 1983 Act. Detained patients have a right to appeal against detention through the Mental Health Review Tribunal (MHRT). This independent body considers whether the criteria for detention continue to be met, and hospital managers now have a duty to refer all detained patient cases to the MHRT where the patient has not appealed but remains detained in hospital six months after their admission (section 68). Hospital managers are also empowered to conduct their own reviews of detention and to order discharge where they unanimously agree that detention conditions are not met (section 23).

2. Enhanced civil and social status

This principle was advocated mainly on therapeutic rather than legal grounds. One way the law was able to implement this principle was through the right to vote. Non-compulsorily detained inpatients were given the right to vote by allowing them to register their entitlement using a previous address (Representation of the People Act 1983). Detained patients did not have the right to vote until it was granted by an **amendment** to the House of Lords Reform Act 2001, although this right is still subject to patients' capacity to decide.

3. Ideology of entitlement

The principle of **ideology** of entitlement promoted access to aftercare services as a legal right for patients who have been detained for treatment. Health and social services have a duty to continue to provide aftercare for such patients until it appears to them the patient is no longer in need (section 117). Patients cannot be charged for these aftercare services (R v Ealing DHA ex parte Fox [1993]).

4. Least restrictive alternative

Any use of formal powers under the 1983 Act must be based on the least restrictive means of meeting the needs of the patient. In making decisions on compulsory admission, the Approved Mental Health Professional (AMHP) has a duty to ensure that the person is actively resisting admission to hospital and that compulsory admission is the most appropriate method of dealing with the person, and must certify that the detention order used is the least restrictive method of meeting the needs of the patient.

5. Multidisciplinary review of medical decisions

The AMHP plays a central role in compulsory admission of patients under the MHA 1983, Part 2. Their role is to ensure that the person appears to be suffering from a mental disorder that warrants compulsory, as opposed to voluntary, **confinement**. This initial safeguard ensures that people who do not have a mental disorder or those who do not actively resist admission are not detained improperly.

Further **multidisciplinary** reviews of medical decisions under Part 4 of the 1983 Act provide safeguards concerning consent to treatment in certain cases. For example, patients who are subject to the consent to treatment provisions have a legal right to be supported through the treatment process by an Independent Mental Health Advocate (MHA 1983, section 130A).

The Mental Health Act Commission

The Mental Health Act Commission (MHAC) is an independent body that oversees the implementation of the 1983 Act; it specifically safeguards and promotes the rights of patients subject to the Act's compulsory powers. The MHAC is able to make both announced and unannounced visits to and inspections of every mental health facility. The purpose and roles of the MHAC are outlined in Box 14.2.

Scope of the Mental Health Act 1983

Part 1, section 1 of the MHA 1983 makes it clear that the Act shall have effect with respect to *the reception, care and treatment of mentally disordered patients, the management of their property and other related matters'*. From the outset it is

Box 14.2 Purpose and role of the Mental Health Act Commission

- To keep under review the operation of the MHA 1983 in respect of patients detained or liable to be detained under that Act.

- To visit and interview, in private, patients detained under the MHA 1983 in hospitals and mental nursing homes.

- To consider the investigation of complaints where these fall within the Commission's remit.

- To appoint registered medical practitioners and others to give second opinions in cases where this is required by the MHA 1983.

- To publish and lay before Parliament a report every two years.

- To monitor the implementation of the Code of Practice (DH 2008) and propose amendments to Ministers.

clear that the 1983 Act applies only to people who suffer from a mental disorder.

Definition of mental disorder

Mental disorder is the legal term used by the 1983 Act to establish who can be made subject to its provisions. It is defined (MHA 1983, section 1(2)) as:

'Any disorder or disability of the mind'

As the definition is very broad, two safeguards are included to narrow the scope of the Act. A person with a learning disability cannot be admitted compulsorily for treatment or guardianship unless their disability is associated with abnormally aggressive or seriously irresponsible conduct (section 1(2A)). Furthermore, dependence on alcohol or drugs alone cannot be considered a mental disorder for the purpose of the Act (MHA 1983, section 1(3)).

Principles of compulsory detention

The process of compulsory detention aims to ensure that the only people made subject to the compulsory provisions of the 1983 Act are those who:

- are or appear to be suffering from a mental disorder, and
- are actively resisting admission to hospital.

Deprivation of liberty

Compulsory detention means that a person is deprived of their liberty. Detention on the grounds that a person is suffering from a mental health problem is not in itself unlawful as long as it is in accordance with wider law (Council of Europe 1950). Such detention must be based on the following conditions (Winterwerp v The Netherlands [1979]):

- It is an emergency
- The person is reliably shown by objective medical evidence to be suffering from a mental disorder, and

- The disorder is of a nature or degree that warrants continued compulsory confinement.

Compulsory admission

Decisions to detain patients compulsorily are the responsibility of three key people:

1 Approved Mental Health Professionals (AMHPs), and

2 Registered Medical Practitioners (RMPs), and

3 The patient's nearest relative.

Approved Mental Health Professionals

AMHPs include nurses and social workers who have been approved by the local authority as having appropriate competence in dealing with people who have mental disorder (MHA 1983, section 114). The AMHP generally makes the application for detention once they are satisfied that the person is suffering from a mental disorder and is actively resisting admission to hospital. They have a duty to conduct a suitable interview with the person before making an application. The AMHP's role is to provide a safeguard against misuse of detention powers. They solely have this role and cannot be directed by their local authority or employer to apply for a person's detention.

Registered Medical Practitioners

Reliable, objective medical evidence is a fundamental requirement of lawful detention and all applications for detention must be founded upon two medical recommendations (one in an emergency). One doctor must also be an **approved clinician** recognized by the primary care trust as being competent in the diagnosis of mental disorder.

The medical recommendations must indicate that the person is suffering from a mental disorder of a nature or degree that warrants continued compulsory confinement.

✖ Practice Example

In St George's Healthcare NHS Trust v S [1998] a pregnant woman with pre-eclampsia was detained under section 2 of the MHA 1983 when she refused hospital treatment for this life-threatening physical condition. The decision of the court was that her detention was unlawful because she did not have a mental disorder and the 1983 Act cannot be used to detain someone just because their thinking seems unusual, irrational, or contrary to public opinion.

The degree of the disorder is its current severity. The nature of the disorder is its prognosis and the person's past history, including previous admissions and compliance with treatment. Only one of these criteria needs to be satisfied to meet the requirements for detention.

The nearest relative

The nearest relative is a statutory friend allocated to a detained patient. The person is drawn from a hierarchy of relatives set out under section 26 of the 1983 Act, with the person in the highest category becoming the nearest relative unless someone lower down the list either ordinarily resides with or cares for the patient. The rights of the nearest relative are set out in Box 14.3. A nearest relative may be removed from this role by the county court if they act unreasonably or are otherwise unsuitable. The patient, another relative, a person living with the patient, or an AMHP can apply to have a nearest relative removed and replaced.

Detention

The properly completed forms are sufficient authority to detain a patient and to take and convey them to a named hospital. Once in hospital, the managers have a duty, usually delegated to a registered nurse, to inform the patient of the conditions of detention and their right to appeal or complain. Under the civil detention provisions (sections 2, 3, and 4), a person can be detained either for assessment (sections 2 and 4) or treatment (section 3). Where a person is detained for treatment, appropriate medical treatment must be available. This is defined as '*medical treatment appropriate to the patient's case taking into account the nature and degree of the mental disorder and other circumstances of his case*'.

A summary of the key detention provisions under Part 2 of the MHA 1983 can be found in Table 14.1.

Informal admission

A person can enter hospital for assessment and treatment of their mental disorder without the need to be detained—referred to as 'informal admission'. Since 1959, formal admission to hospital has been reserved for those who actively resist admission. Informal admission is used for those who consent, those who are incapable of deciding on admission, and those who come into hospital voluntarily.

Holding powers

Informal patients who wish to leave hospital against medical advice can be made subject to the holding powers under section 5 of the 1983 Act. The approved clinician or their nominated deputy can detain a previously informal patient for up to 72 hours to allow for assessment to occur with a view to them being detained under section 2 or 3. Where the immediate attendance of an approved clinician cannot be secured, a **nurse of the prescribed class** may hold the person for up to six hours or until the clinician arrives on the ward (see Table 14.1).

✖ Practice Example

In Reid v United Kingdom [2003], a patient appealed against his detention when he was returned to hospital having been absent without leave for a year with no medical intervention. Whilst the court agreed that the degree of his disorder did not warrant detention, the nature of his disorder, which had shown he deteriorated rapidly and became a danger to the public by making explosive devices, did warrant his continued confinement.

✖ Practice Example

In Reid v United Kingdom [2003] a patient argued he was unlawfully detained as he was not having medical treatment. The Court held that treatment could include control and supervision to prevent harm to himself or others because of his abnormally aggressive behaviour.

Box 14.3 Rights and powers of the nearest relative

Nearest relative means:

- Husband, wife, or civil partner
- Son or daughter
- Mother or father
- Brother or sister
- Grandparent
- Grandchild
- Uncle or aunt
- Nephew or niece
- A person who is not a relative with whom the patient has been living for not less than five years.

The nearest relative has rights to:

- Make applications to admit a person under Civil Admission provisions (sections 2, 3, and 4). The AMHP has to take reasonable steps to inform the nearest relative about an application, and is required to have regard to any wishes expressed by them
- Veto an application for treatment (section 3) and guardianship (section 7)
- Be given information by the hospital managers about the patient's detention and discharge unless the patient objects
- Apply for discharge of their relative from detention under section 2 or section 3 by giving 72 hours' notice to an authorized person at the hospital. (Discharge can be barred by the responsible clinician and a further application cannot be made for six months. The nearest relative then has 28 days to make an application to a Mental Health Review Tribunal for discharge.)
- Apply to the Mental Health Review Tribunal for discharge in respect of a patient detained by a criminal court under section 37 of the Act
- Make a formal complaint to the hospital manager and the MHAC
- Be involved in any consideration as to the after-care needs of a patient unless the patient objects.

Mentally disordered people who commit offences

Where a person commits an offence when suffering from a mental disorder, the Crown Prosecution Service and police must, wherever possible, take steps to divert the person away from the criminal justice system and arrange for appropriate care and treatment (Crown Prosecution Service 2004). Even where prosecution is in the public interest because of the seriousness of an offence, the courts have a range of options under the MHA 1983 to enable the person to be assessed and to receive care and treatment. Similarly, prison inmates who are in need of care and treatment can be transferred to hospital. These provisions are summarized in Table 14.2.

Consent to treatment

Admission and treatment under the MHA 1983 are dealt with separately. Detention under the Act does not necessarily mean compulsory treatment. Section 56 of the MHA 1983 specifically excludes most of the emergency provisions and holding powers from the consent to treatment provisions (Box 14.4). Even though the provisions of the MHA 1983 allow for compulsory treatment without consent, it is essential that care and treatment are given in a climate of consent with respect for the rights and dignity of the patient. Treatment under the provisions of the MHA 1983 is defined as '*nursing, psychological intervention and specialist mental health habilitation, rehabilitation and care*', the purpose of which is to '*alleviate or prevent a worsening of the disorder or its symptoms*' (MHA 1983, section 145(1) and (4)). This recognizes treatment as a whole approach to mental disorder and allows for the treatment of a wide range of symptoms, including the forced feeding of a patient refusing to eat and the taking of blood samples to monitor therapeutic levels of medication. Compulsory treatment for a patient's mental disorder is allowed where it is given by or under the direction of the approved clinician.

The European Convention on Human Rights places a **negative obligation**—a duty not to breach a patient's human rights—on mental health professionals. Treatment for mental disorder can engage rights under Article 3 (the right to be free from torture, inhuman and degrading treatment) and Article 8 (the right to respect for a private and family life that includes respect for personal autonomy and dignity).

Table 14.1 Civil detention powers

Section number and purpose	Method	Conditions for detention	Duration	Can the patient apply to MHRT?	Can nearest relative apply to MHRT?	Automatic MHRT referral?	Do consent to treatment rules apply?
Section 4: Emergency admission for assessment	Application by AMHP or nearest relative founded on one medical recommendation	As for section 2, but AMHP or nearest relative must certify that it is of urgent necessity for the patient to be admitted and that complying with section 2 would involve undesirable delay	72 hours. Can be converted to ordinary admission for assessment if a second medical recommendation is received during this time	No but an appeal under section 2 can begin	No	No	No
Section 2: Ordinary admission for assessment	Application by AMHP founded on two medical recommendations, one of which is from an approved clinician	Suffering from mental disorder of a nature or degree that warrants the detention of the patient in a hospital for assessment (or for assessment followed by medical treatment) for at least a limited period; and person ought to be so detained in the interests of his own health or safety or with a view to the protection of other persons	28 days, not renewable. Will be extended to the date of the hearing where a nearest relative is being displaced by the county court	Yes within first 14 days	Yes	No	Yes

Table 14.1 *Continued*

Section number and purpose	Method	Conditions for detention	Duration	Can the patient apply to MHRT?	Can nearest relative apply to MHRT?	Automatic MHRT referral?	Do consent to treatment rules apply?
Section 3: Admission for treatment	Application by AMHP founded on two medical recommendations, one of which is from an approved clinician	Person is suffering from mental disorder of a nature or degree that makes it appropriate for them to receive medical treatment in a hospital; and it is necessary for the health or safety of the patient or for the protection of other persons that they should receive such treatment and it cannot be provided unless they are detained under this section; and appropriate medical treatment is available	6 months. Can be renewed under section 20 for a further 6 months, then yearly	Yes within first 6 months then once in each period of detention	Yes	Yes, if a completed appeal has not occurred in first 6 months	Yes
Section 5(2)	Report from a doctor or approved clinician in charge of the patient's treatment	Inpatient in a hospital who appears to a registered medical practitioner or approved clinician in charge of their treatment to need detention under this Part of this Act	72 hours, not renewable	No	No	No	No

Section number and purpose	Method	Conditions for detention	Duration	Can the patient apply to MHRT?	Can nearest relative apply to MHRT?	Automatic MHRT referral?	Do consent to treatment rules apply?
Section 5(4)	Report from a nurse of the prescribed class	Appears to a nurse of the prescribed class that a patient who is receiving treatment for mental disorder as an inpatient in a hospital (a) is suffering from mental disorder to such a degree that it is necessary for his health or safety or for the protection of others for him to be immediately restrained from leaving the hospital; and (b) that it is not practicable to secure the immediate attendance of a practitioner or clinician to furnish a report under section 5(2)	6 hours, not renewable	No	No	No	No

Table 14.2 Summary of powers available to the police, courts, and prison service

Section name and number	Duration	Application to MHRT?	Nearest relative application to MHRT?	Automatic referral to MHRT?	Do consent to treatment provisions apply?
Section 35: Remand to hospital for psychiatric report	28 days. May be renewed by the court for further periods of 28 days to a maximum of 12 weeks	No	No	No	No
Section 36: Remand to hospital for treatment	28 days. May be renewed by the court for further periods of 28 days to a maximum of 12 weeks	No	No	No	Yes
Section 37: Hospital order by the court	6 months, renewable for further 6 months, then yearly	In second 6 months, then in each period of detention	In second 6 months, then in each period of detention	After 3 years if patient remains in hospital and has not made an appeal of their own	Yes
Section 37: Guardianship order by the court	6 months, renewable for further 6 months, then yearly	Within first 6 months, then in each period of detention	Within first year, then yearly	No	No
Section 37/41: Hospital order with restriction	Without limit of time. Discharge and leave of absence restricted by the Home Office	In second 6 months, then in each period of detention	No	If one has not been held, Home Secretary will refer the case to the MHRT every 3 years	Yes
Section 38: Interim hospital order	12 weeks. May be renewed in 28-day periods to a maximum of 1 year	No	No	No	Yes
Section 45A: Hospital and limitation direction	Without limit of time	In first 6 months, second 6 months, then yearly	No	Home Secretary will refer case every 3 years if one has not been held	Yes

Section name and number	Duration	Application to MHRT?	Nearest relative application to MHRT?	Automatic referral to MHRT?	Do consent to treatment provisions apply?
Section 46: Transfer to hospital of patient in custody during Her Majesty's pleasure	Without limit of time	Within first 6 months, then once in each period of detention	No	Home Secretary will refer case every 3 years if one has not been held	Yes
Section 47: Transfer to hospital of a person serving a prison sentence	6 months, a further 6 months, then a year at a time	Within first 6 months, then once in each period of detention	No	Hospital managers will refer case every 3 years if one has not been held	Yes
Section 47/49: Transfer with restrictions	Restriction lapses on earliest release date from prison	In second 6 months after transfer, then yearly	No	Home Secretary will refer case every 3 years if one has not been held	Yes
Section 48: Transfer of other prisoners for urgent treatment	According to treatment needs of the patient	Within first 6 months, then once in each period of detention	No	Home Secretary will refer case every 3 years if one has not been held	Yes
Section 48/49: Transfer with restriction	Restriction will lapse on earliest release date	In second 6 months, then in each period of detention	No	Home Secretary will refer case every 3 years if one has not been held	Yes
Section 136: Police power in places to which the public have access	72 hours, not renewable	No	No	No	No
Section 135: Warrant to enter and search for a person with mental disorder	72 hours, not renewable	No	No	No	No

Box 14.4 Detention powers *excluded* from the consent to treatment provisions

Patient detained by virtue of:

• an emergency application (section 4)

• holding powers under section 5(2) or (4)

• remand to hospital for a report on their mental condition (section 35)

• detention by the police (section 135 or 136)

• detention in a place of safety (section 37(4) or 45A(5)).

*They will also **not apply** to a patient:*

• conditionally discharged and not recalled to hospital (section 42, 73, or 74)

• who is a community patient and not recalled to hospital (section 17A)

• subject to guardianship (section 7).

Safeguards

Some treatment under the MHA 1983 may be given only where provisions safeguarding patients have been met. There are three categories of safeguard:

1 Treatments that require consent **and** a second opinion; this includes psychosurgery, and both the consent of the patient and an agreeable second opinion from a doctor appointed by the MHAC are needed.

2 Treatments that require consent **or** a second opinion; this includes the giving of medication for mental disorder beyond three months from when it was first administered, with either the consent of the patient or an agreeable second opinion from an appointed doctor required.

3 ECT cannot be given:

• without the consent of a capable patient, or

• without agreement from an appointed doctor where the person is incapable

• to an incapable patient with a valid and applicable advanced directive refusing health care, or

• a person who can refuse consent to ECT under a Lasting Power of Attorney or Court Deputy cannot have ECT authorized by an appointed doctor.

When asked to sanction treatment for a patient, 'second opinion appointed doctors' must consult with two people about the patient's condition: one a nurse, and one who cannot be a doctor or a nurse. The role of the mental health nurse as consultee is outlined in Box 14.5. Patients who initially consent to treatment may withdraw that consent. Treatment would have to cease unless it could be justified as urgent as set out in section 62 of the MHA 1983.

Rehabilitation and aftercare

Leave of absence

Testing a patient's response to treatment by allowing controlled periods away from hospital is an important element of the rehabilitation process. An approved clinician may grant a detained patient a leave of absence from hospital. The leave may be subject to any conditions the approved clinician considers necessary. The period of leave granted is also at the discretion of the responsible clinician and can range from hours to seven days. A detained patient on leave of absence may be recalled to hospital if they do not fulfil the conditions set out when the leave was granted.

✖ Practice Example

In Herczegfalvy v Austria [1993] the European Court of Human Rights held that mental health care called for increased vigilance in complying with the Convention. Nevertheless, as a general rule, a measure that is considered a therapeutic necessity cannot be regarded as inhuman or degrading. That is, the treatment must be in accordance with a responsible body of professional opinion and be in the patient's best interests.

In R (On the application of PS) v RMO(DR G) and SOAD(DR W) [2003] the Court held that it was not a breach of Article 8 of the Convention to require a patient detained for treatment to take medication for his mental disorder, as it could be justified as necessary for the patient's health and for the protection of others from harm.

Box 14.5 Role of the mental health nurse as consultee

The consultee must be a person who has been professionally concerned with the patient's medical treatment. The nurse will have had direct knowledge of the person's history and condition, and be in a position to comment on the issues affecting the patient including:

- the proposed treatment and the patient's ability to consent to it
- other treatment options
- the way in which the decision to treat was arrived at
- the facts of the case, progress, etc.
- the patient's relatives' view of the proposed treatment
- the implications of imposing treatment on a non-consenting patient
- the reasons for the patient's refusal of treatment
- any other matter relating to the patient's care on which the consultee wishes to comment.

Community treatment orders

Where long-term leave (more than seven days) is contemplated, the responsible clinician must first consider the use of a community treatment order (CTO). Such orders allow an approved clinician to test the rehabilitation of a patient detained for treatment by discharging the patient subject to their being recalled to hospital if they do not continue with treatment in the community. A patient subject to a CTO is known as a 'community patient'. A community patient cannot be made to take treatment by force in the community. Where compulsory treatment is deemed necessary, recall to hospital would be necessary. A summary of the provisions of a CTO is set out in Box 14.6.

Aftercare

Patients detained for treatment under the MHA 1983 have a right to aftercare. It is the duty of statutory health and social services to provide the aftercare services that they consider necessary for the patient. As aftercare is a right, the services provided cannot be charged for. The provision of aftercare

Box 14.6 Summary of CTO provisions

The responsible clinician may make a CTO for a patient detained under sections 3, 47, or 48 of the MHA 1983, if satisfied the criteria are met and an AMHP agrees that a CTO is appropriate for that patient. The criteria and provisions are:

- The patient must need medical treatment for their mental disorder for their own health or safety, or for the protection of others.
- It must be possible for the patient to receive the treatment they need without having to be in hospital.
- The patient may be recalled to hospital for treatment should this become necessary.
- Appropriate medical treatment for the patient must be available whilst living in the community.
- The responsible clinician must state the conditions of the order that have been agreed with the AMHP.
- Where the patient does not comply with the conditions, this can be taken into account when considering a recall to hospital.
- The responsible clinician may also recall a community patient to hospital if they require medical treatment in hospital for mental disorder, and there would be a risk of harm to the health or safety of the patient or to other persons if they were not recalled to hospital for that purpose.

must continue as long as the health and social services consider the patient requires it. The decision to end aftercare services must be a joint one.

Guardianship

Guardianship provides an alternative to detention for treatment by requiring a person with a mental disorder to:
- live at an address specified by the Guardian
- provide access to people named by the Guardian, such as a doctor, nurse, or social worker
- attend any place the Guardian may specify for medical treatment, occupation, education, or training.

No treatment may be given to patients subject to Guardianship without consent. Guardianship is administered by the local social services authority, which will name a social worker as guardian or accept a person known to the patient such as a relative who is suitable and willing to act in the role.

The Mental Capacity Act 2005

Respect for autonomy is a fundamental principle of health care. Adult patients are assumed to have the ability to make decisions about their health care, and their consent to treatment is required before it can proceed (see exceptions under Part 4 of the MHA 1983 above). Where the patient lacks decision-making capacity, the Mental Capacity Act 2005 and its guiding principles are intended to ensure that their rights and interests are at the centre of the decision-making process (Box 14.7).

Assessing decision-making capacity

Generally mental health nurses will be able to presume that a patient aged 16 years or more can make decisions concerning their care and treatment. Only where doubt over a patient's decision-making ability occurs will there be a need to go on to assess decision-making capacity. A person lacks capacity where an impairment or disturbance of the mind or brain affects their ability to make a particular decision. It does not

---

Box 14.7 Guiding principles of the Mental Capacity Act 2005

- A person must be assumed to have capacity unless it is established that they lack capacity.

- A person is not to be treated as unable to make a decision unless all practicable steps to help them to do so have been taken without success.

- A person is not to be treated as unable to make a decision merely because they make an unwise decision.

- An act done, or decision made, under this Act for or on behalf of a person who lacks capacity must be done, or made, in their best interests.

- Before the act is done, or the decision is made, regard must be had to whether the purpose for which it is needed can be as effectively achieved in a way that is less restrictive of the person's rights and freedom of action.

---

matter whether the lack of capacity is permanent or temporary. A person will not be considered capable of making a decision where they are unable to:

- understand the treatment information relevant to the decision, or

- retain the information long enough to make a decision, or

- use or weigh the information as part of the process of arriving at a decision, or

- communicate that decision by any means.

Figure 14.1 outlines a summary of the framework for assessing decision-making capacity.

Designated decision-makers

The Mental Capacity Act 2005 has two formal powers that allow a third party to make decisions on behalf of a person who lacks decision-making capacity. These powers can give the designated decision-maker the right to consent to or refuse medical treatment on behalf of the patient. Where a designated decision-maker with authority is in place for a patient, their consent must be obtained before care and treatment can lawfully be given.

Personal welfare lasting power of attorney

A power allowing another to consent on behalf of a person who lacks capacity can be created through a personal welfare lasting power of attorney. The power must be created by the person (the donor) when they are capable and can come into force only when the person lacks capacity and the power of attorney has been registered with the Office of Public Guardian. A person can also create a lasting power of attorney that allows another to manage their property and affairs. Figure 14.2 outlines the process for designated decision-making.

Court of Protection deputy

When continuing decisions need to be made on behalf of a person who lacks capacity and there is not lasting power of attorney, the Court of Protection may appoint a person, called a deputy, to make personal welfare decisions on behalf of the incapable patient that can include the right to consent to or refuse treatment. The Court must be satisfied that the deputy is willing and able to fulfil the role and that appointing a deputy is a proportionate response to the needs of the patient.

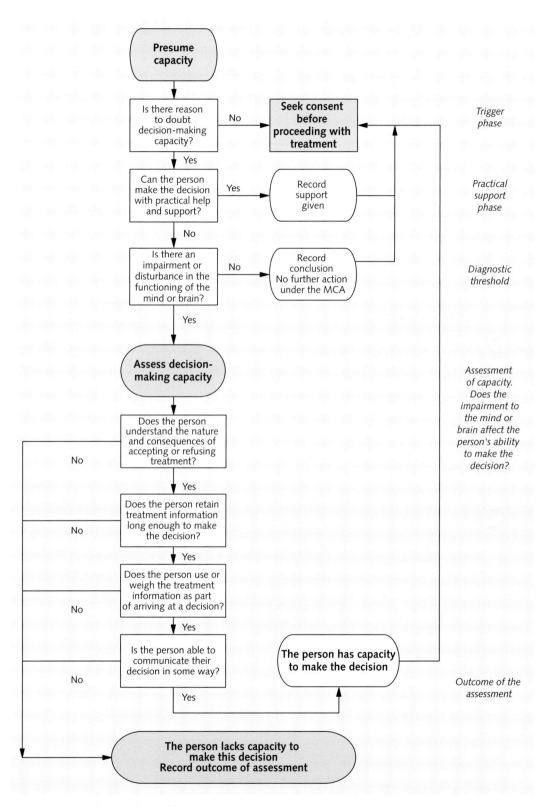

Figure 14.1 Assessing decision-making capacity.

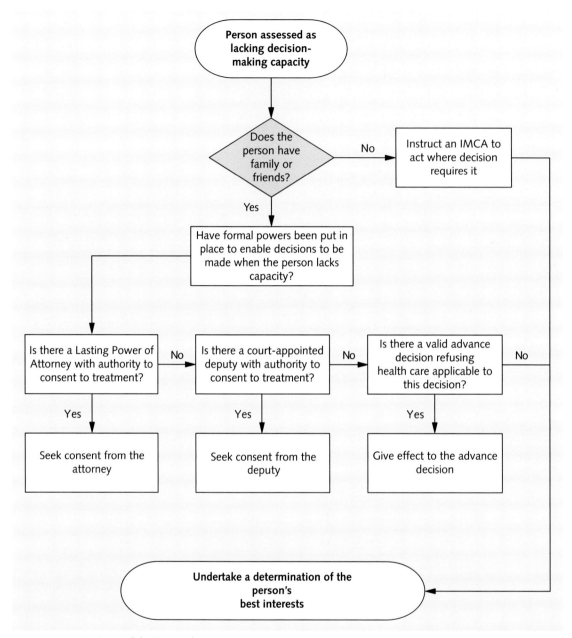

Figure 14.2 Designated decision-makers.

Advance decisions refusing health care

As well as having designated decision-makers able to give consent to treatment decisions, a person can make an advance refusal of treatment. Where a valid applicable advance refusal is in place, the wishes of the patient must be respected and treatment withheld. Compulsory treatment for mental disorder, other than ECT, can override a valid and applicable advance decision refusing health care. Figure 14.2 summarizes the main requirements for a valid advance decision.

Best interests

The Mental Capacity Act 2005 provides a checklist of factors that must be considered when determining whether care and treatment are in the best interests of a patient who lacks capacity. This holistic approach to best interests ensures that the wishes of the patient and the views of those caring for the patient are taken into account. Figure 14.3 outlines the checklist of factors for determining the best interests of an incapable adult.

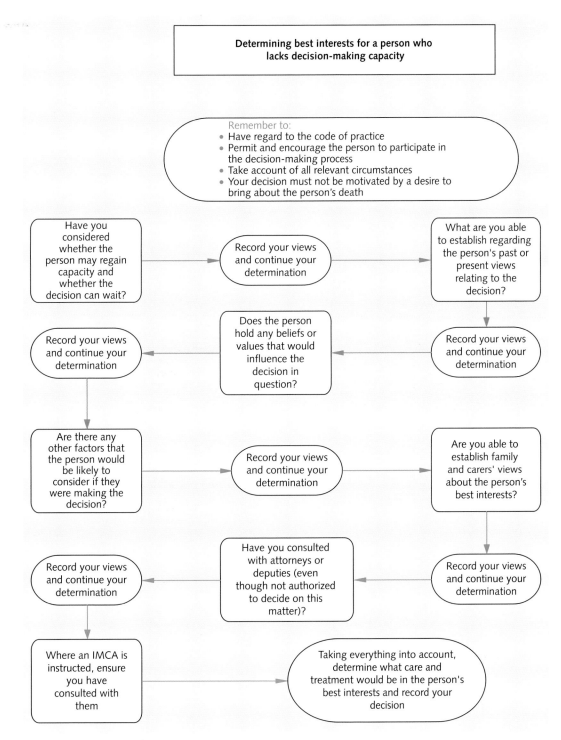

Figure 14.3 Determining best interests.

Independent Mental Capacity Advocate (IMCA)

There is a duty to instruct an IMCA where an incapable adult has no friends or relatives who can be consulted about their best interests. The IMCA will make representations about the person's wishes, feelings, and beliefs, and call the decision-maker's attention to the factors relevant to their decision.

IMCAs will be involved only where the decision concerns:

- **serious medical treatment**
- a change in the person's accommodation where it is provided by the NHS or local authority, or
- authorized detention under the deprivation of liberty safeguards.

Protection from liability

Where care and treatment for an incapable adult proceeds following an assessment of capacity and determination of best interests, the caregiver is protected from liability in the law relating to consent.

Restraint

Restraint is defined in the Mental Capacity Act 2005 as:

> *'the use or threat of force where the person is resisting and any restriction of liberty of movement whether or not the person resists'.*

This wide definition includes even mild forms of restraint, such as holding an incapable person's hand to prevent them wandering away and holding an arm to keep it still when taking a blood sample. Restraint is permitted, but only when the person using it reasonably believes it is necessary to prevent harm to the incapable person. The restraint used must be proportionate both to the likelihood of the harm and to the seriousness of the harm.

Deprivation of liberty safeguards

There may be occasions where a person who lacks decision-making capacity is deprived of their liberty in their best interests when in hospital or a care home. To ensure that the person's human rights are respected the **deprivation of liberty** must be authorized through an assessment by two health and social care professionals, including mental health nurses, to ensure that:

- the adult lacks decision-making capacity due to an impairment or disturbance of the mind or brain
- it is in their best interests to be deprived of their liberty taking into account any objections against such a finding, and
- the person is not or would not be better protected by being subject to compulsion under the MHA 1983 such as Guardianship.

Where those undertaking the assessment agree that the person should be deprived of their liberty in their best interests, this can be authorized for any period up to 12 months. A representative will be appointed who can ask for the issue to be reviewed (Ministry of Justice 2008).

Court of Protection

The Court of Protection is a specialist court that specifically hears cases and settles matters concerning people who lack capacity. The Court can also appoint deputies and give them powers to make ongoing decisions for incapable adults.

Office of Public Guardian

The Office of the Public Guardian is responsible for the supervision of deputies appointed by the Court and for supporting deputies in their role. It also has a role in protecting people subject to the Court's powers from abuse or exploitation by:

- keeping a register of lasting powers of attorney
- keeping a register of orders appointing deputies
- supervising deputies appointed by the Court
- receiving reports from attorneys
- dealing with enquiries and complaints about deputies or attorneys.

Research with incapable adults

Research involving people who lack capacity, other than clinical trials for new medicines, is regulated by the Mental Capacity Act 2005, section 31, which requires researchers to:

- satisfy a research ethics committee as to why subjects who lack decision-making capacity are to be used in the study
- seek the permission of a relative or friend of the incapable adult who can veto the person's participation in the research
- remove the person from participation in the study if during the study they show any resistance or distress for whatever reason.

▲ Conclusion

The position of the patient with mental health problems and disorder is now more legalized than ever before. The MHA 1983, Human Rights Act 1998, and Mental Capacity Act 2005 all regulate the care and treatment that people with mental health problems and disorders receive. To practise their skills effectively, it is essential that mental health nurses inform their practice by reference to the law. This will ensure that their patients are cared for with respect and due regard for their fundamental rights and freedoms.

w Website

You may find it helpful to work through our scenarios intended to help you to develop and apply the skills in this chapter. Please go to:

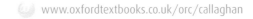 www.oxfordtextbooks.co.uk/orc/callaghan

➤ Further reading

Bartlett, P. (2005). *Blackstone's Guide to The Mental Capacity Act 2005*. London: Oxford University Press.
A readable guide to the provisions of the Mental Capacity Act 2005.

Department of Health. Mental Health Law page.
www.dh.gov.uk/en/Policyandguidance/
Healthandsocialcaretopics/Mentalhealth/index.htm

Jones, R. (2007). *Mental Health Act Manual*. London: Sweet and Maxwell.
A comprehensive guide to mental health law—the mental health professional's law 'bible'.

Ministry of Justice. Mental Capacity Act 2005.
www.justice.gov.uk/whatwedo/mentalcapacity.htm

✦ References

Council of Europe (1950). *European Convention on Fundamental Human Rights and Freedoms*. Rome: Council of Europe.

Crown Prosecution Service (2004). *Code for Crown Prosecutors*. London: CPS.

Department for Constitutional Affairs (2007). *Mental Capacity Act 2005 Code of Practice*. London: The Stationery Office.

Department of Health (2008). *Code of Practice to the Mental Health Act 1983*. London: HMSO.

Herczegfalvy v Austria [1993] (A/242B) 15 EHRR 437.

Ministry of Justice (2008). *Deprivation of Liberty Safeguards: Code of Practice to Supplement the Main Mental Capacity Act 2005, Code of Practice*. London: The Stationery Office.

Nursing and Midwifery Council (2008). *Code of Professional Conduct: Standards for Conduct, Performance and Ethics*. London: NMC.

R v Ealing DHA ex parte Fox [1993] 3 All ER 170.

R (On the application of PS) v RMO(DR G) and SOAD(DR W) [2003] EWHC 2335 QBD.

Reid v United Kingdom [2003] 37 EHRR 9.

St George's Healthcare NHS Trust v S [1998] 3 WLR 936 (CA).

Winterwerp v The Netherlands [1979] 2 EHRR 387.

(15) Risk assessment and management

Sarah Eales

▼ Introduction

This chapter is designed to assist you in understanding and implementing effective risk assessment and management. The focus of the chapter is on adult mental health care. However, many of the principles can be applied to other groups. The chapter includes reference to government guidelines, research evidence, and good practice. Risk assessment must be undertaken systematically and risk management should set out clear strategies including the rationale and intended outcomes. The emphasis is on individualized care that engages the service user and their carers throughout.

This chapter is written in a climate where risk assessment and management remains at the heart of mental health care. There are those who feel that too much emphasis is placed on the topic; however, until each inquiry—both local internal inquiries and external regional/national inquiries—is able to uncover comprehensive, well documented, and defendable practice, risk assessment and management will continue to take centre stage. However, it is important to acknowledge that risk is dynamic and is not entirely preventable. In fact, we will be promoting positive risk-taking with service users as we progress through the chapter.

Learning outcomes

By the end of this chapter you should be better able to:

1 Understand research evidence and best practice guidance in risk assessment and management

2 Demonstrate core skills and competencies required to undertake effective risk assessment and management under supervision.

Definitions

There is a plethora of definitions for risk assessment and management. Risk assessment can be defined as:

> *'the systematic collection of information to determine the degree to which harm to self or others is likely at some point in time'*
>
> O'Rourke and Bird (2001, p. 4)

Morgan (2000, p. 2) defines risk management as:

> *'A statement of plans, and an allocation of individual responsibilities, for translating collective decisions into actions. This process should name all the relevant people involved in the treatment and support, including the service user and appropriate informal carers. It should also clearly identify the review date for the assessment and management plan.'*

Both of these definitions are emphasizing a systematic and structured collection of information that holds individuals accountable for their risk assessment and management plan. Morgan's definition also helpfully reminds us that the process of risk assessment and management must include the service user and carer. Recent evidence from the collection of data for inquiries suggests that carers are frequently not taken seriously when they express concern about an increased risk (Maden 2006).

Policy and guidance

During the past ten years a great number of initiatives have been instigated by the Department of Health (DH) that look at the incidence of suicide and deliberate **self-harm** (DSH) as well as aggression and violence amongst people with mental health problems. Self-neglect has not formed part of the DH's risk considerations.

The public image is one of core failure for the severely mentally ill. Policy responses have been to set national standards that include, in the UK, the National Service Framework for Mental Health (NSFMH) (DH 1999a). This reflects government policy on treating mental health as a national priority. The NSFMH specifies seven standards, the aim of these standards, and how they will be measured. It does not specify how the standards should be implemented. Standard 7 deals with a national reduction in suicide levels by 20% by the year 2010, and the latest reports suggest that overall suicide rates in England are falling (NIMHE 2007). However, in Scotland, Wales, and Northern Ireland, rates of suicide for women are not currently falling (National Statistics 2007). Standard 6 of the NSFMH deals with the involvement and needs of carers. Risk assessment training needs of staff working in mental health services are identified in a number of the standards. The NSFMH was followed in 2002 by the *National Suicide Prevention Strategy* (DH 2002), which sets out broad targets for high-risk groups, promotion of mental well-being, availability of methods, media reporting, and research priorities. The National Institute for Health and Clinical Excellence (NICE) has more recently produced good practice clinical guidelines for the management of self-harm, which include a systematic review of literature and a project detailing service users' experiences of health care following self-harm (NICE 2004). Suicide prevention strategies in the UK are mirrored in other countries such as Australia, although the most recent Australian suicide strategy was published more recently in 2007 (Commonwealth of Australia 2007).

The UK National Confidential Inquiry into Homicides and Suicides last reported in 2006 (University of Manchester 2006). This Inquiry is a government-funded initiative and provides a detailed and comprehensive report that identifies key lessons that can be learned in relation to people with mental health problems. A summary of recommendations is provided in Box 15.1.

NICE has also produced guidelines on the management of disturbed/violent behaviour in psychiatric inpatient settings (NICE 2005). Good practice is considered under the headings of prediction, prevention, interventions, post-incident review, working with service users, and training needs. Guidance on observation in inpatient settings, which is relevant to violence, vulnerability, and deliberate self-harm, is included in the document. Working with risk assessment and management, as all mental health practitioners do, you must be alert

Box 15.1 Recommendations for risk management of homicides and suicides (University of Manchester 2006)

The specific areas highlighted to improve future prevention of both homicide and suicide are:

Absconding from in patient wards (suicide)

- Understand trigger factors
- Greater use of technology (e.g. swipe cards)

Transition from in patient to community (suicide)

- Repeated risk assessment during discharge planning
- Plans to address stressors during leave
- Contacts for a crisis during leave
- Early follow-up on discharge including immediate telephone contact
- Support arrangements for self-discharge

Use of Care Programme Approach (CPA) and management of risk (suicide and homicide)

- Greater alignment of CPA and risk, ensuring assessment at CPA review
- Ensuring enhanced CPA is used for high-risk groups
- Joint review with all teams involved in care

Responding when a care plan breaks down (suicide and homicide)

- Robust use of CPA, including working with families
- Assertive outreach for patients with a history of disengagement
- Use of modern drug treatment as first-line therapy

Attitudes to prevention (suicide and homicide)

- All inpatient suicides should be seen as preventable
- The culture of blame imposed on those in clinical practice must be lifted to prevent a self-protective reaction of inevitability in cases of serious incidents.

Greater emphasis on risk management in older people's services and development of services for patients with a dual diagnosis are also given as recommendations in the summary section of the report, but not expanded upon.

to the publication of new inquiry reports and the impact any recommendations could have upon your own practice. Public inquiries regarding your local Trust can be accessed on the Trust website or via the Strategic Health Authority website.

Expectations of mental health nurses

All standards for mental health practitioner competency or training standards contain references to risk assessment and management (DH 2006a); for example, many of the Ten Essential Shared Capabilities (DH 2004) are relevant to the areas of risk assessment and management, not just the specific capability of 'promoting safety and positive risk taking'. Box 15.2 shows the key competencies from a variety of competency documents relevant to mental health nursing.

Box 15.2 Competencies of mental health nurses in risk assessment and management

Ten Essential Shared Capabilities (DH 2004)

Promoting safety and positive risk taking:

'Empowering the person to decide the level of risk they are prepared to take with their health and safety. This includes working with the tension between promoting safety and positive risk taking, including assessing and dealing with possible risks for service users, carers, family members, and the wider public.'

National Occupational Standards (Skills for Health 2007)

MH16: Assess individuals' needs and circumstances and evaluate the risk of abuse, failure to protect, and harm to self and others.

MH17: Assess the need for intervention and present assessments of individuals' needs and related risks.

MH49: Enable people who are a risk to themselves or others to develop control.

From Values to Action: The Chief Nursing Officer's Review of Mental Health Nursing (DH 2006b)

Recommendation 6: All mental health nurses will be able to comprehensively assess and respond to service users' individual needs and identified risks.

Recommendation 12: All individuals receiving inpatient care will receive a service that is safe, supportive, and able to respond to individual needs.

From these examples the mental health nurse should see that an individualized approach to assessment and management of risk that engages all relevant parties, most importantly the service user and carers, from the outset is the expectation in relation to their skills and knowledge base.

Step-by-step guidelines

Concern for safety and the assessment and management of risk are core components of the Care Programme Approach (CPA) (DH 1999b); however, we know that risk assessment and management are not always fully aligned with CPA (University of Manchester 2006). Of particular importance in ensuring that risk assessment and management and CPA are aligned are the following areas:

1 The assessment of risk

2 The documentation of risk

3 The communication of risk

4 The adoption of appropriate risk management strategies based on assessment.

For each service user and each change in their risk presentation it is important to ask yourself whether you have completed the four tasks listed above. Each of these aspects is now considered.

The assessment of risk

It is important to remember that risk cannot be eliminated entirely and that it is dynamic and fluctuates over time; therefore it requires ongoing assessment. Risk can be general, specific, or both. General risks might include a history of a previous behaviour. A specific risk might include an increase in drinking when feeling low in mood. The person might present an increased risk of suicide both because they have a history of suicide attempts (general risk) and because they are drinking as they feel this helps with their low mood (specific risk). Risk assessment will include elements of clinical judgement, and these cannot be absolutes. We will return to this idea later in the chapter.

Good risk assessment cannot be performed in isolation; ideally risk assessment should be a multiprofessional, multi-agency collaboration. Good practice also demands that service users and their carers are involved in the assessment of risk at the earliest opportunity (DH 2007). Engaging service users with risk assessment and management should be the norm—exceptions to this should be justified clearly—rather than the current situation where the inclusion of service users and carers seems to be an infrequent activity (Langhan and Lindow 2004).

When undertaking a risk assessment there are various sources and techniques for obtaining information. Box 15.3 gives some examples.

Having collected together the risk information, it can be very helpful to consider the factors that increase or decrease risk under the following headings.

Statistical risk factors are background/historical factors statistically known to increase the likelihood of the risk behaviour occurring. The presence of statistical risk factors does not mean the risk is bound to happen, rather their presence heightens the general probability that the given risk may be realized; for example, gender or age may increase risk (NICE 2004, 2005).

Clinical risk factors are critical factors and are dynamic. The presence of these factors occurring against a background of statistical factors increases the likelihood of the potential risk becoming reality for the individual concerned. Clinical risk factors are those that affect the mental state of the service user. An example of a clinical factor would be a service user receiving command hallucinations to harm a specific person (NICE 2005).

Contextual/trigger risk factors are the social and environmental factors that increase the likelihood of a risk behaviour occurring, for example loss of a key support mechanism (e.g. keyworker off sick, relationship breakdown, recent homelessness). These factors are also sometimes known as situational factors (DH 2007).

Overlap may occur between the different categories of factors; however, clinical and contextual factors are those on which the management plan should focus. Their dynamic nature gives the service user, carers, and professionals the opportunity to intervene to reduce risk.

Box 15.3 Assessment techniques used in risk assessment

- Access to past records from relevant sources
- Self-reports at interview
- Observing discrepancies between verbal and non-verbal cues
- Reports from significant others, formally and informally
- Rating scales/descriptive reports
- Intuitive gut feelings
- Recognizing repeat patterns of behaviour

Morgan (2000)

When to undertake a risk assessment

All service users new to a service should receive an initial risk assessment, the aim of which should be to indicate whether a more detailed risk assessment process is needed. By the definition and nature of some services, all service users will require a detailed risk assessment (e.g. assertive outreach service users). Once a detailed risk assessment has been completed it is important to set up a review date; however, there are times when a review will be needed before the specified date; some examples are given in Box 15.4.

When making an assessment of risk the following areas should be considered.

History

The strongest predictor of future behaviour is past behaviour, and therefore a known history of risk behaviour should be documented carefully. Relevant information should be obtained from health records and referral letters, as well as asking service users themselves and carers/relatives.

The **recency, severity, frequency,** and **pattern** of any previous identified risk should be examined:

- **Recency**: the more recent the incident relating to risk, the more alert the assessor should be.
- **Severity**: the more severe the incident relating to risk, the more alert the assessor should be.

Box 15.4 When to review a risk assessment

- When the service user, carer, or professional observes an actual or potential increase in risk, for example using an early signs monitoring process or during a period of enhanced observation
- When transferring a service user to another service/department or service provider (e.g. a service user who has been under the care of the community mental health team and is then admitted to hospital, or vice versa)
- Prior to the service user going on leave
- Prior to discharge
- Immediately after a clinical incident (e.g. following a suicide attempt, self-harm, violence, absconding episode)
- During multidisciplinary reviews including CPA meetings

- **Frequency**: the more frequently the incident relating to risk has occurred in the past, the more alert the assessor should be.
- **Pattern**: of any incidents, e.g. deliberate self-harm occurring as a result of alcohol abuse.

Ideation and mental state

What is the person thinking or feeling now? Are there particular aspects of their mental state that increase the risks, for example evidence of threat/control, thought disorder symptoms, factors that could potentially place the person in a vulnerable situation, low mood, or hopelessness? It is advisable to complete a full mental state examination each time risk is reviewed.

Intent and planning

A statement from the person that they intend to engage in risk behaviour is the strongest indicator of risk and should never be dismissed (NICE 2004). If the person admits that they have thoughts about engaging in risk behaviour, the next thing is to consider how they might do so. The presence of a plan as to how they might engage in particular risk behaviour indicates higher risk. If the person has **access to the means** for carrying out that plan, the degree of risk rises still higher.

Service user's awareness of risk

In considering the service user's awareness of risk, issues to explore include the person's capacity to recognize, understand, and manage risks, to summon help, and their willingness to engage with support services where necessary.

Carers

When formal inquiries of risk behaviours are undertaken, a frequent criticism is the extent to which the concerns of service users' carers were taken into consideration. When a carer is expressing a concern about a service user's mental state, it should be explored and documented (Maden 2006).

The chapters that follow this one give more specific information about assessing and managing specific types of risk. Wherever an evidence-based tool is available to assist in the assessment of risk, this should be used (see Chapters 17 and 18 for examples). The DH guidance on *Best Practice in Managing Risk* (DH 2007) offers a summary of many available tools and their evidence base. During mental health nurse training it is unlikely that the training needed to utilize many of these tools will be offered.

However, it is sensible to familiarize yourself with the tools available and observe their use in clinical practice wherever possible. Once the tool has been completed you can use the results to assist you in making your structured clinical judgement about the likelihood of a risk occurring and when it might occur. Although a risk assessment tool may have good reliability and validity, this does not account for the dynamic nature of risk as highlighted above, therefore does not offer an individualized approach to risk assessment. This is why it is important to also include your clinical judgement (DH 2007).

The documentation of risk

The art of concise, yet informative, documentation is more challenging than many professionals think. The key to this concise documentation is the ability to devise a formulation/summary of the risk. Box 15.5 identifies the questions a formulation of risk should answer for the reader.

All documentation related to risk assessment should contain a section that allows for a formulation/summary of the risk. Each time you attend a new practice area you should familiarize yourself with where you can find this information in the service user's notes.

The communication of risk

Good communication is a key component of the effective management of risk. There have been a series of public inquiries where communication failure has been identified as being a primary cause of the breakdown of effective care. The formulation and management plan should be agreed with the multidisciplinary team. The plan should be discussed and agreed with the service user and, where applicable, with carers/relatives. The importance of involving the service user in the

---

Box 15.5 Formulation of risk

- Is there a risk of harm?
- What sort of harm, and of what likely degree?
- How likely is it that harm will occur?
- What is its immediacy or imminence?
- How long will the risk last?
- What are the factors that contribute to the risk?
- How can the factors be modified or managed?

Brooks (1984), cited in Vinestock (1996)

process cannot be stressed enough. If a person is involved in the risk assessment and producing the risk management plan, it may decrease their fears, therefore aiding implementation of strategies to reduce risk and promote recovery.

Risk assessment and management is a multi-agency activity and to be effective must be communicated to all agencies involved in a service user's care on a **need-to-know basis**. Make sure any changes in circumstances that may alter the context of risk are recorded and communicated to others who need to know; show evidence of this in your documentation.

It is important that you are familiar with your local and regional policies on information sharing. The key to information sharing is the maintenance of the service user's confidentiality, which is enshrined in both common law and the Human Rights Act 1998. Every professional governing body places a responsibility on the individual practitioner to maintain confidentiality; you should be familiar with the most up-to-date version of the Nursing and Midwifery Council guidance on confidentiality and information sharing (NMC 2006).

Many inquiry reports highlight the need for appropriate and timely information sharing. Accurate record keeping is key to ensuring that all relevant parties are safe and providing effective interventions. Morgan (2000) offers a helpful guide to good practice in information sharing which is provided in Box 15.6.

The most basic principles of sharing service user information with a third party are that explicit consent has been obtained from the service user. In order to give/withhold consent, the service user must understand the purpose of the sharing of information, not simply that information will be shared.

When wishing to share information with a third party, it is

important that you ensure the third party will afford the same level of respect to the information with which you and your organization comply. The third party must know why the information is being shared with them and they must use the information only for that specific purpose.

There are a number of instances when you may have to disclose confidential information without obtaining consent or where consent has been withheld (NMC 2006). The consideration is whether the public interest outweighs the right of the individual to privacy. With regard to risk assessment and management, this is most likely to be where there is a concern or a serious concern that harm might occur to the service user or another party. The decision to disclose or not to disclose information must be clearly documented. Most organizations will provide forms to be completed in these instances. Wherever possible, these decisions should not be taken by a single individual but in discussion with the person's supervisor and responsible members of the service user's multidisciplinary team. Non-disclosure, as well as inappropriate disclosure, can potentially lead to prosecution of the individual and/or the organization.

The adoption of appropriate risk management strategies based on assessment

The management plan should change the balance between risk and safety, bearing in mind that some risks cannot be totally eliminated. Interventions should be comprehensively documented and should identify specific care inputs rather than generalities. Care inputs should be regularly reviewed and this should be accurately recorded in the notes. The plan should take into account any need for further specialist assessment, and levels of observation or monitoring.

The needs of children whose parent(s) have mental disorder merit special consideration; care coordinators need to give consideration to involving children's teams and/or invoking the safeguarding children procedure where appropriate. Similarly, women who are pregnant or men whose partners are pregnant, have to receive consideration that takes into account the risk to the unborn child (www.everychildmatters.gov.uk).

Engagement of service users in the management of risk is one potential aspect of working within the recovery model (NIMHE 2004); see Chapter 9 for more information on the recovery model. When the service user is engaged in the process of identifying and managing risks through active engagement in risk assessment, crisis planning, and intervention such as problem solving, the professional is working to the recovery model. The partnership working that this entails facilitates the trusting honest relationship required to implement positive risk taking (DH 2007).

Box 15.6 Good practice in information sharing

- Close liaison with all agencies

- Full and accurate information

- Collaborative inter-agency management plans

- Information shared; no missing key historical information

- Taking a collaborative stand with the service user from the outset

- Learning the language of other agencies

- Joint training and common procedures/leaflets for agencies

Morgan (2000)

✖ Practice Example

Below is a brief summary about a service user called Maureen. By referring to this and to Chapter 17 on self-harm and suicide, can you complete a formulation for Maureen?

Case study: Maureen

Maureen lives with her current partner, who also has a diagnosed mental illness. Maureen is 50 years old and has a current diagnosis of bipolar disorder. She has a history of suicide attempts, her first being in 1975; this brought her to the attention of mental health services. She is prescribed lithium carbonate and she has also been prescribed antidepressants in the past. She has had six previous suicide attempts, all by overdose. Some of these attempts have led to general hospital admission, including a brief period in intensive care when she took her prescribed amitriptyline ten years ago.

Maureen smokes heavily and has a number of physical health problems, including asthma. She has two grown-up daughters, one of whom also has a diagnosis of bipolar disorder. Despite her daughters growing up mainly in the care of their father and paternal grandmother, they have recently made contact with Maureen and are visiting her every month.

When Maureen is hypomanic she presents as very grandiose, and this has led to altercations with family members, with members of the public, and with staff and patients during admissions. Maureen has suffered a number of losses in recent years, including an older sister with whom she was very close; her sister died from cancer at this time of year three years ago.

Maureen has not had a hospital admission for three years and has been quite stable. Her care coordinator has recently left the CMHT. Maureen's partner's mental health is currently unstable. Maureen does not have a history of substance misuse, except that she may drink heavily when she is either hypomanic or depressed. Some of her suicide attempts have been impulsive whilst under the influence of alcohol.

Box 15.7 offers an example of a formulation for Maureen.

Box 15.7 Formulation: Maureen

Maureen presents with a risk of harm to herself. This could take the form of a suicide attempt or self-neglect. There is a long-term risk of both a suicide attempt and self-neglect. There are a number of dynamic, primarily contextual factors that potentially increase the current likelihood of self-neglect or a suicide attempt occurring. The risk will last until these dynamic factors are addressed by Maureen and her care team. The factors currently contributing to risk are:

Static: statistical	Dynamic: contextual
History of suicide attempts	Physical health needs
History of bipolar affective disorder	Recent regained contact with adult daughters
	Anniversary of death of sister
	Care coordinator has left CMHT
	Partner's mental health is unstable

The **management plan** is to:

1 Allocate a new care coordinator.

2 Care coordinator to offer supportive time to talk about the contact with Maureen's daughters and the anniversary of the loss of her sister. Referral/offer of formal counselling if needed.

3 Liaise with Maureen's partner's care coordinator and have a joint meeting to discuss Maureen's support needs as a carer for her partner.

4 Maureen and new care coordinator to monitor her mental state for possible increase in hypomanic symptoms or symptoms of depression, e.g. grandiose ideas, irritability and arguments increasing at home, suicidal ideation, or evidence of low mood. Also monitor levels of drinking, because this is an early sign of deteriorating mental state.

5 Offer support with smoking cessation, and help Maureen to seek support from primary health care services for her physical health needs.

6 Should Maureen's mental health deteriorate, drinking increase, and suicidal ideation, intent, and planning increase, Maureen would like to be considered for home treatment or respite care rather than admission to an inpatient mental health unit.

▲ Conclusion

Effective risk assessment and management relies on the risks being clearly identified through the use of structured clinical judgement. Risk must be articulated clearly, both in documentation through the use of a formulation but also through effective communication with relevant people on a need-to-know basis. In order to engage in effective risk assessment and management, the service user and carer must be involved from the outset. When a risk is identified, the clinical and contextual factors should form the basis for intervention. Plans to manage the risk should include measurable goals for improvement. Positive risk taking is possible when risk has been shown to have reduced; early warning signs of risk increase are described overtly. All risk assessment and management plans should include contingency plans for intervention when risk is increasing; advanced decisions on the part of service users can help in risk management (DH 2007).

w Website

You may find it helpful to work through our short online quiz and scenario intended to help you to develop and apply the skills in this chapter. Please go to:

 www.oxfordtextbooks.co.uk/orc/callaghan

✚ References

Commonwealth of Australia (2007). *Living is for Everyone: A Framework for Prevention of Suicide in Australia.* www.health.gov.au/internet/wcms/ publishing.nsf/Content/CEA901E9FE08EC4ECA25737 60083A127/$File/frame.pdf [accessed 17 Jan 2008].

Department of Health (1999a). *A National Service Framework for Mental Health.* London: DH. www. dh.gov.uk/en/Publicationsandstatistics/Publications/ PublicationsPolicyAndGuidance/DH_4009598 [accessed 17 Jan 2008].

Department of Health (1999b). *Effective Care Co-ordination in Mental Health Services: Modernising the Care Programme Approach—A Policy Booklet.* London: DH. www.dh.gov.uk/en/ Publicationsandstatistics/Publications/ PublicationsPolicyAndGuidance/DH_4009221 [accessed 17 Jan 2008].

Department of Health (2002). *National Suicide Prevention Strategy for England.* London: DH. http:// www.dh.gov.uk/assetRoot/04/01/95/48/04019548. pdf [accessed 17 Jan 2008].

Department of Health (2004). *The NHS Knowledge and Skills Framework (NHS KSF) and the Development Review Process.* London: DH. www.

dh.gov.uk/en/Publicationsandstatistics/Publications/ Publications-PolicyAndGuidance/DH_4090843 [accessed 17 Jan 2008].

Department of Health (2006a). *Best Practice Competencies and Capabilities for Pre-registration Mental Health Nurses in England: The Chief Nursing Officer's Review of Mental Health Nursing.* London: DH. www.dh.gov.uk/en/Publicationsandstatistics/ Publications/PublicationsPolicyAndGuidance/ DH_4135647 [accessed 17 Jan 2008].

Department of Health (2006b). *From Values to Action: The Chief Nursing Officer's Review of Mental Health Nursing.* London: DH. www.dh.gov.uk/en/Publication- sandstatistics/Publications/PublicationsPolicy- AndGuidance/DH_4133839 [accessed 17 Jan 2008].

Department of Health (2007). *Best Practice in Managing Risk: Principles and Evidence for Best Practice in the Assessment and Management of Risk to Self and Others in Mental Health Services.* London: DH. www.dh.gov.uk/en/Publicationsandstatistics/ Publications/PublicationsPolicyAndGuidance/ DH_076511 [accessed 17 Jan 2008].

Langhan, J. and Lindow, V. (2004). *Living with risk. Mental Health Service User Involvement in Risk Assessment and Management.* Bristol: The Policy

Press. www.jrf.org.uk/knowledge/findings/socialcare/414.asp [accessed 17 Jan 2008].

Maden, T. (2006). *Review of Homicides by Patients with Severe Mental Illness.* London: National Institute for Mental Health.

Morgan, S. (2000). *Clinical Risk Management. A Clinical Tool and Practitioner Manual.* London: The Sainsbury Centre for Mental Health.

National Institute for Health and Clinical Excellence (2004). *Self-harm. The Short Term Physical and Psychological Management and Secondary Prevention of Self-harm in Primary and Secondary Care. Clinical Guideline 16.* London: NICE. www.nice.org.uk/guidance/index.jsp?action=byID&o=10946 [accessed 17 Jan 2008].

National Institute for Health and Clinical Excellence (2005). *Violence—The Short-term Management of Disturbed/Violent Behaviour in In-patient Psychiatric Settings and Emergency Departments. Clinical Guideline 25.* London: NICE. www.nice.org.uk/guidance/index.jsp?action=byID&o=10964 [accessed 17 Jan 2008].

National Institute for Mental Health in England (2004). *Emerging Best Practice in Mental Health Recovery.* London: NIMHE.

National Institute for Mental Health in England (2007). *National Suicide Prevention Strategy for England. Annual Report on Progress 2006.* Leeds: NIMHE. www.nimhe.csip.org.uk/silo/files/national-suicide-prevention-strategy-for-england-annual-report-on-progress-2006.pdf [accessed 17 Jan 2008].

National Statistics (2007). *Corrected Suicide Rates for the UK 1991–2004.* www.statistics.gov.uk/downloads/theme_health/Corrected_suicide_data_22Feb07.xls [accessed 17 Jan 2008].

Nursing and Midwifery Council (2006). *A–Z Advice Sheet: Confidentiality.* London: NMC. www.nmc-uk.org/aFrameDisplay.aspx?DocumentID=1560 [accessed 17 Jan 2008].

O'Rourke, M. and Bird, L. (2001). *Risk Management in Mental Health. A Practical Guide to Individual Care and Community Safety.* London: Mental Health Foundation.

Skills for Health (2007). *Skills for Health Competence Application Tools: Mental Health Framework.* http://www.skillsforhealth.org.uk/tools/view_framework.php?id=62 [accessed 17 Jan 2008].

University of Manchester (2006). *Avoidable Deaths: Five Year Report of the National Confidential Inquiry into Suicides and Homicides by People with Mental Illness.* www.medicine.manchester.ac.uk/suicideprevention/nci/Useful/avoidable_deaths.pdf [accessed 17 Jan 2008].

Vinestock, M. (1996). **Risk assessment. 'A word to the wise'?** *Advances in Psychiatric Treatment* 2, 3–10.

(16) Practising safe and effective observation

Julia Jones   Sarah Eales

▼ Introduction

This chapter addresses the core skill of **observation.** It is quite confusing for everyone (nurses, service users, carers) that there is no universal term used to describe the procedure of observation. Instead the procedure is known by a number of different terms in different places and countries. Here is a list of some of the terms you may encounter in your reading and practice: nursing observation; formal observation; close observation; special observation; maximum observation; continuous or constant observation or supervision; suicide watch or precaution; 15-minute, timed, or intermittent checks; specialing; one-to-one nursing; within eyesight; within arm's length. In this chapter, for purposes of consistency, the simple term of 'observation' is used.

The main purpose of observation is to keep people safe when they are acutely mentally ill and disturbed. It is a commonly used intervention for service users 'at risk' of harming themselves or others, or at risk of being harmed or exploited by others. The procedure of observation is generally carried out according to prescribed 'levels' of observation, which vary in intensity according to the degree of perceived risk. Service users assessed to be at greatest risk of harming themselves or others are nursed on the highest level of observation, with service users never being left alone by nurses, and with the nurse often within 'arm's reach' of the service user.

The Chief Nursing Officer's (CNO) Review of Mental Health Nursing (Department of Health [DH] 2006) identified risk and risk management as a key area requiring good practice guidance, with the ultimate aim of improving outcomes for service users. Regarding observation specifically, the CNO review specifies that mental health nurses are required to:

'Demonstrate an understanding of the benefits and limitations of the use of levels of observation to maximise therapeutic effect on inpatient units'

DH (2006, p. 29)

As noted in this extract from the CNO report, observation is designed to be a therapeutic intervention, yet it is acknowledged that there are benefits, limitations, and challenges involved. The challenge for nurses who conduct observation is to maintain the safety of 'high risk' service users, whilst maintaining their dignity, privacy, and autonomy.

Learning outcomes

By the end of this chapter you should be better able to:

1 Be aware of the current research evidence and best practice guidance regarding observation

2 Understand the core skills and competencies required to observe service users 'at risk' in an effective and supportive way

3 Understand the potential benefits and limitations of conducting observation at different levels of intensity

4 Be aware of service users' accounts of the experience of being observed by nurses.

The evidence base

There is very little evidence regarding the effectiveness of observation. There are various policies and good practice documents regarding observation, at both national and local levels. However, many of the current policies and guidance are based on expert guidance and recommendations, rather than actual research 'evidence'. This is because there has been very little research conducted that tells us for sure how therapeutic, effective, and 'safe' observation really is. In this section, the main principles of observation are described and the current evidence base discussed.

What is observation?

Observation is a commonly used mental health nursing intervention for service users who are assessed to be at risk of harming themselves or others, or at risk of being harmed or exploited by others (Bowers and Park 2001). It involves the allocation of one nurse (although sometimes two or even more nurses—up to five—have been reported) to one service user for a prescribed length of time in order to provide intensive nursing care. A widely used definition of observation is from the practice guidance *Safe and Supportive Observation of Patients at Risk,* from the Standing Nursing and Midwifery Advisory Committee (SNMAC) report *Addressing Acute Concerns* (DH 1999b). This definition is shown in Box 16.1. As highlighted by this quotation, a great challenge for nurses who conduct observation is to maintain the safety of 'high risk' service users, whilst minimizing the custodial nature of the intervention.

Observation can be used as an intervention in a number of different situations, as highlighted in Box 16.2. Some studies have demonstrated that particular characteristics of service users, in terms of their age, sex, and diagnosis, can also make some individuals more likely to require intensive forms of observation (Childs et al. 1994, Phillips et al. 1977), for example

---

Box 16.1 Definition of observation

Observation is defined as:

'Regarding the service user attentively while minimising the extent to which they feel that they are under surveillance'

Department of Health (1999b, p. 2)

Box 16.2 Main reasons for observation

Observation is typically used for service users who are:

- Suicidal or actively interested in harming themselves
- Aggressive and who pose a danger to staff or other service users
- Vulnerable
- Likely to abscond
- Sexually disinhibited.

Derived from Bowers and Park 2001, Bowers et al. 2000

---

young male schizophrenia sufferers who are deemed to be suicidal or who have behavioural problems; depressed older and suicidal female service users; and service users suffering from a personality disorder.

Observation and suicide

As indicated in Box 16.2, service users who are suicidal or at risk of self-harm are a particular group who may require observation. The purpose of observing service users who are suicidal or at risk of self-harm is to keep service users safe, and to also support service users in **feeling** safe. Indeed, research that asked service users about observation demonstrated that the interpersonal aspect of observation is important, with supportive interactions with staff enhancing service users' feelings of safety and hope (Cardell and Pitula 1999, Jones et al. 2000a,b, Pitula and Cardell 1996). However, an influential report *Avoidable Deaths* (National Confidential Inquiry into Suicide and Homicide by People with Mental Illness 2006) has shown that a minority of service users do not remain safe in hospital, even when they are being observed closely by nurses. This study found that out of all suicides in England and Wales during that period, 27% (6367 individuals) were by current or recent mental health inpatients. Some 856 of these individuals had actually committed suicide whilst in hospital, and of these 185 (22% of all inpatient suicides) were at the time (or supposedly) under observation, with 18 (3%) of these cases reported to be under the most intensive one-to-one observation when the suicide occurred. Although these figures may seem relatively small, it clearly demonstrates that observation is not 100% effective in preventing inpatient suicides.

Observation and disturbed/violent behaviour

Observation is a primary intervention in the recognition, prevention, and therapeutic management of violence (National Institute for Health and Clinical Excellence [NICE] 2005, UK Central Council for Nursing, Midwifery and Health Visiting [UKCC] 2002). The NICE guidance recommends the use of observation as an intervention for the short-term management of disturbed/violent behaviour in both mental health and emergency department settings.

Observation levels

A key component of all observation policies is the prescribed 'level' of observation. This section describes current good practice guidance regarding observation levels in England, Wales, and Scotland. Despite national initiatives to standardize observation policies and procedures, it is still largely the case that observation policies are developed and implemented at the local level, i.e. within an individual hospital or Trust. There remains variation and debate in different places and between experts regarding the number, terminology, and nature of levels to be used.

In England and Wales, the SNMAC practice guidance recommends four levels of observation (DH 1999b) (Box 16.3). These levels have since been adopted by the NICE (2005) guideline on the short-term management of disturbed/violent behaviour.

In Scotland, a good practice statement regarding nursing observation has been in existence since 1995 and was revised in 2002 by the Clinical Resource and Audit Group (CRAG 2002). The CRAG (2002) Good Practice Statement has three levels of observation: general, constant, and special (Box 16.4).

A significant difference between the practice guidance in England and Wales, compared with the good practice statement in Scotland, is that the SNMAC guidance recommends the use of intermittent observation, whereas the CRAG good

practice statement does not. This difference is a significant one and represents differences in opinion amongst many mental health practitioners regarding the usefulness of intermittent observation. CRAG (2002) state that timed observations do not contribute to the safety of service users. Similar concerns are highlighted in the *Avoidable Deaths* report, in response to the 185 inpatient deaths among service users who were under observation when they committed suicide. However, research reported by Bowers et al. (2007) found that the more intermittent observation used on a ward, the lower the rate of self-harm.

Are there alternatives to observation?

Some commentators have called for a review of the practice of observation *per se* because they believe that observing service users has become primarily a custodial task, rather than a therapeutic intervention (Barker and Cutcliffe 1999, Cutcliffe and Barker 2002, Dodds and Bowles 2001). '*Despite the rhetoric of "supportive observation", the nurse is often construed as a custodian, if not simply the doorman*', wrote Barker and Cutcliffe (1999, p. 11). It is clearly not good practice simply to 'watch or guard' service users (CRAG 2002). Indeed, service users have reported such practices as intrusive, making them feel unsupported (Cardell and Pitula 1999, Jones et al. 2000a). Nurses have also reported the custodial nature of observation as stressful and unrewarding (Cleary et al. 1999, Duffy 1995).

There are no 'proven' effective alternatives to observation. However, there are different kinds of 'evidence' that can be considered on this issue. A good case study to discuss here is the work of Dodds and Bowles (2001) on an inner-city male inpatient admission ward in Bradford, England. The authors report on a 'refocusing' practice development project, implemented to reduce the use of observation. During the project the nursing staff, with support of the rest of the multidisciplinary team, totally reorganized the 'culture' of patient care and nursing practice on the ward, with a structured programme of individualized activity for patients, involving greater patient/service user contact and engagement. As a result, service users were more engaged with their named nurses, better informed, and more involved in their care. Importantly, the project was successful in significantly reducing the use of observation on the ward. Other changes on the ward that have also been evaluated included significant reductions in: incidents of deliberate self-harm; incidents of violence and aggression; absconding; and staff sickness. A positive outcome of the reduction in staff sickness was cost savings, with fewer agency and bank staff required (Dodds and Bowles 2001).

Box 16.3 Four levels of observation recommended in England and Wales (DH 1999b)

Level I

General observation is the minimum acceptable level of observation for all inpatients. The location of all service users should be known to staff, but not all patients need to be kept within sight.

Level II

Intermittent observation means that the service user's location must be checked every 15–30 minutes (exact times to be specified in the notes).

Level III

Within eyesight is required when the service user could, at any time, make an attempt to harm themselves or others. The service user must be kept within sight at all times, day and night.

Level IV

Within arm's length is for service users at the highest levels of risk of harming themselves or others, who may need to have nurses in close proximity. On rare occasions more than one nurse may be necessary.

Box 16.4 Three levels of observation recommended in Scotland (CRAG 2002)

General observation

The staff on duty should have knowledge of the service user's general whereabouts at all times, whether in or out of the ward.

Constant observation

The staff member should be constantly aware of the precise whereabouts of the service user through visual observation or hearing.

Special observation

The service user should be in sight and within arm's reach of a member of staff at all times and in all circumstances.

The work of Dodds and Bowles (2001) in Bradford is considered by many to be innovative and to demonstrate good practice. However, it is important to remember that one must be cautious of making generalizations from such a small case study (i.e. a single ward). Despite this cautionary note, the achievements in Bradford certainly demonstrate that the practice of observation cannot be changed in isolation. In order to reduce the use of observation, the Bradford nursing team totally reorganized the 'culture' of nursing practice on the ward, with dedicated time for patient/service user contact and engagement. Thus, the key principle underpinning this work was not just the nature of the range of activities that occurred on the ward, but their function as a 'gift of time', which we know is highly valued by service users (Jackson and Stevenson 1998). The results of the Bradford project highlight the fact that if the practice of observation is to be challenged and improved it has to involve a cultural shift within the clinical team regarding acute inpatient care *per se*, not just observation in isolation.

Step-by-step description

This section focuses upon some key principles for the actual practice of observation. It is divided into three parts:

1 Before observation—deciding whether or not to use observation)

2 During observation

3 After observation.

Before observation

Decision-making process

The SNMAC guidance and the CRAG good practice statement recommend that, wherever possible, decisions about observation should be made jointly by the multidisciplinary team. Such a decision should be based upon an assessment of risk using an evidence-based risk assessment tool, a consideration of the service user's history, and an interview with the service user and his/her carer or advocate, as requested by the service user (see Chapter 15).

Decisions regarding observation are made at various different stages of the procedure: whether or not observation is required; on which level of observation to place a service user; whether to either increase or decrease the intensity of observation; and when to terminate observation. These decisions should also be reviewed regularly. The SNMAC guidance recommends that a service user's observation status should be reviewed by a doctor and the primary nurse or ward sister/charge nurse every day (including weekends). For the most intensive level of observation—within arm's length—there should be three reviews, two during the day and one during the night shift (DH 1999b).

It is essential that all decisions are recorded in a service user's clinical notes by a member of the multidisciplinary team, including the name of the person conducting the observation, and the time they commenced and concluded their period of observation. It is also recommended that a detailed record of the service user's behaviour, mental state, and attitude to observation be recorded every 15 minutes. The SNMAC practice guidance states that the records should include the information detailed in Box 16.5.

Conducting observation

An essential skill when conducting observation is to engage positively with service users. This involves the development of a two-way relationship, established between a service user and a staff member, that is meaningful, grounded in trust, and therapeutic for the service user (UKCC 2002). Spending time with service users, whether engaged in activities, discussion, or simply 'being' with them, is essential for nurses to conduct an effective assessment and monitor the service user's behaviour and mental state (CRAG 2002).

A care plan should be created to identify the rationale for the current level of observation, including the current risks and the service user's mental state. The therapeutic interventions that

Box 16.5 Documentation of observation decisions (DH 1999b)

- Current mental state
- Current assessment of risk
- Specific level of observation to be implemented
- Clear directions regarding therapeutic approach (i.e. occupation, therapy sessions)
- Timing of next review

the nurse is expected to undertake and also how the service user will be monitored to determine both improvement and also potential deterioration in risk should be included in the care plan. Clear documentation of the nursing role and the interaction with the service user during each period of observation should be made. An effective handover from one observer to another should be carried out before and after every period of observation that includes an evaluation of the care plan. This is important to ensure continuity of care and that the service user is not offered the same interventions for the duration of observation (CRAG 2002).

Therapeutic activities, from assisting with personal hygiene through to supporting the service user to understand the triggers and signs of deterioration in their mental health that have led to the current situation, can serve as an effective method of observing an individual's level of functioning during observation. Some practical ideas for therapeutic activities during observation are provided in the CRAG (2002) *Good Practice Statement* and shown in Box 16.6.

Who should conduct observation?

To date there has been no research conducted to tell us who (qualified or non-qualified staff) is most effective in terms of providing the 'best' and 'safest' observation. Evidence shows that different people perform the 'observer' role, including: qualified nurses; unqualified nurses; nursing and medical students; agency nurses; family members; friends; and volunteers (Bowers and Park 2001).

The SNMAC practice guidance adopts a rather unhelpful position on this issue, stating that '*it is impossible to stipulate exactly who should carry out this task*' (DH 1999b, p. 4). The CRAG (2002) good practice statement states that observation can be delegated to unqualified members of staff who have had the relevant training, but that the qualified nurse in charge must ensure that their unqualified colleague knows why the service user is being

Box 16.6 Practical suggestions for activities during observation (based on CRAG 2002)

- *Activities of daily living:* assist individuals to maintain self-care, maintaining some responsibility and dignity. Assist with bed-making, tidying room, and doing personal laundry. Support to write letters and/or make telephone calls.
- *Social interaction:* respect a patient's right for silence. If a patient wishes to talk, don't talk only about symptoms but introduce general conversation topics. Remember the habit of talking **at** the patient may be due to a staff member's personal difficulty with silence.
- *Clinical interaction:* a spell of uninterrupted contact allows time for brief psychological interventions, focusing on negative or intrusive thought patterns, reality checking and problem solving, or self-harming thoughts. Self-help and guided materials can be used during this time.
- *Ask the service user* what would be helpful to them at that moment in time. Is there anything in the service user's history that could be discussed further with benefit?
- *Respect a service user's wishes* within safety boundaries, within the current level of observation. For example, open the door or sit outside the room if the service user's mental state is deteriorating as a consequence of the close proximity of the observation.
- *Utilize on-ward occupational therapy* to assist service users in engaging in activities.
- *Make an appointment for the service user with their named nurse* to ensure planned contact and to provide service users with a chance to discuss concerns and frustrations.

observed and the purpose of the observation. However, CRAG (2002) cautions the excessive use of temporary and casual staff for this task. A similar standpoint is adopted by the SNMAC guidance, which states: '*it is undesirable for someone who does not know the ward or the service user to be responsible for observing a service user who is suicidal, vulnerable or violent*' (DH 1999b, p. 4). Research from the service user perspective supports this position; service users stated that being observed by someone they didn't know made them feel less safe, and this was particularly the case for suicidal patients (Jones et al. 2000b).

Involving service users and carers

A guiding value of the *National Service Framework for Mental Health* (DH 1999a) is that service users and their carers are involved in the planning and delivery of their care. A major complaint amongst service users who experience observation is the lack of information provided; service users have reported that sometimes they were not informed that they were being observed (Cardell and Pitula 1999, Jones et al. 2000a). It is imperative that every effort is made to involve service users and their carers/friends in the decision-making process regarding observation, and staff must ensure that the procedure and the reasons for its implementation are explained clearly.

The care plan that accompanies any period of observation should also involve the service user. The service user should continue to be engaged through explanation and evaluation of the care plan, to assist in building and maintaining the therapeutic relationship. When appropriate, each handover from one observer to another and each evaluation of the care plan should also include the service user. This ensures that the service user becomes an active participant in the period of observation, able to make their feelings heard about its usefulness (or not) and the effectiveness of the interventions agreed in the care plan. With the service user's permission an explanation of the plan of care, including the rationale for observation, should also be provided to the service user's carer. The carer's feedback on the care plan should be considered, as their knowledge and experience of the service user may help to explain the service user's presentation and inform the choice of appropriate therapeutic interventions.

Gender, ethnicity, and culture

The issues of gender, ethnicity, and culture remain relatively 'invisible' at the present time in the literature on observation. Regarding gender, two studies have shown that women are placed on more intensive levels of observation compared with men (Kettles 2001, Shugar and Rehaluk 1990). However, we know little regarding the reasons to explain these gender differences. A number of reports have highlighted problems around the care and safety of women in acute inpatient psychiatric settings (Mental Health Act Commission 2005, Mind 2004, National Patient Safety Agency 2006). With the recognition of the need to establish better provision for women, it would seem important to ask women (and also men) if they

would prefer an observer of the same or different gender, as far as staffing situations allow. This is particularly important for the more intensive levels of observation, where a nurse may need to accompany a service user to the bathroom. Such awareness of gender issues around observation should certainly be paid greater attention than presently received in the SNMAC practice guidance or the CRAG good practice statement.

It is essential that people from ethnic minority communities receive care that is sensitive to their cultural and religious backgrounds. With regard to observation, for example, the gender or cultural background of a nurse observing a service user from a different cultural or religious background may make the service user feel uneasy because of their particular beliefs or values. In addition, particular dietary or religious activities that a service user may wish to adhere to whilst they are being observed require particular attention and sensitivity by staff. Such issues can be addressed through training and other activities aimed to raise staff's awareness and understanding of the religious and cultural needs of ethnic minority service users. Language is also an important issue; for a growing number of service users, English will not be their first language, and the provision and access to interpreters in many units and Trusts in the UK is variable (Sainsbury Centre for Mental Health 2000). This problem is significant in terms of involving service users in decisions about their care and informing them of what their care may involve and the reasons for any decisions made.

Box 16.7 Topics for discussion with the service user after observation

- The positives and negatives about the experience of observation.

- Ask the service user if they understood the reasons why observation was instigated and any difference between this and the professional's understanding of the purpose.

- What caused the deterioration in mental state that increased risk and required observation?

- What could be done both by the service user and the nurse to prevent the need for observation in future?

- Drawing up advanced decisions about preferences related to observation should the need arise in the future.

After observation

After a period of observation has ceased the service user should be offered the opportunity to explore their feelings about the intervention. Some possible topics to explore are shown in Box 16.7. It should be acknowledged that for some nurses this may prove difficult, particularly if the service user was hostile to observation or the risk of harm was high. Clinical supervision can play an important role in allowing the nurse to debrief and reflect upon undertaking what has already been acknowledged to be a challenging

---

✖ Practice Example

This section contains a case study about a man called Adrian who is admitted to an acute inpatient psychiatric ward and placed on constant (within eyesight) observation because of his risk of suicide. Read the case study and then think about some appropriate therapeutic activities to undertake with Adrian. Then compare your ideas with our suggestions in Box 16.8.

Case study
Adrian is in his early thirties and has a history of schizophrenia since the age of 19. His symptoms are typified by him hearing command auditory hallucinations whose content switches between harming others and Adrian himself. When acutely unwell he believes he has a transmitter inside his head that gives him these instructions. Whilst in the community he has previously self-harmed in attempts to remove the transmitter he believed was in one of his ears. Adrian usually lives with his mother and has no social contacts or activities. His main coping strategy for the voices is listening to music, usually via headphones, but this is not guaranteed to work all of the time. He has a long history of poly-substance abuse and does not understand the need to take medication. He has just been admitted to an acute unit in order to stabilize his schizophrenia, but also because he currently poses a suicide risk. Adrian currently believes that the transmitter is inside his head.

> **Box 16.8** Suggested therapeutic activities whilst observing Adrian constantly (within eyesight)
>
> 1 Explain the meaning of constant observation to both Adrian and his mother. Explain why the level of observation has been prescribed. Provide this information in different formats (e.g. verbal explanation, written information).
>
>   *Rationale:* To ensure the service user and carer both understand the nature and purpose of observation.
>
> 2 Explain what constant observation will involve, for example regular changes in staff, drafting a care plan, handovers from one nurse to another.
>
>   *Rationale:* To ensure both the service user and carer understand what will happen to Adrian during observation.
>
> 3 Plan with Adrian how he would like to spend the next 24 hours, encouraging a combination of activities of daily living, therapeutic relationship building, social interaction, clinical interactions, and time with his named nurse.
>
>   *Rationale:* Engage the service user in the process of observation, offering choice wherever possible.
>
> 4 Clinical interaction might include learning about Adrian's illness from his perspective, exploring early signs to deterioration, learning about current coping strategies, and discussing alternative strategies.
>
>   *Rationale:* Collect information for completion of full assessment of Adrian and his strengths/needs. Begin problem solving and identifying management strategies to reduce risk.
>
> 5 Assessment and monitoring of mental state considering particularly the intensity of auditory hallucinations, whether they remain command, exploration of delusions regarding the transmitter, and ideation, intensity, and plan for self-harm to remove transmitter. Plus assessment of feelings of harm to others.
>
>   *Rationale:* Utilize a method of assessment to identify potential improvement or deterioration in risk that may lead to decreasing or increasing the level of observation.

caring role. CRAG (2002) recommends that in the case of an untoward incident occurring either before or during observation, a thorough critical incident review (CIR) should take place.

▲ Conclusion

This chapter has described the core skills and competencies required to observe service users 'at risk' on acute inpatient psychiatric wards. It is problematic that there is no real 'evidence base' for the effective practice of observation, with a paucity of large-scale research studies on observation. Instead this chapter has referred a great deal to the existing written guidance on observation, specifically the SNMAC practice guidance (DH 1999b) and the CRAG (2002) good practice statement. What is still required is rigorous evaluative research to assess the effectiveness of such practice guidance.

It is undeniable that, for nurses, observing a service user who is deeply distressed and potentially suicidal or aggressive is one of the most difficult and demanding roles to undertake. It involves the challenge of maintaining the safety of service users, whilst minimizing the custodial nature of the intervention. As highlighted by Duffy (1995), conducting observation reveals the inherent tension around service user-focused care, because the aim of 'keeping someone safe' may in reality mean having to stop a service user from doing something they are intent on doing, for example: attempting to harm themselves in some way; attempting to abscond; or behaving aggressively towards others. However, evidence from service users' accounts of the experience of being observed tells us that, when observation is conducted by nurses who engage with them in a supportive way, therapeutic benefits can include feeling cared for, protected, safer, and more optimistic (Cardell and Pitula 1999, Jones et al. 2000a). This is what mental health nurses should strive to achieve in their practice of observation.

W Website

You may find it helpful to work through our short online quiz intended to help you to develop and apply the skills in this chapter. Please go to:

 www.oxfordtextbooks.co.uk/orc/callaghan

✚ References

Barker, P. and Cutcliffe, J. (1999). Clinical risk: a need for engagement not observation. *Mental Health Practice* 2(8), 8–12.

Bowers, L. and Park, A. (2001). Special observation in the care of psychiatric inpatients: a literature review. *Issues in Mental Health Nursing* 22, 769–86.

Bowers, L., Gournay, K., and Duffy, D. (2000). Suicide and self-harm in inpatient psychiatric units: a national survey of observation policies. *Journal of Advanced Nursing* 32(2), 437–44.

Bowers, L., Whittington, R., Nolan P., et al. (2007). *The City 128 Study of Observation and Outcomes on Acute Psychiatric Wards. Report to the NHS SDO Programme*. London: NHS SDO Programme.

Cardell, R. and Pitula, C. R. (1999). Suicidal inpatients' perceptions of therapeutic and nontherapeutic aspects of constant observation. *Psychiatric Services* 50, 1066–70.

Childs, A., Thomas, B., and Tibbles, P. (1994). Specialist needs. *Nursing Times* 90(3), 32–3.

Cleary, M., Jordan, R., Horsfall, J., Mazoudier, P., and Delaney, J. (1999). Suicidal patients and special observation. *Journal of Psychiatric and Mental Health Nursing* 6, 461–7.

Clinical Resource and Audit Group (2002). *Engaging People: Observation of People with Acute Mental Health Problems: A Good Practice Statement*. Edinburgh: Scottish Executive.

Cutcliffe, J. and Barker, P. (2002). Considering the care of the suicidal client and the case for 'engagement and inspiring hope' or 'observations'. *Journal of Psychiatric and Mental Health Nursing* 9, 611–21.

Department of Health (1999a). *A National Service Framework for Mental Health*. London: HMSO.

Department of Health (1999b). *Practice Guidance: Safe and Supportive Observation of Patients at Risk. Mental Health Nursing—Addressing Acute Concerns.* London: HMSO.

Department of Health (2006). *Best Practice Competencies and Capabilities for Pre-registration Mental Health Nurses in England. The Chief Nursing Officer's Review of Mental Health Nursing.* London: HMSO.

Dodds, P. and Bowles, N. (2001). Dismantling formal observation and refocusing nursing activity in acute inpatient psychiatry: a case study. *Journal of Psychiatric and Mental Health Nursing* 8, 183–8.

Duffy, D. (1995). Out of the shadows: a study of the special observation of suicidal psychiatric in-patients. *Journal of Advanced Nursing* 21(5), 944–50.

Jackson, S. and Stevenson, C. (1998). The gift of time from the friendly professional. *Nursing Standard* 12(51), 31–3.

Jones J., Lowe, T., and Ward, M. (2000a). Inpatients' experiences of nursing observation on an acute psychiatric unit: a pilot study. *Mental Health Care* 4(4), 125–9.

Jones J., Ward M., Wellman N., Hall J., and Lowe, T. (2000b). Psychiatric inpatients' experiences of nursing observation—a UK perspective. *Journal of Psychosocial Nursing and Mental Health Services* 38(12), 10–20.

Kettles, A. (2001). *The relationship between self-harming behaviour and the level of observation patients are placed on at the time of admission: an exploratory study.* Conference presentation at the Seventh International Network for Psychiatric Nursing Research Conference, Oxford, UK, September 2001.

Mental Health Act Commission (2005). *In Place of Fear? The Eleventh Biennial Report of the Mental Health Act Commission.* London: The Stationery Office.

Mind (2004). *Ward Watch: Mind's Campaign to Improve Hospital Conditions for Mental Health Patients.* London: Mind.

National Confidential Inquiry into Suicide and Homicide by People with Mental Illness (2006). *Avoidable Deaths: Five Year Report of the National Confidential Inquiry into Suicide and Homicide by People with Mental Illness.* Manchester: University of Manchester.

National Institute for Health and Clinical Excellence (2005). *Violence: The Short-term Management of Disturbed/Violent Behaviour in In-patient Psychiatric Settings and Emergency Departments.* London: NICE.

National Patient Safety Agency (2006). *With Safety in Mind: Mental Health Services and Patient Safety.* London: National Patient Safety Agency.

Phillips, M., Peacocke, J., Hermanstyne, L., et al. (1977). Continuous observation—Part 1. *Canadian Psychiatric Association* 22, 25–8.

Pitula, C. R. and Cardell, R. (1996). Suicidal inpatients' experience of constant observation. *Psychiatric Services* 47(6), 649–51.

Sainsbury Centre for Mental Health (2000). *National Visit 2. Improving Care for Detained Patients from Black and Minority Ethnic Communities.* London: Sainsbury Centre for Mental Health.

Shugar, G. and Rehaluk, R. (1990). Continuous observation for psychiatric inpatients: a critical evaluation. *Comprehensive Psychiatry* 31(1), 48–55.

United Kingdom Central Council for Nursing, Midwifery and Health Visiting (2002). *The Recognition, Prevention and Therapeutic Management of Violence in Mental Health Care,* London: UKCC.

17 Recognition and therapeutic management of self-harm and suicidal behaviour

Martin Anderson   **Keith Waters**

▼ Introduction

In practice, mental health nurses inevitably encounter actions in people of what might seem to be superficial acts of harm to self through to clear attempts to end life. The chapter addresses this by providing background to the subject area and a brief epidemiological overview of the behaviour. Current policy is at the centre of guiding practice; therefore, we shall place this subject into this policy context. At the heart of working with an individual is the assessment of risk in people who **self-harm**. This will support negotiation and participation in ways of working therapeutically with people who are actively suicidal and those who repeat self-harming behaviour. The evidence and guidance in this chapter applies to people of all ages. Clinical scenarios will facilitate exploration of ways of working with different people. We include service user quotes (expressed in italics) to emphasize specific points.

Learning outcomes

By the end of this chapter you should be better able to:

1 Understand and be able to build on knowledge gained in relation to the practice of risk assessment and management of suicidal behaviour (Best Practice reference numbers: 2.4.1K, 2.4.2K, 2.4.3K) (Department of Health [DH] 2002, 2006, National Institute for Health and Clinical Excellence [NICE] 2004)

2 Recognize the need to include a range of health and social care professionals (nurses, doctors, social workers, police, ambulance staff, etc.) in the assessment and ongoing therapeutic work with people who self-harm (2.4.11K)

3 Employ the key principles of a person-centred approach—in particular recognize the ways in which individuals cope and the nature of response to life events and changes (2.4.8K)

4 Implement best practice in the use of the therapeutic relationship when assessing for risk of further **suicide** attempts and in working together with a person who self-harms or who has attempted suicide (2.4.6P and 2.4.8P)

5 Implement mental health promotion activity—mental, physical, and emotional well-being as protective factors in suicide prevention (DH 2002)

Evidence base and guidelines

Prevalence

Self-harm—intentional self-poisoning or **self-injury**, irrespective of the apparent purpose of the act—is a significant health and social issue in England and Wales, with approximately 170 000 hospital admissions each year (Hawton et al. 2006). The problem is prevalent in many other countries around the world (Department of Health and Ageing 2000, Department of Health, Social Services and Public Safety 2006, Ministry of Health 2006, Scottish Executive 2002). It is a major public health problem and an important risk factor for suicide (DH 2002, Johnston et al. 2006).

In the UK, hospital presentations most often involve self-poisoning; as many as 70–80% are **overdoses**. Over the past two to three decades, self-poisoning has become the most common cause of acute admission in females and the second most common reason for admission of males (Hawton et al. 2006). Approximately 1 in 15 people self-harm (Camelot Foundation/Mental Health Foundation 2006). The considerable increase in self-poisoning in recent decades has directed more attention to this problem (Hawton et al. 2004). However, it is hard to present a true picture of the extent of self-harm as data can be generated only for reported episodes of self-harm. The rate of self-harm is likely to be much higher than predictions because much self-harm goes unreported. Self-cutting is often repeated, and those who repeatedly self-harm may have a significant risk of suicide (Hawton et al. 2004).

People who self-harm often use general practitioners and present at emergency departments regularly. Some 15–23% of such people will be seen for treatment of self-harm within one year (3–5% of who may die by suicide within 5–10 years) (Bennewith et al. 2002). Self-harm is most frequently encountered in mental health or specialist mental health services. This includes forensic secure services, child and adolescent mental health services, and acute inpatient mental health services (Wildgoose and Williams 2007). Mental disorder is associated with an 11-fold increase in the risk of suicide. A half of those who complete suicide have previously been referred to mental health services and 25% have been in contact with services in the year before their death (Appleby et al. 2001, Kapur 2006, Lonnvist 2000). *The National Confidential Inquiry* is the formal process of auditing all suicides that occur in mental health services in England and Wales (Appleby et al. 2001). The 2001 report showed that, of 4859 suicides in contact with services, 2308 (47%) had had contact in the previous seven days and 3077 (63%) had a history of previous self-harm (Kapur 2006). Evidence from a case–control study carried out in Manchester adds to the importance of this fact. This work revealed that the most important independent clinical predictors of suicide were a previous history of self-harm and communicating suicidal thoughts in the period between discharge and death (Appleby et al. 1999). Given the strong association with suicide, a number of monitory studies of self-harm have been established as part of national strategies in several countries (Hawton et al. 2006); for example, these include: England (DH 2002), Scotland (Scottish Executive 2002), Ireland (Health Service Executive 2005), and Norway (Norwegian Board of Health 1995).

Suicide

Suicide is a global phenomenon. It is estimated that between 500 000 and 1.2 million people die by suicide each year worldwide. Concern is based on the personal, psychological, social, political, cultural, and economic impact the behaviour has on societies (Anderson and Jenkins 2006). This increase is reflected in the escalation of global suicide rates reported by the World Health Organization (WHO 1999). A 60% increase can be observed between 1950 and 1995, from 10.1 to 16 per 100 000. The distribution of global suicide rates according to age and sex also highlights an increase in most male age groups compared with those of female age groups (WHO 1999). The majority of suicides in England and other countries occur in males aged under 40 years. In comparison to women in the same age group, men are more likely to commit suicide. Most at risk are those in the 30–39 years age group, where there are four male suicides for each female suicide (National Institute for Mental Health in England [NIMHE] 2007). More recent evidence shows that the suicide rate in the general population and in young men in England is on a downward trend, yet, as in other countries, the overall suicide rate continues to cause concern (DH 2005, Ministry of Health 2006). The suicide rate in England is currently 5000 deaths per year.

Policy

National policy on suicide prevention now has an established history in England and other countries. Most recently, *The National Suicide Prevention Strategy for England* (DH 2002) set out the target to reduce the death rate from a baseline rate of 9.2 deaths per 100 000 population in 1995–1997 to 7.3 deaths per 100 000 population in 2009–2011. Arising out of the strategy are useful instruments for practitioners, including the Suicide Prevention Toolkit which is aimed at acute care audit of suicide and suicide risk (Duffy et al. 2003) and the NICE (2004) guidelines on the management of self-harm in primary and secondary care.

Assessing risk of suicide—a contemporary process model

Risk

The assessment of risk is never static: it is ongoing throughout the time of working with someone who has self-harmed or engaged in suicidal behaviour. It is important to recognize that the initial assessment itself can be very therapeutic to the person: '*It* [the person's difficulties] *has become much clearer now I have had the chance to talk.*' This may be the first time the person has been able to discuss their difficulties (Hawton 2000). Yet the process can be viewed as a combination of both **art** and **science**—and to this end it is rather 'inexact' (Cooper and Kapur 2004).

From a **scientific** point of view, psychological autopsy research studies indicate that a significant proportion of people who commit suicide have been in contact with primary care services prior to death. However, many have had no contact with health care services (Appleby et al. 1999). Such findings illustrate the role for the mental health, primary care, social, and voluntary services in the recognition and effective treatment of people who are suicidal (Cooper and Kapur 2004). Knowing what makes a person susceptible to suicide is a fundamental part of assessing risk. Using various data, particularly psychological autopsy studies, we can construct a picture of potential risk factors (Box 17.1). These are useful in practice.

Box 17.1 Risk factors for suicide (Hawton 2000, Cooper and Kapur 2004)

Gender

- Being male

Age

- Younger age group (19–34 years) and older age group (85+)

Health

- Physical health conditions—chronic medical illness

Social factors

- Unemployment and poverty
- Financial difficulties
- Legal problems
- Relationship problems
- Abuse—past, present (sexual, physical, emotional)
- Divorced, widowed, bereavement/loss, retirement
- Loss of parents through divorce or death during childhood
- Being single
- Living alone (also loneliness)/social isolation/social network
- Homelessness
- Social class (1 and 5)
- Occupation (professional groups)
- Being a prisoner/in criminal justice system
- Imitation and contagion—exposure to suicidal behaviour

Experience of mental health

- Previous history of self-harm/suicide attempts (especially where planned delay in discovery has been evident)
- Depression (other common mental health problems)

- Hopelessness (especially feeling of entrapment and unable to solve problems)
- Serious mental health problems
- Alcohol problems and drug misuse
- Personality disorder (co-morbid with other mental health problems)
- Family history of mental health problems (as above)
- Recent contact with mental health services

High intent

- Choice of method—violent (hanging, jumping in front of a train, shotgun)
- Access to means of suicide
- Plans for death (changing of will, family farewells)

However, the **art** is the skill of understanding these risk factors in the context of the individual. An important component of this 'art' is the much heralded expression 'the gut reaction': '*This doesn't feel right*'. If an individual causes concern, or when the picture does not appear to fit the information provided, there is usually a good reason for this. The gut reaction is not simply an intuitive response, but may be occurring at a more unconscious level, when the evidence being presented does not quite fit the picture. This may be a result of non-verbal communications, hidden messages, transferences occurring within the assessment process. Motto (1991) emphasizes the fact that the final decision regarding degree of suicide risk is a subjective one. He argues that it is important to accept that having gathered all the information possible, this 'intuitive sense' is our best guide to predicting risk (Motto 1991). Therefore, although we have assessment tools, scales, and tests to help in assessing risk, the important fact is **not** to rely solely on such devices but to attend to the individual's unique characteristics and circumstances (Hawton 2000).

The attitude and values of the carer

Later, we address some of the research indicating what service users have valued most in the carer during times of feeling suicidal. However, well before a full assessment (and subsequent therapeutic engagement) is planned, it is important for nurses to consider and explore their attitudes towards suicidal behaviour. In different professional groups and specialties, attitudes have been shown to be multifaceted and complex (Anderson and Standen 2007). Some of the fundamental questions are:

- What is my definition of self-harm?
- Should people be given the right to take their own life?
- How do I view people who self-harm?
- Is self-harm attention-seeking behaviour?

There may not be cut-and-dried answers to such questions, but the practitioner needs to consider their position regarding these issues, build self-awareness, and explore what impact this might have on the relationship. This is crucial not only in establishing a therapeutic relationship with the person but also in conducting an effective risk assessment.

Putting 'risk factors' into use

It is important to note that features of risk vary between groups, while circumstances in an individual can alter over time and so vulnerability may fluctuate (Cooper and Kapur 2004). These factors can be considered as individual components, but also viewed within a collective context. For example, clear indications of the 'risk times' are during inpatient admissions (National Confidential Inquiry 2006). The initial period of inpatient stay and the time around discharge are potentially risky times: *'Going home is too much'*. For an individual, it may be that there are many factors that, on their own, may be viewed as less significant, but together may become more influential. The emphasis is not so much on predicting suicide with certainty: it is using or identifying the risk factors that increase the likelihood (Cooper and Kapur 2004).

The mental health nurse needs to be constantly mindful of those situations where 'suicide risk' is present, for example where depression and schizophrenia have been identified (Bolton et al. 2007). There are times during such illnesses where the risks may be greater. For example, a person with severe depression starts to show improvement. This may be a time when the person begins to have the energy to carry through actions that they have previously only thought about, but not been able to carry through: *'I felt too ill before, but now I think I could do it'*. When the improvement starts, they may well be more at risk of acting on these thoughts than previously. In a classic study, Barraclough et al. (1974) found that more than half of the people diagnosed with depressive illness displayed warning signs of suicidal thinking, but the methods of modern psychiatric treatment were not implemented effectively. Therefore, the mental health nurse needs to use a structure in order to assess for **suicidal intent** and so utilize the 'risk factors' (see Box 17.1) effectively.

Barker (1997) offered a set of dimensions for assessment, which we have adapted below.

A: Preparing and setting the scene

Establish a rapport; use initial questions, such as: 'What has brought you to the services?', 'What has been the main problem?'.

B: Suicidal thoughts and person's view of the future

During the assessment we need to know whether the person feels a sense of hopelessness. Are they experiencing difficulty in solving problems? How do they see themselves now and in the future? Have they given up on life? The mental health nurse needs to know about the person's suicidal thoughts, ideas, and indeed plans. However, it may not always be the best approach to be asking directly and concretely whether the person is feeling suicidal or whether they have any plans to take their life. This is a process—we call it **stages of revelation**. Here, we allow the patient to feel at ease to discuss any suicidal thoughts and ideas, whilst also ensuring that they feel the nurse is taking them seriously and acknowledging their difficulties. Therefore, when interviewing a depressed patient it may be a useful starting point to ask: 'Have things been getting too much for you to cope with?'. This may lead the nurse to ask: 'Have you ever thought that you would prefer not to face a future event?', or 'Have you ever thought that you would prefer not to face the next day or your current problems and difficulties?'.

C: Clear 'gestures' at suicide

From here, the nurse then needs to check for signs of suicidal intent. Has the person prepared for this suicide attempt? Have plans been put into place? Was a suicide note included? Have wills recently been finalized? Have financial arrangements been made?

The line of questions in process (B) above can be followed by: 'Have you considered any ways in which you may wish to escape from the difficulties?'. The nurse can then check: 'Have you made some plans about this, preparations for it?'. They can also check whether indeed the person had wanted to die in order to feel an escape from the situation, and how they felt and dealt with these thoughts and ideas. If as a result of this the patient reveals various levels of **suicidal ideation**, this should be included in the risk assessment.

D: History of suicidal behaviour

Ask about previous attempts on life: What went on? What were the circumstances? What methods were used?

E: Family history of suicide

Check for a history of mental health problems, self-harm, suicidal behaviour. Are there any key events in family background that might be important?

F: Mental health difficulties

Ask and observe whether the person is suffering from depression, serious mental health problems (schizophrenia), other? For how long? How problematic?

G: Withdrawal and isolation

Does the person have a family or social network? Does the person live alone? Are they homeless?

H: Instruments to help the clinician during the assessment process

As mentioned earlier, the clinician's experience and subjective view will be crucial to the decision on risk of suicide in a person. Having a structure to work within is also fundamental. Evidence-based assessment tools and instruments can help in this process. These tools help to facilitate an objective and subjective assessment. For example, a number of scales developed by Aaron T. Beck continue to be favoured by clinicians; these scales have been subjected to validity test studies to demonstrate their effectiveness in practice (Beck and Weishaar 1990). The most commonly used scales are:

- **Beck Depression Inventory**—this is a 21-item self-report questionnaire. Each item contains statements that reflect increasing levels of intensity of a depressive symptom.
- **Suicide Intent Scale**—this is a clinical interview and rating scale for people who have recently attempted suicide. The scale helps to evaluate the severity of the person's psychological intent to die at the time of recent attempt at suicide. The scale examines aspects of the person's behaviour and thinking before, during, and after the attempt to end

their life. It also assists in identifying reasons behind the person's actions.

- **Scale for Suicidal Ideation**—this scale allows an assessment of the person's current thinking related to suicidal behaviour. It is a 19-item structured interview/rating scale that helps to assess the frequency, duration, and intensity of suicidal thoughts. It covers what might protect against suicide, history of suicide, final acts (leaving a note), ease of access to method, and the person's views on their wish to live or die.
- **Beck Hopelessness Scale**—this 20-item scale is a true–false self-report questionnaire that assesses the level of pessimism and negative views about the future.

These scales remain important and useful today, owing to the evidence that hopelessness, specific ideas, and plans increase risk in people who experience depression (Cooper and Kapur 2004). Such factors are essential in recognizing the risk of suicide. It is important for the clinician to be able to determine how these relate to other feelings and experiences, such as fatigue, anxiety, insomnia, confusion, anger, etc. (Williams et al. 2005).

The assessor's objective will be, where appropriate, to combine the results of the one-to-one assessment and the use of a suicide assessment scale. This will assist in the formulation of an overall risk assessment strategy and plan, particularly focusing on contingency arrangements (Hawton 2000). Screening and risk assessment tools provide a focus for the nurse, encouraging most of the known risk areas to be explored, measured, and recorded. This record is not only useful for the nurse at the time, but also forms part of the clinical record and thus will help inform others at future times, regarding the factors that were established. This will highlight aspects or areas of the person's life that may have helped to reduce risk previously, that is 'protective factors'. The student of methods of risk assessment should look further into the predictors of suicidal behaviour and use this knowledge when observing assessments being undertaken by experienced practitioners.

This work requires experience and is not for the novice. However, under close supervision it is possible to observe and practise. It is important to build on these skills. For mental health nurses, in most settings, a significant part of a risk assessment process is consultation and sharing. Therefore, good supervision and mentorship are required for risk assessment work.

Working with and supporting people who engage in self-harming and suicidal behaviour

Once a risk assessment has been completed, the mental health nurse will need to consider what options there are for further support and therapeutic management. Applying the above process, the following clinical examples provide an overview of some of the possible therapeutic/caring actions required in each case.

Remember that 'suicidal risk' is not static: the degree of suicidal ideation, plans, and associated risk can fluctuate at any time. When conducting assessments it is important to consider the contextual factors of the risk, identifying those aspects that will increase the risk, but also the more protective factors. These are important in formulating a care plan and actions to reduce the risk factors present. It is worth looking at the *Pathways to Suicide* described by Kerkhof and Arensman (2001), and to consider these in relation to the Practice Example of Darren below. Consider the points made in the section on 'risk' above. Use of appropriate evidence, such as psychological autopsy studies, will help clinicians to build a 'picture' of the pathway relating to an individual. What are the telling signs of Darren's vulnerability?

It is important to ensure the immediate safety of the person who may be at risk of suicidal behaviour once admitted to an inpatient unit. There is an important need for clear terminology and procedure in the use of observation when someone is at risk of suicidal behaviour (Bowers et al. 2000). Risk of self-harm and suicide is most often the reason for this intervention, but it is important to be sure of Trust policy, particularly for processes such as record-keeping. What the mental health nurse does when working with the person who has self-harmed or is at risk of suicide is crucial. Samuelsson et al. (2000) found that what patients on an inpatient ward valued most were: being cared for, receiving understanding, and confirmation. Being listened to without prejudice, establishing trust, and respect for personal integrity are also essential experiences for such patients (Talseth et al. 2001). Safety, care, compassion, and sensitivity are essential qualities during interventions (Sun et al. 2006). Being involved in 'own care' and 'protected time' for therapeutic work is important to people with mental health problems in inpatient mental health services (Brimblecombe et al. 2007).

Health promotion

Strategies for mental health promotion underpin suicide prevention work. This is seen clearly in the structure of national suicide prevention policies (Anderson and Jenkins 2006). Mental health nurses have a key role in working with colleagues in primary care and public health in order to promote mental health, for example: promoting mental health and well-being in schools and colleges; stress management at work; exploring opportunities for social integration; expression of health and mental health in art and literature. Some of these activities have evidence of effectiveness as part of national strategies (WHO 2004). Building coping/problem-

---

✖ Practice Example: Darren

Darren is a 24-year-old male, admitted to the psychiatric unit following a serious attempt to hang himself on the banister of his girlfriend's house. He was an only child and his parents separated when he was around six years of age. At school, Darren remained rather quiet and isolated. During his teenage years he began self-cutting, but this was usually in private and not known to anyone else. After school he became a mechanic and moved out of his mother's home two years ago to stay with his fiancée. About 18 months ago, his mother died in a road traffic accident, as a result of a brake failure. Darren blamed himself as he had recently worked on his mother's car. He became withdrawn, isolated, had a reduced libido, started drinking heavily, and began to self-harm again. His GP diagnosed depression and prescribed SSRIs. By chance, his father-in-law returned home with Darren's girlfriend and managed to cut Darren down. He was admitted to hospital.

In working with Darren, the steps outlined in Table 17.1 —maintaining an assessment of suicidal thinking; managing mental health issues; keeping the person safe; working with the individual—form the basic essential structure of practice.   »

» **Table 17.1** Steps for working therapeutically with Darren

Maintaining an assessment of suicidal thinking	Managing mental health issues	Keeping the person safe	Working with the individual
Establish a rapport (see Chapters 5–7). Carry out a risk assessment (in coordination with column 2: Managing mental health issues). Take into account risk factors in Box 17.1. Use process model to establish background to suicidal risk (A–C). Explore level of depression, feelings of hopelessness, and view of the future. Use appropriate suicide assessment scale where possible.	Carry out an assessment of mental health problems (in coordination with column 1: Maintaining an assessment of suicidal thinking).	Create a safe environment. Check room for any **ligature** points, check items for use as a possible ligature. Make all medications safe and locked away. Check for any other possible methods of self-harm (e.g. sharp objects, razor blades). Observation: use carefully and diligently. Follow guidelines for observation of people at risk. Ensure the unit has undergone a suicide audit using the NIMHE Suicide Prevention Audit Toolkit (Duffy et al. 2003).	Establish an ongoing trusting therapeutic relationship with the person; key/basic qualities of care, compassion, sensitivity. Work with the person and acknowledge previous factors and how they will affect the relationship and rapport development. Negotiate and collaborate on planning (medium and longer term), with involvement of family, friends, local networks (where possible). Follow general NICE guideline principles for all health care professionals (NICE 2004).

✖ Practice Example: Zoe

Zoe is a 13-year-old girl who was admitted to the local A&E department on Friday evening after taking ten paracetamol tablets. This is third time she has been admitted into hospital over the past year. The previous two admissions were for lacerations to her arms and a suspected overdose. Zoe lives with her mother and two older brothers. She has been bullied at school and continues to do poorly in course work. There has been an allegation that her oldest brother sexually abused Zoe when she was nine years old. Zoe has very few friends and her mother is unable to offer adequate support as she drinks heavily and also suffers from depression. Zoe herself has begun to drink regularly. She recently had a boyfriend, whom she cared about, but the two argued frequently. Zoe is about to be seen by nurses from the local child and adolescent mental health team.

In this example, it is important to ensure that all precipitating and ongoing risks of repetition are discussed with the

»

» young person. In working with Zoe, the steps outlined in Table 17.2—maintaining an assessment of suicidal thinking; assessing the personal, social, and family situation; managing self-harm; liaising with the multidisciplinary services—form the basis of practice.

Table 17.2 Steps for working therapeutically with Zoe

Maintaining an assessment of suicidal thinking	Assessing the personal, social, and family situation	Managing self-harm	Liaising with the multidisciplinary services
Establish a rapport.

Carry out a risk assessment (in coordination with column 2: Assessing the personal, social, and family situation).

Take into account risk factors in Box 17.1.

Use appropriate suicide and depression risk scales for younger people. | The assessment process detailed earlier can be used. However, in practice this will need to be modified. For example, it would be important to include identification of exposure to suicide and self-harm by others and risk of repetition and of suicide.

As column 4 indicates, the family, guardian, and others need to be included in the assessment of the young person.

It is important to explore factors leading to the self-harm, such as family problems, relationship problems, school problems, alcohol use, drug use, bullying, physical abuse, sexuality, trouble with the police, friends engaging in self-harm, family member engaging in self-harm, trauma such as bereavement, media and internet influences (Hawton and Rodham 2006). | There are a number of options for the treatment of young people who self-harm.

In the short term, though, it is important to ensure that the person is safe and has adequate support and care. This may mean discussing safe storage of drugs at home, for example.

Ongoing work will depend on the nature of the circumstances surrounding each case. Evidence supports the use of problem-solving therapy and crisis intervention, cognitive behavioural therapy, and family therapy, and there is growing evidence for the benefit of group psychotherapy. | Parents, other guardians, friends, teachers, and other professionals involved in the care of the young person. The GP, for example, should be asked to supplement the information given by the young person. |

solving skills will help protect against suicide. However, health promotion stretches further into policies to reduce discrimination of people with mental health difficulties and stigmatizing portrayals of suicide in the media (which can also fuel further suicide acts in the community) (Hawton and Williams 2005). Mental health nurses are also best placed to work directly with service users and voluntary groups on issues that contribute to reducing suicidal behaviour.

▲ Conclusion

People who engage in self-harming and/or suicidal behaviour present some of the most challenging issues in the work of mental health nurses. The profession is at the centre of suicide prevention work. Nurses are required to gain experience in developing assessment skills, drawing not only upon clinical experience but also on knowledge of the evidence relating to risk of suicide. However, the crux of the assessment and ongoing management of people who self-harm and those who are suicidal involves not relying on lists of risk factors but recognizing the individual and seeing each act of self-harm or suicidal behaviour as unique.

w Website

You may find it helpful to work through our short online quiz and scenario intended to help you to develop and apply the skills in this chapter. Please go to:

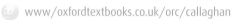 www/oxfordtextbooks.co.uk/orc/callaghan

✚ References

Anderson, M. and Jenkins, R. (2006). The National Suicide Prevention Strategy for England: the reality of a national strategy for the nursing profession. *Journal of Psychiatric and Mental Health Nursing* 13, 641–50.

Anderson, M. and Standen, P. J. (2007). Attitudes toward suicide among nurses and doctors working with children and young people who self harm. *Journal of Psychiatric and Mental Health Nursing* 14, 470–7.

Appleby, L., Dennehy J. A., Thomas, C. S., et al. (1999). Aftercare and clinical characteristics of people with mental illness who commit suicide: a case control study. *Lancet* 353, 1397–400.

Appleby, L., Shaw, J., Meehan, J., et al. (2001). *Safety First: Five Year Report of the National Confidential Inquiry into Suicide and Homicide by People with Mental Illness.* London: DH.

Barker, P. (1997). *Assessment in Psychiatric and Mental Health Nursing: In Search of the Whole Person.* London: Stanley Thornes.

Barraclough, B., Bunch, J., Nelson, B., and Sainsbury, P. (1974). A hundred cases of suicide: clinical aspects. *British Journal of Psychiatry* 125, 355–73.

Beck, A. T. and Weishaar, M. E. (1990). Suicide risk assessment and prediction. *Crisis* 11(2), 22–30.

Bennewith, O., Peters, T., Evans, M., and Sharp, D. (2002). General practice based intervention to prevent repeat episodes of deliberate self harm: cluster randomised controlled trial. *British Medical Journal* 324, 125.

Bolton, C., Gooding, P., Kapur, N., Barrowclough, C., and Tarrier, N. (2007). Developing psychological perspectives of suicidal behaviour and risk in people with a diagnosis of schizophrenia: We know they kill themselves but do we understand why? *Clinical Psychology Review* 27, 511–36.

Bowers, L., Gournay, K., and Duffy, D. (2000). Suicide and self harm in in-patient psychiatric units: a national survey of observation policy. *Journal of Advanced Nursing* 32(2), 437–44.

Brimblecombe, N., Tingle, A., and Murrells, T. (2007). How mental health nursing can best improve service users' experience and outcomes in in-patient settings: a response to a national consultation. *Journal of Psychiatric and Mental Health Nursing* 14, 503–9.

Camelot Foundation/Mental Health Foundation (2006). *Truth Hurts: National Inquiry into Young*

People and Self Harm. London: Mental Health Foundation.

Cooper, J. and Kapur, N. (2004). Assessing suicide risk. In: *New Approaches to Preventing Suicide: A Manual for Practitioners* (ed. D. Duffy and T. Ryan), pp 20–38. London: Jessica Kingsley.

Department of Health (2002). *National Suicide Prevention Strategy for England*. London: HMSO.

Department of Health (2005). *National Suicide Prevention Strategy for England. Annual Report on Progress 2004*. London: HMSO.

Department of Health (2006). *Best Practice Competencies and Capabilities for Pre-registration Mental Health Nurses in England: The Chief Nursing Officer's Review of Mental Health Nursing*. London: DH.

Department of Health and Ageing (2000). *Living is for Everyone: A Framework for the Prevention of Suicide and Self Harm in Australia (LIFE Framework)*. Canberra: DHA.

Department of Health, Social Services and Public Safety (2006). *Protect Life: A Shared Vision: The Northern Ireland Suicide Prevention Strategy and Action Plan 2006–2011*. Belfast: DHSSPS.

Duffy, D., Ryan, T., and Purdy, R. (2003). *Preventing Suicide: A Toolkit for Mental Health Services*. London: National Institute for Mental Health in England.

Hawton, H. (2000). General hospital management of suicide attempters. In: *The International Book of Suicide and Attempted Suicide* (ed. K. Hawton and K. van Heeringen), pp 519–37. Chichester: John Wiley.

Hawton, K. and Rodham, K. (2006). *By Their Own Young Hand: Deliberate Self Harm and Suicidal Ideas in Adolescents*. London: Jessica Kingsley.

Hawton, K. and Williams, K. (2005). Media influences on suicidal behaviour: evidence and prevention. In: *Prevention and Treatment of Suicidal Behaviour. From Science to Practice* (ed. K. Hawton), pp 293–306. Oxford: Oxford University Press.

Hawton, K., Bale, L., Casey, D., Shepherd, A., Simkin, S., and Harris, L. (2006). Monitoring deliberate self harm presentations to general hospitals. *Crisis* 27(4), 157–63.

Hawton, K., Harriss, L., Simkin, S., Bale, E., and Bond, A. (2004). Self cutting: patients' characteristics compared with self poisoners. *Suicide and Life Threatening Behaviour* 34(3), 199–208.

Health Service Executive, The National Suicide Review Group, and Department of Health and Children (2005). *Reach Out: National Strategy for Action on Suicide Prevention 2005–2014*. Dublin: Health Service Executive.

Johnston, A., Cooper, J., Webb, R., and Kapur, N. (2006). Individual- and area-level predictors of self harm repetition. *British Journal of Psychiatry* 189, 416–21.

Kapur, N. (2006). Suicide in the mentally ill. *Psychiatry* 5(8), 279–82.

Kerkhof, A. and Arensman, E. (2001). Pathways to suicide: the epidemiology of the suicidal process. In: *Understanding Suicidal Behaviour: The Suicidal Process, Approach to Research, Treatment and Prevention* (ed. K. van Heeringen), pp 15–39. London: John Wiley.

Lonnvist, J. K. (2000). Psychiatric aspects of suicidal behaviour: depression. In: *The International Book of Suicide and Attempted Suicide* (ed. K. Hawton and K. van Heeringen), pp 117–20. Chichester: John Wiley.

Ministry of Health (2006). *The New Zealand Suicide Prevention Strategy 2006–2016*. Wellington: Ministry of Health.

Motto, J. (1991). An integrated approach to estimating suicide risk. *Suicide and Life-Threatening Behaviour* 21(1), 74–89.

National Confidential Inquiry (2006). *Avoidable Deaths: Five Year Report of the National Confidential Inquiry into Suicide and Homicide by People with Mental Illness*. Manchester: University of Manchester.

National Institute for Health and Clinical Excellence (2004). *Self Harm: The Short Term Physical and Psychological Management and Secondary Prevention of Self Harm in Primary and Secondary Care*. Leicester: British Psychological Society.

National Institute for Mental Health in England (2007). *National Suicide Prevention Strategy for England: Annual Report on Progress 2006*. London: NIMHE.

Norwegian Board of Health (1995). *The National Plan for Suicide Prevention 1994–1998*. Oslo: National Board of Health.

Samuelsson M., Wiklander, M., Asberg, M., and Saveman, B.-I. (2000). Psychiatric care as seen by the attempted suicide patient. *Journal of Advanced Nursing* 32(3), 635–43.

Scottish Executive (2002). *Choose Life: A National Strategy and Action Plan to Prevent Suicide in Scotland*. Edinburgh: Scottish Executive.

Sun, F.-K., Long, A., Boore, J., and Tsao, L.-I. (2006). A theory for the nursing care of patients at risk of suicide. *Journal of Advanced Nursing* 53(6), 680–90.

Talseth, A., Jacobsson, L., and Norberg, A. (2001). The meaning of suicidal psychiatric in-patients' experiences of being cared for by physicians. *Journal of Advanced Nursing* 34(1), 96–106.

Wildgoose, A. and Williams, D. (2007). *Managing Self Harm: A Training Pack for People Working with Individuals who Self Harm*. Brighton: Pavilion Publishing.

Williams, J. M. G., Crane, C., Barnhofer, T., and Duggan, D. (2005). Psychology and suicidal behaviour: elaborating the entrapment model. In: *Prevention and Treatment of Suicidal Behaviour: From Science to Practice* (ed. K. Hawton), pp 71–89. Oxford: Oxford University Press.

World Health Organization (1999). *Figures and Facts About Suicide*. Geneva: WHO.

World Health Organization (2004). *For Which Strategies of Suicide Prevention is there Evidence of Effectiveness?* Copenhagen: WHO Regional Office for Europe's Health Evidence Network.

18 Prevention, recognition, and therapeutic management of violence

Richard Whittington   **David Riley**

▼ Introduction

In this chapter we look at the key skills needed to work safely and effectively with service users who may be violent whilst receiving mental health nursing care. There are three interrelated sets of skills to be considered here: recognizing that a service user is likely to become violent in the imminent future; working with this service user to prevent their anger or resentment turning into **violence**; and, if this does not work, therapeutically managing the actual violent behaviour that takes place (Box 18.1).

These skills form a sequence over time in that good recognition means prevention may not be needed and good prevention, in turn, means that management may not be needed. They are only one aspect of the overall interaction between the nurse and the service user. It is better to think in terms of violent incidents rather than violent service users, as the nurse's behaviour has a dramatic effect, for better or worse, on the service user's feelings, thoughts, and responses at times of crisis and despair (Whittington and Richter 2005). In addition, the skills can be deployed effectively only within the context of an overall caring relationship where a collaborative approach and joint decision-making with the service user is emphasized as much as possible. Working **with** rather than **on** the service user is vital to the recognition and prevention of violence, and should remain the aim even during coercive interventions such as restraint (National Institute for Health and Clinical Excellence [NICE] 2005).

To start with, it is important to keep the problem of violence in proportion so that the nurse avoids fear on the one hand and complacency on the other. Common stereotypes of people with mental health problems almost always include the assumption that mental illness is strongly associated with dangerous and violent behaviour. Anybody

Box 18.1 Core values and skills underpinning violence recognition, prevention, and management

Core values

- Empathy, caring
- Respect, realistic trust
- Self-awareness
- Active listening
- Collaborative approach
- Awareness of service user's strengths
- Judgement of proportionality
- Ability to balance needs for safety and autonomy
- Awareness of the principle of 'least intrusiveness'

Recognition

- Antecedents
- Risk factors
- Warning signs

Prevention

- Observation
- Engagement
- De-escalation

Therapeutic management

- Physical restraint
- Rapid tranquillization
- Seclusion

working as a registered nurse will have sufficient experience and knowledge to know that this is a false belief that increases the social exclusion experienced by many service users. However, the same registered nurse will also know that certain personal and social attributes (e.g. sex) are associated with an increased risk, either alone or in combination with mental health problems.

Learning outcomes

Most registered mental health nurses will encounter violence by a service user at some point in their career. Depending on the chosen specialism, many will witness such violence directed at their colleagues or other service users, and some will be the target of assaults themselves. More importantly, though, most nurses will at some point use their skills to be successfully involved in preventing

anger from becoming **aggression**, aggression becoming violence, or low-level violence (e.g. pushing) becoming something more serious.

The learning outcomes and key skills that the registered nurse needs in this area are listed in Box 18.2. In this chapter, the focus is on the skills set out in criterion 2, although it is possible here only to give some awareness of the relevant specific skills.

Another useful reference point for what the registered nurse needs to know is provided by the UK National Health Service (NHS) Counter Fraud and Security Management Service (NHS CFSMS 2003). This body is responsible for designing a national syllabus for conflict resolution training that must be attended by all NHS staff shortly after starting in a new post. As can be seen in Box 18.3, the syllabus covers the three areas of recognition, prevention, and management considered here.

All good training programmes should have the principle of **proportionality** running through them. This means ensuring that those working with service users choose the right level of intervention when there appears to be a **risk** of violence in the near future. At all times, the least intrusive and coercive intervention that maintains safety should be used. In other words, it is bad practice to overreact to

---

Box 18.2 Knowledge and performance criteria relating to the recognition, prevention, and management of violence

Knowledge criteria

The registered mental health nurse should be able to demonstrate knowledge of:

1 The reasons for violence and aggression within mental health services

2 Measures for the recognition, prevention, and reduction of violence and aggression

Performance criteria

The registered mental health nurse should be able to:

3 Apply effective, evidence-based interventions that minimize risk of harm to others through violence

4 Recognize signs and circumstances associated with aggression and violence

5 Show an awareness of prevention and risk reduction strategies for aggression and violence

6 Contribute to the prevention and management of abusive and aggressive behaviour

7 Work as a member of the therapeutic team in making a safe and effective contribution to the de-escalation and management of anger and violence

(Adapted from Department of Health 2006)

Box 18.3 The ten objectives of the national conflict resolution training syllabus

1 Describe common causes of conflict

2 Describe the two forms of 'communication'

3 Give examples of how communication can break down

4 Explain three examples of 'communication models' that can assist in conflict resolution

5 Describe patterns of behaviours you may encounter during different interactions

6 Give examples of the different warning and danger signs

7 Give examples of impact factors

8 Describe the use of distance when dealing with 'conflict'

9 Explain the use of 'reasonable force' as it applies to conflict resolution

10 Describe different methods for dealing with possible conflict situations

(Source: www.cfsms.nhs.uk/training/crt.html)

relatively minor disruptions or distress and, equally, to underreact to imminent danger. The first response to angry shouting, for example, should be **de-escalation** rather than restraint; however, open questions and active listening are of secondary importance if somebody is actually under physical attack.

The evidence base

Recognition of the potential for violence

The first step that you must take is to develop skills for identifying when a service user is likely to act violently. Service users, like everybody else, vary hugely in terms of what is experienced as anger provoking and how angry feelings are expressed. The top priority, therefore, in recognizing potential violence is getting to know the individual service user as soon as possible. Individual trigger factors and warning signs should be identified as early as possible in the admission. A large number of common factors have been identified through research (Box 18.4) and an awareness of these should inform any discussion with the service user without the assumption that they all apply to everybody.

The classical presentation of somebody who is at high risk of imminently being violent is the well known pattern of agitation and barely controlled anger or resentment. These classical signals include shouting, pacing, clenching fists, and slamming doors, and most people—nurses or otherwise—will recognize this is behaviour that requires some immediate intervention such as soliciting information on what has made the service user angry. It is important to note, though, that people differ individually and culturally in how they express angry feelings and that nurses differ as well, in terms of how they 'read' individual service users. Some service users will become withdrawn and silent before acting aggressively and, conversely, some, who appear to you to be agitated, may actually have no intention of becoming violent. The golden rule, as always, is to get to know the service user as an individual as well as possible, and work with him or her in identifying the important issues.

Self-awareness is also an important skill when working with any service user. As well as recognizing the signals of stress and strain from the service user, you should be able to recognize personal signs of stress. You should be aware of negative feelings you have toward the service user (either as an individual or as a member of a particular social group). Your feelings of fear, anger, dislike, or exhaustion may lead to unfair expectations of the service user and may impair effective

---

Box 18.4 Selected risk factors for violence in a mental health context

Demographic factors

- Male
- Young age
- Lack of social support
- Employment problems
- Criminal peer group

Background history

- Childhood maltreatment
- History of violence
- First violent at young age

Clinical history

- Psychopathy
- Substance abuse
- Schizophrenia
- Non-compliance with treatment

Psychological and psychosocial factors

- Anger
- Impulsivity
- Suspiciousness
- Command hallucinations
- Lack of insight

Current 'context'

- Threats of violence
- Availability of weapons

(Department of Health 2007, Farrington 2001, MacArthur Research Network 2005)

---

communication. Basic things, such as adopting the wrong tone of voice, can have a massive impact on the service user's feelings and may trigger escalation.

Prevention

All nurses, be they on a practice placement or qualified, need to be aware of the local Trust policy for dealing with violent incidents. This will set out the organization's approved approaches to preventing and managing violence. These are likely to vary from employer to employer with regard to particular issues such as dealing with weapons. Enhanced **observation** is often the first response to a service user who is felt to be at risk of acting violently. The ability intelligently to observe people at risk and make sense of their behaviour is an important nursing skill. The minimum expectation for every service user in hospital is that staff know their location at all times and they are met with at least once every shift (NICE 2005). Beyond that, for those at risk, there are three further levels of enhanced observation: intermittent (checked every 15–20 minutes); within eyesight; and within arm's length. One-way observation on its own, the aptly called 'clinical gaze' (Foucault 1973, Stevenson and Cutcliffe 2006), is clearly not enough in a therapeutic relationship and it is vital that the observing nurse engages with the service user at the same time as observing. Service users will vary significantly in how comforting or irritating they find the experience of being observed, and this reaction should be discussed explicitly. The right way to engage is also something to be judged within the context of the specific relationship at the time and may include attentive silence, phatic (ordinary, everyday) conversation (Burnard 2003), or more personal and focused talk.

When working with the potentially violent service user, engagement may at some point move into the more proactive skills required for de-escalation (Cowin et al. 2003, Jonikas et al. 2004, Paterson and Leadbetter 1999, Richter 2006). Practising these skills should be a central part of any conflict resolution training programme. As with observation and engagement, many of these skills, such as active listening, establishing rapport, and asking open questions, are core to any effective mental health nursing practice, but the major new challenge here is to be able to use these skills in a rapidly changing, highly charged situation where the nurse may well feel afraid or angry themselves. Again, all service users are individuals and will respond differently to different styles of de-escalation. Knowing the service user well and maintaining a sense of empathic caring in the face of even verbal abuse and threats will help the nurse to tailor their response effectively, and may resolve the situation without resort to the more coercive measures of therapeutic violence management. More detailed examples of de-escalation skills are given in the two scenarios later in the chapter.

Therapeutic management

Moving from prevention to management of violence involves a major step into the unknown for both the service user and the nurses who take that step. The decision physically to restrain, forcibly to medicate, or to seclude a service user must

only be taken when the safety of other people is in imminent jeopardy and when all other attempts to prevent violence have failed. The experience of being forcibly touched, held, moved around, and injected is likely to evoke very strong feelings in the service user (e.g. terror, humiliation, rage) (Cusack et al. 2003, Johnson 1998, Wynn 2004). The nurse involved in these interventions is likely to feel strong emotions, such as fear. They will put themselves and the service user at risk of physical harm, jeopardize the trust they may have built up with the service user, and may experience a profound challenge to what they considered to be their ethical values. Fortunately, in most settings, the decision to use coercive measures is relatively rare and is almost always made by senior staff, where possible in consultation with other care team members.

It is highly undesirable for student nurses to participate in **physical interventions**, but occasionally in some situations of imminent violence this principle may be overridden. The only physical skill required of the newly qualified nurse operating on his or her own is the ability to **break away** from dangerous situations (Wright et al. 2005). Usually this is provided as part of induction training, which will be offered as soon as possible after starting a new job. Ideally, in addition, any nurse involved in the more demanding coercive procedures described here must also have attended specialist training from their Trust beyond that provided in pre-registration training (NICE 2005).

The skills required to carry out physical restraint, **rapid tranquillization**, and **seclusion** safely and effectively are both technical and human. The technical skills such as ways of holding, drug dosages, and resuscitation, should only ever be used in combination with the human and personal skills outlined in Box 18.1: the core nursing activities of cultivating empathy, caring, rapport, and a desire to minimize the distress of the service user during the procedure. As with de-escalation, but even more so, the major challenge for the nurse is to maintain these states of mind during a physical struggle.

Working with violence in the community

Some skills, especially the core values and recognition skills outlined in Box 18.1, apply to both inpatient and community mental health work. However, managing violence in the community is not really an option and most of the techniques discussed above are not relevant. A judgement must be made on when the prevention skills should be used and when exiting the situation is the priority. The community worker is usually alone and operating on the service user's territory with no prospect of immediate back-up. In this setting the emphasis is on staying safe by developing a good environmental aware-ness (e.g. escape routes) and being prepared to leave quickly when perceived danger crosses a particular personal thresh-old. Joint visits should be arranged whenever possible, and the nurse's location should be known by other members of the team at all times. Above all, physical interventions should never be used in community settings except in rare and extreme situations where there is an immediate, life-threaten-ing risk.

Health promotion

The successful prevention of violence can play a key role in promoting the overall health and opportunities of the serv-ice user who is prone to act violently at times of crisis. Enabling the service user to develop new strategies for cop-ing with feelings of fear or anger can lead to them having more satisfactory relationships with other people. It also will

✖ Practice Examples

Peter

A female staff nurse, who has recently qualified, is in charge of a busy mental health admissions unit. She becomes aware of shouting from the corridor outside the office and goes out to find a service user, Peter, complaining angrily about the theft of a bar of chocolate from his bedside table—the third occasion since admission that this has happened to him. The nurse requests that a member of staff escort Peter to the bed area to get an account of exactly where the item was taken from.

The nurse goes to Peter's notes because she is aware that he has completed an advance statement about how he would like to be cared for if he becomes aggressive or angry. It emphasizes that Peter finds the presence of too many male nurses provocative at these times. It also states that he is antagonized if staff suggest medication as a solu-tion at these times. The document also suggests people whom Peter can contact by phone if he is getting angry.

At this point a young male nursing assistant walks into the office and states: 'I think Peter is going to blow about this chocolate. Do you want me to stick around him just in case?'. The nurse says 'no' to this and reassures her col-league that she does not think that he will be required.

Peter then enters the office and angrily says that he wants to talk to the nurse in charge about the issue. The nurse is welcoming, relaxed, and highly supportive. She then employs a range of verbal and non-verbal interven-tions to reduce Peter's arousal and reassure him about the situation. Half way through the discussion she is aware of the male nursing assistant outside the office stating: 'She is taking a chance in there, she needs to get some PRN into him fast'. The nurse responds quickly and decisively to this by going out on to the corridor and politely but firmly ask-ing the nursing assistant to go to the dayroom and engage with other service users. She clearly asserts that she is man-aging the situation and thanks him for his concern.

She returns to Peter and sets out her response to his frus-tration. She states that she will make all of the other staff aware of these problems and ask them to be extra vigilant. She records this request in the staff communication book in front of Peter. She also states that she will make the issue a priority at the service users' meeting that she will be facili-tating the next day. The nurse asks Peter if he would like to use the office phone to ring anybody about this issue. Peter declines to do so, but does ask if he can use the phone later to ring his brother. The nurse happily agrees to this.

Peter leaves the office, still quite angry, but appreciative of the help and support he has received. Table 18.1 shows the mental health nursing practice skills used in this scenario.

Susan

A newly qualified male staff nurse is in sole charge of a reha-bilitation ward. A female service user, Susan, has had a par-ticularly disturbed period, during which she has assaulted other service users and staff. Susan looks forward to a visit from her sister, who brings the service user's young nephew. Susan is particularly fond of her nephew, and staff reinforce positively the value of the visits with Susan.

The nurse in charge receives a phone call from Susan's sister, who tells him that she will not be able to visit her on this particular day because her son, Susan's nephew, is feel-ing unwell. The nurse in charge is concerned that, on hear-ing this news, Susan will be immensely disappointed and concerned, respond aggressively, and put herself, other service users, and staff at risk.

The nurse has a lot to consider. He is determined to impart this negative information to Susan in a way that dis-plays sensitivity and an acknowledgement of the distress it will cause. At the same time he will have to ensure that safety for all involved is maximized. The possibility of

»

» **Table 18.1** Skills used to prevent, recognize, and manage violence with Peter

Establishing the risk	Managing the environment	Verbal/non-verbal communication	Non-verbal communication
Risk factors: Take into consideration actuarial (historical) risk factors and clinical variables at that particular time.	*Other service users:* Ensure that the staff remove other service users from the area and potential involvement in the incident.	*Tone and volume:* Staff should avoid interacting with agitation and maintain a calm and concerned tone. Volume of interaction should remain low to model an appropriate response.	*Positive body language:* Staff should avoid accidentally sending out a dismissive, confrontational message with negative body language. Folded arms can suggest guardedness, hands on hips a confrontational attitude. Open-handed gestures can communicate receptiveness and an open, honest approach.
Advance directives: Establish presence of advance directive and specific guidance around service user's preferred strategies to manage their aggression.	*Noise and heat:* Reduce environmental stimuli to help facilitate a sense of calm. Reduce noise and ensure that the area is well ventilated to avoid high temperatures that add to agitation.	*Active listening:* The nurse should be able to summarize and repeat back to the service user their perception of the difficulties.	
Relationship factors: Be aware of interpersonal relationships between staff and service users, and integrate these considerations into your strategy. Staff with a good therapeutic relationship with the service user will be utilized ahead of physically bigger staff by the confident, therapeutically focused, staff nurse. The risk of physical violence should not be over-assessed at the expense of a preventive strategy.	*Weapons:* Ensure that there are no items left lying around that could be used as a potential weapon.

Accessing exit: In case of an escalation of the situation, it should be ensured that the member of staff is situated closest to the door to facilitate a rapid exit if required.

Staff support: Other staff may be required to stay in the vicinity at these times, but ideally they should be as unobtrusive as possible in order not to be an intimidating presence for the service user. | *Positive:* Staff should maintain a positive attitude and seek to collaborate with the service user to come to a mutually agreeable solution.

Empathy: The ability to empathize with the service user is recognized as a key component of the process. The ability to say to an angry person, 'I'm not in your position, but if I was I think I would be angry too,' can be a critical skill in forging an alliance with the service user. | *Personal space:* An angry individual needs an expanded area of personal space in order to feel secure. Staff standing too close can be mistakenly perceived as a threat by the angry individual. Staff should be aware of varying requirements around personal space depending on the person's cultural background.

Eye contact: Sustained eye contact should be avoided with an aroused person because it can be seen as challenging. The use of intermittent eye contact can convey sincerity and interest without being seen as confrontational. |

»

»
physical intervention has to be acknowledged and planned for, although the nurse remains upbeat and optimistic that this can be avoided. He is aware of Susan's advance statement that records her resistance to male staff intervening with her if she becomes agitated. He is aware that any obvious increased staff presence may be intimidating for Susan and unduly alarm her, but he does want to make sure that the real possibility of physical confrontation is managed with as little harm as possible being caused.

He decides that a consistent and well-coordinated staff response is essential, so decides to speak to all of the staff on duty to outline their particular responsibilities when Susan hears this news. He also recognizes the need to utilize the experience and resources from other wards nearby. One of his colleagues suggests (only half joking) that he 'leaves it for the next shift to tell Susan'. The staff nurse rejects this option completely. He sees this as a real opportunity to demonstrate his organizational and risk management skills.

After carefully planned measures to minimize risk, the message from Susan's sister is passed on to her. She responds with frustration and anger but does not become aggressive and violent. Her concerns for the well-being of her nephew are accommodated with patience and empathy by the staff assigned to pass on the information to her. Table 18.2 shows the mental health nursing practice skills used in this scenario.

Table 18.2 Skills used to prevent, recognize, and manage violence with Susan

Demonstrating leadership	Managing the environment and resources	Verbal/non-verbal communication	Contemplating physical intervention
Role model: It is vital that the nurse projects an image of calm and composure at these times. Junior staff will take a lead from your reactions. *Maintaining composure:* Slowing down and avoiding impulsive reactions and decisions is key at these times. Unless there is a particular risk that demands a prompt response, most challenges of this kind can be considered, discussed, planned. A confident nurse will resist the temptation to 'get it over with'. *Controlling anxiety:* It is perfectly understandable to be anxious in anticipation of potential violence. Controlling your	*Choosing a room:* It is important that real consideration is given to the room where the information is going to be passed over. It should be as welcoming and as informal as possible, but set out in a way that maximizes safety for all. A ward office, for example, would be inappropriate, because it is generally a formal setting that can symbolize the staff authority role. It is also often cluttered and cramped. *Environmental factors:* The room should be clear of items that could be picked up and thrown, but not 'stripped out' in a way that makes it seem harsh and unwelcoming. It should be ensured that noise levels	*Facial expression:* It is essential that the member of staff who is deployed to undertake verbal interaction expresses appropriate concern through their facial expression. Staff should be careful not to smirk, through anxiety, or grimace and frown at what is being said to them. A calm and concerned expression recognizes the distress the service user will feel at this news. *Eye contact:* The use of eye contact is very powerful, and staff should be careful during periods of service user anger and agitation to ensure that any prolonged eye contact is not perceived as a threat or challenge. At	*Constitution of staff:* It is essential that the nurse looks to utilize the minimum number of staff deemed necessary for any potential intervention. Excessive staff numbers can create an intimidatory presence that might lead the service user wrongly to conclude that a physical intervention is inevitable. *Physical presence:* A confident practitioner will not simply look to utilize staff of a large physical stature but will consider which staff are able to provide a calm and reassuring presence for the service user in the event of a distressing physical intervention being required.

»

» **Table 18.2** Skills used to prevent, recognize, and manage violence with Susan (*continued*)

Demonstrating leadership	Managing the environment and resources	Verbal/non-verbal communication	Contemplating physical intervention
breathing and the use of positive self-statements (such as 'I can handle this situation' or 'It's a real opportunity to prove myself') can help. *Gather opinions of senior staff:* Asking for help where appropriate is an indication of a good level of self-awareness and in no way contradicts the point about assertiveness made earlier. There may be senior staff and experts in particular fields who would appreciate the opportunity to give advice at these times. *Assign roles:* Any potential incident of this kind should be no surprise to any of the staff on the unit when it occurs. Staff should be briefed on the potential for an incident and the role that is required of them in each possible eventuality. The staff assigned to a potential physical intervention should be told that their input is by no means inevitable.	are kept to a minimum and that the room is not too hot. *Choosing the member of staff to convey the information:* The person to pass on the information should be fully appraised of all the information available. Advance statements would be a consideration when choosing the member of staff. Obviously a member of staff with a good relationship with the service user is less likely to antagonize the situation accidentally. The choice of the right member of staff should not be based on the role of the member of staff within the hierarchy—simply the person best equipped to pass on the news compassionately.	the same time, constant avoidance of eye contact on the part of the staff may be interpreted as displaying disinterest or insincerity. *Positive statements:* Despite negative information being passed on to the service user, it is important that the member of staff maintains a positive perspective and a sense of optimism about the future. *Offer choice:* Service user frustration and anger can often stem from a lack of empowerment and a sense that other people are making choices for them. Asking the service user to identify potential options to deal with the difficulty in question gives a sense of control.	*Therapeutic relationship:* It has to be recognized that, for a number of reasons, not all nursing staff have an ideal therapeutic relationship with the service user. Wherever possible, the nurse in charge should assign them to other duties and keep them away from an area where a physical intervention may be required. *Least intrusive interventions:* If physical intervention is utilized, it should be the minimum required to deal with the harm that needs to be prevented. This means that it should be ensured that the minimum number of staff utilize physical interventions and, crucially, that physical intervention should be carried out in the seated or standing position. Physical intervention on the floor should be considered only as an absolute last resort when all other ways of keeping the situation safe have been exhausted.

enable the service user to be less stigmatized and socially excluded when in the community. The **post-incident review** can play a part in this learning process. It is good practice to hold such a review after every episode of violence, and this should include an open discussion with the service user on the triggers for the incident and alternative ways of expressing strong or uncomfortable feelings. Whilst violent tendencies are usually quite fixed and require intensive therapeutic work to change, these reviews provide an opportunity to work collaboratively with the service user and attempt to repair damage that the therapeutic relationship has sustained as a result of the incident.

Conclusion

Most mental health nurses will encounter aggression by a service user at some point in their career and, with practice, supervision, and experience, will develop effective strategies for dealing confidently with it. Confidence means being able to judge what level of intervention is needed when, and then implementing the intervention safely and humanely. It is as important to hold on to the core values of mental health nursing when relating to the aggressive service user as it is in less charged interactions. The aggressive incident is one episode within the ongoing relationship between nurse and service user, and this relationship should have the capacity to withstand the sense of conflict and breakdown that may occur during the incident. The technical skills of restraint can be learned and used efficiently, but they become nursing skills only when they are used within the context of the human skills that have been emphasized here.

w Website

You may find it helpful to work through our short online quiz and scenario intended to help you to develop and apply the skills in this chapter

 www.oxfordtextbooks.co.uk/orc/callaghan

➤ Further reading and URLs

National Institute for Health and Clinical Excellence (2005). *Clinical Practice Guidelines for Violence: The Short Term Management of Disturbed/Violent Behaviour in Psychiatric In-Patient Settings and Emergency Departments*. London: NICE. http://guidance.nice.org.uk/CG25/quickrefguide/pdf/English. This is the current statement of best practice in this area by NICE based on a systematic review of evidence and extensive consultation with experts. The full review is available but this link is for the quick reference guide.

National Institute for Mental Health in England/Care Service Improvement Partnership. http://www.nimhe.csip.org.uk/our-work/risk-management-programme.html. This links to the English National Risk Management Programme website with a range of resources for assessing and managing the clinical risk of harm.

NHS Security Management Service (2004). *Conflict Resolution Training: Implementing the National Syllabus*. London: NHS CFSMS. http://www.cfsms.nhs.uk/doc/crt/crt.implementing.syllabus.pdf. This document outlines the situation with regard to the national conflict resolution training programme that is currently being implemented across England.

Richter, D. and Whittington, R. (ed.) (2006). *Violence in Mental Health Settings: Causes, Consequences, Management*. New York: Springer. This edited book has contributors from across Europe and takes a multidisciplinary and research-focused approach. It covers many relevant aspects of the problem including de-escalation, coercive interventions, and post-incident management.

✤ References

Burnard, P. (2003). Ordinary chat and therapeutic conversation: phatic communication and mental health nursing. *Journal of Psychiatric and Mental Health Nursing* 10(6), 678–82.

Cowin, L., Davies, R., Estall, G., Berlin, T., Fitzgerald, M., and Hoot, S. (2003). De-escalating aggression and violence in the mental health setting. *International Journal of Mental Health Nursing* 12, 64–73.

Cusack, K. J., Frueh, B. C., Hiers, T., Suffoletta-Maierle, S., and Bennett, S. (2003). Trauma within the psychiatric setting: a preliminary empirical report. *Administration and Policy in Mental Health* 30(5), 453–60.

Department of Health (2006). *Best Practice Competencies and Capabilities for Pre-registration Mental Health Nurses in England*. London: DH.

Department of Health (2007). *Best Practice in Managing Risk: Principles and Evidence for Best Practice in the Assessment and Management of Risk to Self and Others in Mental Health Services*. London: DH.

Farrington, D. P. (2001). Predicting adult official and self-reported violence. In: *Clinical Assessment of Dangerousness. Empirical Contributions* (ed. G. F. Pinard and L. Pagani), pp 66–88. Cambridge: Cambridge University Press.

Foucault, M. (1973). *The Birth of the Clinic. An Archaeology of Medical Perception*. London: Tavistock Publications.

Johnson, M. (1998). Being restrained: a study of power and powerlessness. *Issues in Mental Health Nursing* 19, 191–206.

Jonikas, J. A., Cook, J. A., Rosen, C., Laris, A., and Kim, J. B. (2004). A program to reduce use of physical restraint in psychiatric inpatient facilities. *Psychiatric Services* 55(7), 818–20.

MacArthur Research Network on Mental Health and the Law (2005). *MacArthur Violence Risk Assessment Study: Update of the Executive Summary*. www.macarthur.virginia.edu/risk.html [accessed 1 Jun 2007].

National Institute for Health and Clinical Excellence (2005). *Violence: The Short Term Management of Disturbed/Violent Behaviour in Psychiatric In-Patient Settings and Emergency Departments*. London: NICE.

NHS Counter Fraud and Security Management Service (2003). *Protecting Your NHS: A Professional Approach to Managing Security in the NHS*. London: NHS CFSMS.

Paterson, B. and Leadbetter, D. (1999). De-escalation in the management of aggression and violence: towards evidence-based practice. In: *Aggression and Violence: Approaches to Effective Management* (ed. J. Turnbull and B. Paterson), pp 95–123. London: Macmillan.

Richter, D. (2006). Non-physical conflict management and de-escalation. In: *Violence in Mental Health Settings: Causes, Consequences, Management* (ed. D. Richter and R. Whittington), pp 125–44. New York: Springer.

Stevenson, C. and Cutcliffe, J. R. (2006). Problematizing special observation in psychiatry: Foucault, archaeology, genealogy, discourse and power/knowledge. *Journal of Psychiatric and Mental Health Nursing* 13(6): 713–21.

Whittington, R. and Richter, D. (2005). Interactional aspects of violent behaviour on acute psychiatric wards. *Psychology, Crime and Law* 11(4), 377–88.

Wright, S., Sayer, J., Parr, A. M., Gray, R., Southern, D., and Gournay, K. (2005). Breakaway and physical restraint techniques in acute psychiatric nursing: Results from a national survey of training and practice. *Journal of Forensic Psychiatry and Psychology* 16(2), 380–98.

Wynn, R. (2004). Psychiatric inpatients' experiences with restraint. *Journal of Forensic Psychiatry and Psychology* 15, 124–44.

Working with people with substance misuse problems

Peter Phillips   Patrick Callaghan

 Introduction

Substance misuse is a growing and serious public health problem that continues to affect individuals, communities, and families. Apart from the immediate effects of substance use on health and social functioning, there are important short- and long-term psychological and psychiatric issues, physical health problems, and criminality associated with continued use.

Looking back at the training and preparation of mental health nurses over the past 20 years, substance misuse has often occupied either an 'elective' or 'specialist placement' role, and the volume of curriculum teaching on the subject has generally been low. However, there is a growing recognition that patients with substance misuse problems frequently use all parts of the health and social care services, not least the mental health services, which are often charged with providing 'treatment' for both patients with substance misuse problems, and those with substance misuse **and** mental health problems (commonly known as **dual diagnosis** or co-morbidity). Mental health nurses working across the range of hospital-based, community, or specialist mental health services—be they for working age adults, older people, forensic patients, or children and adolescents—will inevitably work with patients who misuse drugs or alcohol.

Working with substance misuse problems is a **core skill** for all mental health nurses, and requires a comprehensive understanding of theoretical issues pertinent to substance misuse (e.g. development of substance use problems, drug effects, relevant legal issues, transtheoretical model of change, physical and psychological correlates of use), alongside a set of evidence-based therapeutic working strategies (e.g. harm minimization, motivational interviewing, and relapse prevention). You will encounter people with substance misuse and mental health problems in many mental health settings.

In this chapter you will learn about the prevalence of substance misuse, evidence- and values-based interventions that help people recover, what skills you require to care for people you encounter, and how you can best demonstrate these skills in your work with service users.

Learning outcomes

By the end of this chapter you should be better able to:

1 Understand the prevalence of substance misuse

2 Describe evidence- and values-based interventions that help people recover from substance misuse problems

3 Apply the skills you require to care for people with substance misuse problems

4 Demonstrate these skills in your work with service users.

The evidence base

Prevalence of substance misuse in the general population

Estimating the prevalence of problematic substance use in the general population is fraught with methodological, definitional, and practical problems: what is considered misuse, and by whom? How and where is substance misuse recorded as problematic? Do most patients with substance misuse problems tend to report them when seeking help? Despite these concerns about the reporting of substance (mis)use estimates overall, there is robust epidemiological evidence concerning substance use across the European Union (EU) area, including the UK, which makes it clear that substance use is a very common phenomenon. Data from the 2006 European Monitoring Centre on Drugs and Drug Addiction (EMCDDA) annual report (EMCDDA 2006) states that

65 million adults in Europe (approximately 20%) have used cannabis at least once, with 12 million Europeans using the drug regularly. Ten million adults (3% of European adults) have used amphetamine at least once, with 2 million using it within the past year. Eight and a half million European adults (2.6%) have used ecstasy at least once, with more than a million using in the past month. Cocaine is Europe's second most commonly used illicit drug, with at least 10 million adults having ever used the drug, with over 1.5 million uses of the drug in the past month. Opioid users (largely heroin) account for what the report calls 1.7 million 'problem drug users' resident within the EU area. Opioid use was responsible for over 7000 acute drug deaths in 2003, and was the principal drug of misuse in more than 60% of all requests for help or treatment. More than 500 000 opioid users received substitution therapy (such as methadone or buprenorphine) in 2003 (most recent data).

Prevalence of substance misuse amongst people with mental health problems

The co-morbidity of substance misuse and mental illness has been recognized as a significant clinical issue within the past 15 years, in Europe and internationally (Phillips and Johnson 2003). Large-scale North American epidemiological studies suggest that about 50% of the mentally ill also have substance use problems, and that the prevalence is higher amongst inpatients and in emergency service settings (Regier et al. 1990).

The Epidemiological Catchment Area study (Regier et al. 1990) also found that this rate was increased to 64% in drug users who were engaged in drug treatment (detoxification and rehabilitation). Various reviews and UK national policy documents have illustrated some of the complex clinical problems presented by people with these problems. A common factor appears to be a higher level of 'multi-problems', which are not solely medical, psychological, or psychiatric, and this can challenge traditional health care roles. These patients often present to services in crisis with problems relating to social, legal, housing, welfare, and 'lifestyle' matters with which medically oriented services are not always ready or able to help directly. These problems and difficulties often reflect the social stigma that persons with dual diagnosis face, in that they are not only drug users but are also mentally ill—perhaps two of the most socially stigmatized groups in society. These and other issues have raised the profile of substance misuse amongst the mentally ill in the past decade (particularly) and it has subsequently been recognized as an important clinical problem in service provision for the severely mentally ill (Farris

et al. 2003, McCrone et al. 2000, Smith and Hucker 1994, Timko and Moos 2002). A number of significant clinical issues are associated with dual diagnosis and there is equivocal evidence, reported largely from North American studies, that associates dual diagnosis with a range of poor outcomes including: relapse of psychotic illness, exacerbation of psychotic symptoms, poor medication compliance and efficacy, (increased) contact with the criminal justice system, engagement and retention in (mental health or substance misuse) treatment, poor social functioning, increased prevalence of serious physical health problems such as viral hepatitis, HIV, venous thrombosis, and cardiac disease in intravenous injectors, respiratory disease including pneumonia in those who smoke drugs, incidence of suicide, increased service utilization, and problems in the management of residential mental health facilities (Cantwell 2003, Dixon 1999, Gearon et al. 2001, Murray et al. 2002, Smith and Hucker 1994).

In response to these issues, a range of policy and workforce initiatives have been developed, including widespread training programmes for the current workforce and the integration of skills-based approaches to substance misuse in pre-registration health curricula. Policy in England (Department of Health [DH] 2002) and a review of evidence in Scotland (Skellington Orr and Shewan 2006) has focused on the provision of services for the greatest number of patients with dual diagnosis, and guidance published in 2002 (DH 2002) recommends local determination of what constitutes dual diagnosis, and the mainstreaming of individuals with this co-morbidity into mental health service care (as opposed to substance misuse services).

Attitudes towards working with patients with substance misuse issues

Harmful substance use is one behaviour in a spectrum of behaviours that can be understood by others as harmful: people drive too fast, smoke cigarettes. Attempts to increase health professionals' knowledge and skills in working with patients with substance use problems are a critical aspect of improving patients' experiences in health care settings. However, the personal and professional attitudes of health care professionals towards drug and alcohol use (and users) are equally important as they mediate whether and how knowledge and skills are utilized by such staff. Professional attitudes in this context refers to concerns over professional and practice issues, including role legitimacy (is it appropriate to respond to drug use issues in professional health care settings?), while personal attitudes concern beliefs and feelings that originate from understandings of substance use within the popular culture (stigma, anger, and blaming) (National

Council for Education and Training on Addiction [NCETA] 2006). Negative attitudes towards drug users tend to be rooted in beliefs about the deservingness of substance misuse patients' access to appropriate medical and psychological care and treatment, and have been widely recognized as an important factor in addressing staff approaches to this group (DH 2002, NCETA 2006).

From a client perspective, research evidence demonstrates that therapeutic attitude is a key indicator of effective engagement and overall 'treatment' efficacy (Albery et al. 2003).

How are substance use disorders defined and categorized?

Terminology used to describe the use of, and problems relating to, substance use are manifold, and often varies from country to country, and between the general population and those whose professional or family life brings them into contact with substance users. Some of the terms commonly used are based in diagnostic language (misuse, dependence), whereas others have a clearly pejorative meaning (junky, addict, misuser, clean vs. 'dirty'). Within the two psychiatric classification systems (the ICD-10 and the DSM-IV) there are two major groups of diagnoses that relate to ongoing severe and problematic drug and alcohol use; these are **harmful use** and **dependence syndrome**. The ICD-10 (World Health Organization [WHO] 1992) describes harmful use as a pattern of psycho-active substance use that is causing damage to the individual's health. The damage may relate to either physical health (as in the case of hepatitis from injection drug use behaviours) or mental health (as in depressive disorder secondary to heavy alcohol use), or indeed both.

The ICD-10 identifies four main criteria for **harmful use**; these are:

1 Clear evidence that the substance use was responsible for (or substantially contributed to) physical or psychological harm, including impaired judgement or dysfunctional behaviour.

2 The nature of the harm should be clearly identifiable (and specified).

3 The pattern of use has persisted for at least one month, or has occurred repeatedly within a 12-month period.

4 The disorder does not meet criteria for any other mental or behavioural disorder related to the same drug in the same time period (except for acute intoxication).

Dependence syndrome is a cluster of behavioural, cognitive, and physiological phenomena that develop after repeated substance use, and usually includes a strong subjective desire to take the substance, difficulty in controlling its use, persisting in its use despite harmful consequences, a higher priority given to substance use than to other activities and obligations, increased tolerance, and sometimes physical withdrawal states. The dependence syndrome may be present for a specific psycho-active substance (e.g. diazepam), or for a class of substances (e.g. opiates), or for a wide range of pharmacologically different substances.

The International Classification of Mental and Behavioural Disorders (ICD-10) (WHO 1992) identifies six main criteria in dependence, of which three must be present for a period of at least one month or, if persisting for periods of less than one month, should have occurred together repeatedly within a 12-month period:

1 A strong subjective desire or compulsion to take the substance.

2 Impaired capacity to control substance taking behaviour in terms of its onset, termination, or levels of use, as demonstrated by the substance being taken in larger amounts or over a longer period than intended, or by a persistent desire or unsuccessful efforts to reduce or control substance use.

3 A physiological withdrawal state when substance use is reduced or ceased, followed by further substance use in order to relieve or avoid withdrawal symptoms.

4 Evidence of tolerance to the effects of the substance(s), so there is a need for significantly increased amounts of the substance(s) to achieve intoxication or the desired effect, or a markedly diminished effect with continued use of the same amount of the substance.

5 A preoccupation with substance use, as manifest by important alternative pleasures, interests, or activities being given up or reduced because of substance use; or a great deal of time spent in obtaining, taking, or recovering from the effects of the substance.

6 Persistent substance use despite clear evidence of harmful consequences of such use of which the individual is subjectively aware.

The Diagnostic and Statistical Manual of Mental Disorders (DSM-IV) (American Psychiatric Association 1994) also uses the same broad criteria in categorizing substance use disorders (substance dependence and substance misuse), using the term substance misuse in place of harmful use, as employed in the ICD-10. Both classification systems also have diagnoses for **intoxication** for each substance (e.g. in the ICD-10, acute intoxication due to use of **opioids** [F11.0]), and for **withdrawal** for each substance (e.g. in the DSM-IV, alcohol withdrawal [291.8]).

Step-by-step description of the skills required to care for people with substance misuse

Assessment of substance misuse problems

Comprehensive assessment of substance use problems and behaviours is an essential prerequisite in the provision of high-quality, collaborative, and patient-focused care and management. Service settings and priorities can impact on the purpose and type of assessment that is provided (e.g. you may be in a setting where you see the patient only once, or you may have an ongoing relationship). Issues surrounding confidentiality are also crucial in assessing people with substance use problems. Much drug use is illegal in nature, and patients may not feel comfortable in disclosing use to health service staff. **This means you should be explicit with patients about the parameters of confidentiality in your relationship**. Thinking through under what circumstances the patient's confidence can be broken is important, as well as considering your statutory and legal duties. Discussing these issues with colleagues from substance misuse services can be helpful.

As substance use can affect all aspects of an individual's functioning, assessment must be broad and inclusive, focusing on a full range of domains. Box 19.1 shows the areas that you should cover when assessing people with substance misuse.

Evidence-based interventions for caring for people with substance misuse problems

There are a large number of models, interventions, and physical treatments tailored for working with people with substance use problems, ranging from **harm reduction** approaches and self-help, to medical detoxification. The approach to each individual will depend on their needs and circumstances, and on your service setting and approach. However, without the basics of a therapeutic alliance between helper and individual, any approach is likely to be ineffective. This means offering empathy and support to patients, within a professional helping relationship with clear boundaries. Responsibility for change should be left with the client, whilst continuing to support efficacy for change by reinforcing self-worth and self-esteem.

Success should be measured on client terms, and not by professional measures—meaning that making positive changes to substance use behaviours does not always mean complete cessation of substance use (a common goal for

Box 19.1 Assessing the person with substance misuse problems

Substance use

- Full history (what used and when started, progression)
- Use over past week, month, and year (what used and how: volume, frequency, and route—oral, injection, other?)
- Which is primary substance?
- Any prescribed drugs? Home storage and safety
- Urine drug screen
- Use with others or alone?
- Ever abstinent? (Why?)
- Control over use (dependent?)

Physical health

- Known medical problems
- Route related—abscesses, septicaemia, thrombosis
- Overdosed in past?
- Blood-borne viruses—hepatitis A, B, C, and HIV status known?
- Respiratory and cardiac assessment
- Sexual health and contraception issues

Psychological and psychiatric issues

- Previous or current mental health service contact?
- Evidence of current mental illness?
- Association between use and psychiatric symptoms (exacerbation or relief? risk?)
- What do they see as their primary concerns?
- Motivation to change, and stage of change?
- Reasons/motivations for substance use

Social and personal circumstances

- Key personal relationships—users/non-users?
- Support and social network
- Education and qualifications
- Housing
- Benefits/income
- Children—ages and location
- Employment history

Box 19.1 *Continued*

- Use of time
- Interests outside substance use

Risk issues

- Injection use ever?
- Skill in injection use?
- Ever shared injecting equipment (include partner)?
- Storage of methadone, etc. at home? Safety
- Safer sex? Condoms?
- How obtains needles?
- Use and aggression/disinhibition
- Risk of overdose?

Legal and forensic issues

- Outstanding charges?
- Funding of current use
- Contact (current or past) with criminal justice system?
- Types of offence (acquisitive, violent, etc.)
- Probation service involvement

health professionals). For example, stabilizing substance use by not using, or reducing substance use on top of a substitution prescription (such as methadone or buprenorphine) can be as much of a success as an individual stopping all substance use. This is working on client terms.

Understanding change in substance misuse behaviours

The Stages of Change model

Substance use behaviours develop, in most users, over a prolonged period of time during which they are reinforced and become part of a user's coping patterns or daily lifestyle, or provide some other function to the user. Making longlasting changes to substance use behaviours, then, is not something undertaken rapidly, but rather over a period, considering a range of psychological stages. A useful model of change has been developed by Prochaska and DiClemente (1982) which demonstrates these aspects or stages of change, and is used widely in working with problem substance users, and others who want to make changes to behaviour. The chronic and relapsing nature of substance use problems are represented

by the cyclical depiction of the model in Figure 19.1. Stages are not time limited, and each individual's course around the cycle may vary enormously, taking months or years before moving from one stage to another. Whilst helpers can assist in helping individuals to identify issues, it is important that issues and material discussed in stages of change work come from individuals themselves.

Caring for people with substance misuse problems: matching interventions to stage of change

The process of change starts in **pre-contemplation**, where the user has no active interest in making changes. In the context of substance use problems, the person may be aware that other people (e.g. spouse, family, employers, and medical and health care staff) feel and think their substance use is problematic, but they do not understand it to be problematic themselves. This means that when you challenge the person about their substance use in a confrontational way it has little or no effect. The skills you require in pre-contemplation are to raise concern **within the individual themself** as to the nature and effects of their continued substance use, and to help reduce harms of continued use. This is important in terms of the continuing relationship with the patient, and in encouraging the patient to move towards **contemplation**.

The skills you require during the contemplation stage are to assist the person to analyse the pros and cons of his or her continued substance use, and weigh up the costs and benefits of change (this can be undertaken very usefully and simply by using a decision matrix) in order to reach a decision to make changes (or not!). Contemplation is not to be confused with persuasion, and the issues raised in contemplation must be **person centred, not introduced directly by the helper**.

In **decision**, the person makes a choice to change their substance use behaviours (this does not necessarily mean stopping altogether, but could be reducing use, for example); the skills you require in this stage are to increase the person's commitment to change, and to help make a practical plan of actual change that the person will put into place.

In **action**, the substance use behaviours are changed, and a new pattern of behaviour emerges. The skills required in this stage are to help the person sustain the new pattern of behaviour.

Maintenance occurs when the new pattern of behaviour (in this case substance use) has been sustained for a period. The skills required during this stage are helping the person develop practical strategies to maintain the change, such as developing drug refusal skills, and awareness of environmental issues and relapse risk factors.

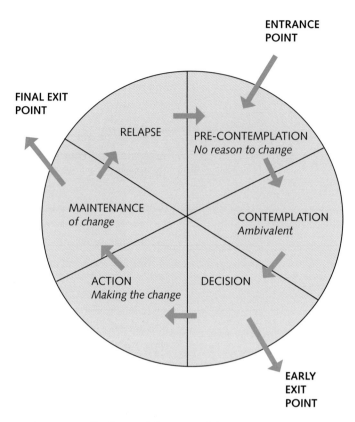

Figure 19.1 The Stages of Change model.

When **relapse** occurs, you require skills in helping the person to try to deconstruct what actually happened, using a behavioural **antecedent–behaviour–consequence** analysis approach, so that the individual can learn from the experience and not view it as total failure. Relapses can be helpful in identifying situations and environments that present a high risk for individuals who are attempting to stop using altogether.

Motivational interviewing

Motivational interviewing (MI) is a style of interacting with people, as opposed to a particular set of interventions or techniques, that borrows heavily from cognitive psychology (Miller and Rollnick 1991). The role of the helper in MI approaches is to take the lead from the individual, so that interactions are based on thoughtful, and sometimes provocative (e.g. using devil's advocate position), open-ended questions. In MI, the nurse's urge to influence, advise, and guide individuals is resisted, with the adoption of a neutral position in relation to the individual's substance use. The avoidance of lecturing, blaming, and provoking guilt is important, as these positions are likely to lead to patient defensiveness. The principles of MI involve addressing behaviours the patient wants to change to begin with, not trying to force the patient to change—and locating the responsibility for change clearly with the patient, assessing readiness and preparedness to change (using the Stages of Change model as discussed earlier), and raising and reflecting the patient's own motivation to change. A useful way to demonstrate your skill in applying MI is to use a decision matrix (Figure 19.2) by completing a cost–benefit analysis with the patient, identifying what are the costs of change and benefits of staying the same.

Demonstrating skills in using the principles of motivational interviewing with the person who misuses substances

Table 19.1 shows you how to demonstrate your skills in caring for a person who misuses substances using the principles of motivational interviewing.

✖ Practice Example

David has been using illicit substances for many years and has made several attempts to get off drugs and remain 'clean', mostly without success. After his most recent attempt he managed to get to the maintenance stage, but relapsed soon afterwards. Box 19.2 shows you how to demonstrate skills in caring for David using the antecedent–behaviour–consequence approach to help David understand why he relapsed.

Box 19.2 Using the antecedent–behaviour–consequence approach

Antecedent

Ask David to list the factors that may have triggered his relapse (e.g. feeling down, having little to do, breaking up with his partner, losing his job).

Behaviour

For each of the triggers, ask David to list how he responded to these factors (e.g. went to the local bar that has a reputation for being a place to buy drugs easily).

Consequence

Ask David to discuss what were the consequences of his behaviour (e.g. met some old friends who are substance users and who sold him some drugs).

Harm reduction approaches

Harm reduction approaches to substance use began to appear in the late 1970s and early 1980s in the Netherlands (where drug policy is based on public health and sociomedical approaches, and was led by organizations such as the Junkiebond) and in the UK (where they were led by health workers who established needle and syringe exchange programmes [NSEPs]). The approach was motivated initially by the increasing numbers of people infected with the HIV virus,

Costs of changing, reducing, or stopping substance use	Benefits of changing, reducing, or stopping substance use
Benefits of continued substance use	Costs of continued substance use

Figure 19.2 Decision matrix.

Table 19.1 How to use motivational interviewing

Principle	Rationale	Mental health nursing skills
Express empathy	Acceptance facilitates change. Skilful reflective listening is fundamental (see Chapters 7 and 8). Ambivalence is normal.	Be non-judgemental—do not use terms that will indicate your disapproval of the person. Listen actively—do not interrupt, pay attention, be non-judgemental, do not give direct advice, clarify anything that is not clear, provide enough time, do not undermine the person's problem.
Develop dissonance	Awareness of the consequences is important. A discrepancy between present behaviour and important goals will motivate change. Client should present the arguments for change.	Use the antecedent–behaviour–consequence approach. Help client to identify the discrepancies (e.g. 'There appears to be a discrepancy between what you are doing now and what your goals are. What do you think of this?' Ask the person to identify the arguments for change (e.g. 'What are the costs and benefits of change?)
Avoid arguments	Arguments are counterproductive. Defending breeds defensiveness. Resistance is a signal to change strategies. Labelling is unnecessary.	Use verbal skills—paraphrase (i.e. repeat back to the person) what they have said; reflect on the feelings that may underpin any verbal statement. Be empathic—convey your understanding of the impact of what the person is saying. Be non-judgemental—do not use terms that will indicate your disapproval of the person. Listen actively—do not interrupt, pay attention, be non-judgemental, do not give direct advice, clarify anything that is not clear, provide enough time, do not undermine the person's problem. Do a functional analysis (e.g. ask the person what their behaviour represents for them).
Roll with resistance	Momentum can be used to good advantage. Perceptions can be shifted. New perspectives are invited but not imposed. The client is a valuable resource in finding solutions to problems.	Use a collaborative problem-solving approach (e.g. ask person to state specifically the problem that is causing resistance to change). Help the person to identify all possible solutions. Discuss the advantages of each solution. Prioritize agreed solutions. Ask the person to imagine using the solutions to deal with resistance. Help the person apply the solutions.
Support self-efficacy	Belief in the possibility of change is an important motivator. The client is responsible for choosing and carrying out personal change. There is hope in the range of possibilities available.	Assess level of self-efficacy using a recognized measure (e.g. www.uri.edu/research/cprc/Measures/). Ask the person to focus on those issues where their self-efficacy is particularly low. Use a collaborative problem-solving approach with the person; this will help them to improve their self-efficacy levels.

and the desire to prevent widespread transmission into the wider community through injecting drug users (one of the early groups infected with HIV). This was summed up by the Advisory Committee on the Misuse of Drugs (ACMD), which stated that the risk to public health from HIV was greater than that posed by drug misuse.

Harm reduction approaches were initially employed with injecting drug users, although the approach can be modified to work with the full range of substances. There is no universally accepted definition of harm reduction, but Riley and O'Hare (2000) have defined it as having several main characteristics: pragmatism (accepting that substance misuse exists, and that rather than ignoring, condemning, or criminalizing individuals who use substances we should work towards minimizing their harmful effects, acknowledging that some ways of using drugs are safer than others); humanistic values (avoiding moralistic judgements about drug use, and supporting the dignity of the user); focus on harms (whether an individual uses or not is important, but harms to individual and community health, social, and economic functioning are the focus; the priority is to reduce harms of drug use to users and others, not necessarily drug use itself); environment (acknowledging that poverty, social class, racism, social isolation, gender discrimination, and inequalities affect vulnerability to and capacity for managing substance-related harms).

These approaches are manifest in NSEPs, the prescribing of methadone and other opiate substitution therapies, educational and outreach programmes, and law enforcement policies that understand substance use as a health issue, and not primarily a criminal justice matter.

Health promotion

Health promotion plays an important role in working with people who misuse substances, especially in relation to physical health. As a mental health nursing student you are well placed to address health promotion issues with clients with substance misuse problems. The issues that you might find helpful include: promoting the wider benefits of being drug free on the client's physical, mental, and social health and wellbeing; promoting physical health (e.g. regular physical health check-ups, attendance at blood-borne virus services, advice on safer injecting practices for intravenous drug users maintaining their habit); and promoting the value of social support to enable people to sustain positive changes.

 ## Conclusion

This chapter has introduced you to some of the basic issues relevant to the development of nursing skills and approaches in working with people with substance use problems. Working with people with substance use problems is challenging, but the mental health nursing skills described in this chapter can help you to enable people living with substance misuse problems to effect lasting change in their behaviour so that they may recover from their problems, or manage them in a way that does not overwhelm them and allows them to lead satisfying lives.

w   Website

You may find it helpful to work through our short online quiz and scenario intended to help you to develop and apply the skills in this chapter. Please go to:

  www.oxfordtextbooks.co.uk/orc/callaghan

+   References

Albery, I. P., Heuston, J., Ward, J., et al. (2003). Measuring therapeutic attitude among drug workers. *Addictive Behaviours* 28, 995–1005.

American Psychiatric Association (1994). *Diagnostic and Statistical Manual of Mental Disorders*, 4th edn. Washington, DC: APA.

Cantwell, R. (2003). Substance use and schizophrenia: effects on symptoms, social functioning and service use. *British Journal of Psychiatry* 182, 324–9.

Department of Health (2002). *Mental Health Policy Implementation Guide: Dual Diagnosis Good Practice Guide*. London: DH.

Dixon, L. (1999). Dual diagnosis of substance misuse in schizophrenia: prevalence and impact on outcomes. *Schizophrenia Research* 25(suppl), S93–100.

European Monitoring Centre on Drugs and Drug Addiction (2006). *The State of the Drugs Problem in Europe. Annual Report 2006*. Lisbon: EMCDDA. http://www.emcdda.europa.eu/

Farris, C., Brems, C., Johson, M., Wells, R., Burns, R., and Kletti, N. (2003). A comparison of schizophrenic patients with or without coexisting substance use disorder. *Psychiatric Quarterly* 74(3), 205–22.

Gearon, J. S., Bellack, A. S., RachBeisel, J., and Dixon, L. (2001). Drug use behaviours and correlates in schizophrenia. *Addictive Behaviours* 26 (1), 51–61.

McCrone, P., Menezes, P. R., Johnson, S., et al. (2000). Service use and costs of people with dual diagnosis in South London. *Acta Psychiatrica Scandinavica* 101(6), 464–72.

Miller, W. R. and Rollnick, S. (1991). *Motivational Interviewing: Preparing People to Change Addictive Behaviours*. New York: Guilford Press.

Murray, R. M., Grech, A., Phillips, P., and Johnson, S. (2002). What is the relationship between substance misuse and schizophrenia? In: *The Epidemiology of Schizophrenia* (ed. R. M. Murray, M. Cannon, P. Jones, J. Van Os, and E. Susser), pp 317–42. Cambridge: Cambridge University Press.

National Council for Education and Training on Addiction (2006). *Health Professionals' Attitudes Towards Licit and Illicit Drug Users: A Training Resource*. Adelaide: NCETA, Flinders University.

Phillips, P. and Johnson, S. (2003). Drug and alcohol misuse amongst in-patients with psychotic illnesses in three inner-London psychiatric units. *Psychiatric Bulletin* 27(6), 217–20.

Prochaska, J. O. and DiClemente, C. C. (1982). Transtheoretical therapy: toward a more integrative model of change. *Psychotherapy: Theory, Research and Practice* 19, 276–88.

Regier, D. A., Farmer, M. E., Rae, D. S., et al. (1990). Co-morbidity of mental disorders with alcohol and other drugs of misuse: results from the epidemiological catchment area (ECA) study. *Journal of the American Medical Association* 264, 2511–18.

Riley, D. and O'Hare, P. (2000). Harm reduction: history, definition and practice. In: *Harm Reduction: National and International Perspectives* (ed. J. A. Inciardi and L. D. Harrison), pp 1–26. Thousand Oaks, CA: Sage.

Skellington Orr, K. and Shewan, D. (2006). *Substance Misuse Research: Review of Evidence Relating to Volatile Substance Abuse in Scotland*. Edinburgh: Substance Misuse Research Programme, Scottish Executive.

Smith, J. and Hucker, S. (1994). Schizophrenia and substance misuse. *British Journal of Psychiatry* 165, 13–21.

Timko, C. and Moos, R. H. (2002). Symptom severity, amount of treatment, and 1-year outcomes among dual diagnosis patients. *Administration and Policy in Mental Health and Mental Health Services Research* 30(1), 35–44.

World Health Organization (1992). *The ICD-10 Classification of Mental and Behavioural Disorders: Clinical Descriptions and Diagnostic Guidelines*. Geneva: WHO.

PART 3
A positive, modern profession

Chapters

⑳ Interagency and interprofessional working

Ben Hannigan

▼ Introduction

Mental health nurses never work alone. In hospitals and in the community, nurses practise alongside psychiatrists, social workers, occupational therapists, clinical psychologists, general medical practitioners (GPs), and others. Recently in the UK new groups have appeared in the workforce. These include graduate primary care and support, time, and recovery workers. Different practitioners often work for different employing agencies. In the UK many staff (including most nurses) work in the National Health Service (NHS), whereas others (including many social workers) are employed by local authorities. Contributions to care are also made by staff located in a variety of other statutory and non-statutory agencies (such as criminal justice, housing, and user-led organizations).

The large number of professions and agencies sharing responsibility to provide care makes the mental health field a complex one, with implications for service users and carers. The experience of receiving interagency and interprofessional care can be a disjointed one, and users run the risk of being 'left in limbo' (Preston et al. 1999). This experience may be compounded where resources are scarce. In this context it is vital that mental health nurses have the capabilities to provide and coordinate care across multiple agency, occupational, and organizational boundaries. The UK's regulatory body, the Nursing and Midwifery Council (NMC), refers to standards in relation to this in a number of publications. The Code of Professional Conduct states that registered nurses must work with others in order to promote and protect health (NMC 2008); the NMC's *Standards of Proficiency for Pre-Registration Nursing Education* also determines that registrants should be able to:

> *'demonstrate knowledge of effective interprofessional working practices which respect and utilise the contributions of members of the health and social care team'*
>
> NMC (2004, p. 5)

In addition, the NMC's *Essential Skills Clusters for Pre-registration Nursing Programmes* includes extensive reference to the skills associated with the organization of care. In this context the NMC states that registrants should be able to challenge practice and function in interprofessional settings in order that the following aspiration be met:

> *'Patients can expect to trust a newly registered nurse to be confident in their own role within the multidisciplinary/multiagency team and to inspire confidence in others.'*
>
> NMC (2007, p. 13)

Learning outcomes

The aim of this chapter is to support students of mental health nursing to develop skills for practice in interagency, interprofessional, and complex organizational environments. By working through this chapter and its associated website students will:

1 Understand the prevailing policy context surrounding interagency and interprofessional working

2 Appreciate the practical significance of working across agency, professional, and organizational boundaries in improving the service user experience

3 Be familiar with a range of organizational factors that both help and hinder effective collaboration in practice

4 Recognize the skills required by nurses in working across multiple interfaces with the aim of promoting **continuity of care**.

The evidence base

The policy context

Delivering more 'joined up' services for the benefit of users and carers is a long-held health and social policy aspiration in the UK and internationally. The following extract from a Department of Health discussion document illustrates UK thinking in this area:

> 'All too often when people have complex needs spanning both health and social care good quality services are sacrificed for sterile arguments about boundaries. When this happens people, often the most vulnerable in our society – the frail elderly, the mentally ill – and those who care for them find themselves in the no man's land between health and social services. This is not what people want or need. It places the needs of the organisation above the needs of the people they are there to serve. It is poor organisation, poor practice, poor use of taxpayers' money – it is unacceptable.'
>
> Department of Health (1998, p. 3)

A number of powerful factors increase the likelihood of care failing to be joined up. Some are structural and relate to the characteristics of different agencies. Others relate to the divisions between occupational groups. The need for services to be provided across multiple organizational interfaces can also contribute to care becoming disjointed.

Structural barriers to joint working

Structural factors can be a major barrier to effective interagency working (Hudson et al. 1999). Examples include:

- Differences in the responsibilities of health and social care agencies to commission and provide services
- Different, and sometimes contradictory, policies and priorities
- Unshared geographical and population boundaries
- Differences in agency funding cycles
- Unshared systems for managing information exchange.

Lack of integration between agencies can create opportunities for perverse incentives (Glasby and Lester 2004). For example, hospitals are a particularly expensive way of providing care, and the cost is borne by the NHS. In contrast, the cost of providing services in the community is typically shared between (health care providing) NHS organizations and (social care providing) local authorities. In this context an NHS Trust's wish to discharge service users into the community has the potential to conflict with a local authority's financial incentive for users to remain in hospital and thus consume no scarce social care resources.

Contradictory policies for different agencies can also hinder the provision of collaborative care. It is widely recognized that effective coordination of services is necessary for people with complex health and social care needs. In the UK, the Care Programme Approach (CPA) was specifically introduced as the framework through which integrated care should be provided to individuals in contact with specialist mental health services. Central to the CPA is the role of the care coordinator (often a nurse, or another mental health professional such as a social worker or occupational therapist) whose work involves ensuring that needs are assessed, services provided, and care reviewed. The CPA was introduced as an NHS-led initiative in England in the early 1990s. Local authority led care management was introduced at the same time, however. This was also a system for care coordination, which included an additional mechanism for the management of funded social care packages. Lack of integration of the two systems (Hancock and Villeneau 1997) had implications for service users, with some having both a CPA care coordinator *and* a care manager. Only at the end of the 1990s was clarification forthcoming of the relationship between the CPA and care management (Department of Health [DH] 1999), with the CPA more recently being subjected to a root-and-branch review with the aim of reducing the administrative burden it sometimes places on practitioners (DH 2006).

Various initiatives have been taken to overcome the structural barriers to collaborative working. For example, England's NHS Plan introduced a new type of health and social care provider organization, the Care Trust (DH 2000). Care Trusts have the responsibility to manage and provide combined health and social services, as an alternative to these being provided by separate bodies. Their aim is to promote more stable and integrated provision, and examples of Care Trusts in England include organizations with specific responsibilities in the mental health field. Evidence of the effectiveness of Care Trusts in improving collaboration across the health and social care interface is underdeveloped (Glasby and Lester 2004). One interesting in-depth evaluation has taken place, however, in which the Centre for Mental Health Services Development (CMHSD) investigated the approach taken in Somerset, England, to the joint commissioning and provision of combined health and social services for people with mental health problems (Gulliver et al. 2000a,b, Peck et al. 2001, 2002).

Interprofessional barriers to joint working

Changing structures, such as bringing together separate health and social care organizations into unified bodies as was pioneered in Somerset, does not necessarily result in changed professional practices (Hudson 2002). CMHSD researchers described how, despite large-scale structural changes having taken place in Somerset, cultural differences between different professions persisted. Workshops generated evidence that some staff were concerned that their new organization lacked a clear identity, and that they were uncertain over management arrangements and professional development opportunities (Peck et al. 2001).

Professional groups differ in significant ways. There are differences in the knowledge claimed by nurses, psychiatrists, social workers, psychologists, and others. This is important, as knowledge often underpins professional claims to control particular types of work (Abbott 1988). In mental health care, the profession of psychiatry has been successful in advancing its biomedically based claims to identify mental illness and to oversee treatment (Hannigan and Allen 2006). Social workers, in contrast, claim legitimacy for their work from a knowledge base derived from the social sciences, whereas psychologists claim a place in the mental health workforce by virtue of their knowledge of both healthy and unhealthy psychological functioning. As an aspirant professional group, the knowledge base of mental health nurses is a relatively broad one, borrowing from both the biomedical and the social sciences. For an occupational group competing for space in a crowded division of labour, it is helpful to be able to claim that its underpinning knowledge is distinct. One way in which mental health nurses have attempted to define and defend their place has been through the development of nursing-specific theories and associated practices. The Tidal Model is an interesting recent example of this phenomenon (Barker 2001), and is one that builds on nursing's long-held claim to fulfil a distinct role based on the centrality of the therapeutic interpersonal relationship. In reality, however, nursing roles (and the roles of members of other occupational groups) are impossible to pin down with absolute certainty. In real-life practice settings, the work undertaken by members of staff is likely to reflect immediate contextual factors (such as team composition and patterns of local need) as much as it reflects the specific occupational backgrounds of practitioners.

It is a longstanding axiom that the best way to provide joined up services is to bring together representatives of different groups in unified teams. This thinking lay behind the establishment of interagency and interprofessional community mental health teams (CMHTs) from the mid-1980s onwards. Initially teams of this type were intended to provide comprehensive services to all people with mental health problems living within defined localities. More recently, New Labour's 'modernization' of mental health services in the UK has seen the appearance of new types of team, delivering targeted services to specific user groups. Examples include teams providing crisis resolution and home treatment services (which have, as one of their aims, the responsibility to reduce hospital admissions), assertive outreach, and early intervention for people with psychosis (DH 2001).

Whatever the intended function of interprofessional teams, from the provision of comprehensive services to the delivery of highly focused interventions, it does not necessarily follow that housing representatives of different groups within a single workplace leads to more effective, collaborative care. Teams have the potential to become sites for interprofessional dispute. The roles and responsibilities of different groups may become blurred, and professions vie for control over areas of work. Without care being taken, a lack of clarity may also exist in the contexts of team leadership, management, and accountability arrangements. Claims have been made that early comprehensive locality CMHTs were vulnerable to problems of this type (Galvin and McCarthy 1994). Studies also reveal that professionals in teams report strong adherence to professional cultures, are distrustful of managerial solutions to the problems of working together, and describe joint teams as often lacking shared philosophies (Norman and Peck 1999, Peck and Norman 1999).

Organizational barriers to joint working

One of the features of modern systems of care is that services are typically provided across multiple sites. This can lead to fragmented service user experiences, with people with the most complex needs often being most at risk. For example, people with severe and long-term mental health problems may: use the services of locality CMHTs; make use of new crisis resolution and home treatment teams during periods of acute illness; receive care in hospital; use NHS, local authority, or non-statutory sector day care services; receive services in primary health care settings from GPs and others; receive services from housing agencies; use independent advocacy services; and so on. The potential for a disjointed experience is particularly acute when people move between different sites, as when (for example) users cross the boundary between hospital and community, or between prison and home.

In the example of services provided across the hospital/community interface, effecting smooth hospital discharge requires effective collaboration between inpatient and community nurses. All involved may share an occupational background and work for the same NHS Trust. Despite these agency and professional commonalities, return to the community often remains a poorly managed interorganizational process (Glasby and Lester 2005). For some, discharge involves lengthy delays, whereas for others pressure on scarce hospital resources means that returning home happens prematurely and without adequate planning.

Step-by-step description: skills to improve service user experience

One way of linking structural, interprofessional, and organizational hindrances to joined up working to the experience of service users is by using the concept of continuity of care. As the examples given so far in this chapter demonstrate, common to barriers to collaborative care of all types is their potential for disrupting the smooth provision of services to individuals over time.

Continuity of care is a term used with increasing frequency, but is also one that tends to be employed in different ways for different purposes. Recognizing this in their scoping study undertaken for England's National Coordinating Centre for NHS Service Delivery and Organisation R&D, Freeman and colleagues (2001) recommended a definition that focused unequivocally on the service user experience. Their recommendation was that continuity of care is best defined as:

> 'The experience of a coordinated and smooth progression of care from the patients' point of view.'

> Freeman et al. (2001, p. 7)

They also added that achieving **experienced continuity** of this type requires:

- '*excellent information transfer* (continuity of information)*;*
- *effective communication between professionals and services, and with service users* (cross-boundary and team continuity)*;*
- *care which is flexible and able to accommodate to the changing needs of individuals* (flexible continuity)*;*
- *care from as few professionals as possible, consistent with needs being met* (longitudinal continuity)*; and*
- *the provision of one or more named workers with whom the individual service user can establish and maintain a therapeutic relationship* (relational or personal continuity).'

> Freeman et al. (2001, p. 7)

Nurses, as the largest of the professional groups providing dedicated mental health services, are well placed to take action to improve these different elements of care continuity. To support the 'Skills' section that follows, particular use has been made of a further review completed by Freeman and colleagues, this time focusing specifically on continuity of care for people with severe mental health problems (Freeman et al. 2002).

Skills to improve continuity of information

The large number of agencies, occupations, and organizations with parts to play in the provision of mental health care to individuals makes information exchange vitally important. New technologies have the potential to improve continuity in this area. The introduction of computerized systems of recording and exchanging service user information has clear implications for nurses' technological skills. However, even the most powerful information technology systems have limitations. Systems are typically not compatible between NHS and local authority agencies, or between mental health and primary care teams. More traditional communication skills such as exchanging information in face-to-face forums or through the use of written or telephone media therefore remain important. Face-to-face information exchange has a particularly important part to play at key junctures, such as when service users are making the transition from one part of a system (e.g. inpatient care) to another (e.g. care in the community). Here, the skills of the nurse as care coordinator additionally come to the fore (see below).

Skills to improve cross-boundary and team continuity

The point has been made in this chapter that the people with the most complex needs are often the people most likely to receive services from multiple professionals and organizations. Parts are typically played by NHS and local authority workers, but some service users are also likely to have their needs met by staff working in housing, employment, criminal justice, and other agencies. Nurses often fulfil the role of care coordinator under locally implemented CPA arrangements, and therefore have responsibilities to enhance continuity within and between teams, professions, and agencies. Skills for cross-boundary working include the demonstration of a proactive approach to coordinating care across mental health–primary care, community–hospital, health–social care, and other complex interfaces.

GPs and others in primary care often complain of poor communication with mental health services, although various approaches to improving the organization of care across this boundary exist (Gask et al. 1997). Simple strategies, such as convening care plan reviews at times and places accessible to busy primary care practitioners, may help to improve collaboration.

Community mental health nurses are likely to find that investing in relationship-building with primary care and other colleagues improves communication and continuity across teams. Particular attention again needs to be paid during periods of transition, such as when service users are admitted to or discharged from hospital. In this context it is significant that independent inquiry teams have often implicated poor coordination across boundaries as a factor contributing to tragedies involving people with mental health problems (see, for example, Ritchie et al. 1994).

Skills to improve flexible continuity

The needs of people with mental health problems vary over time. This places a premium on the capacity of nurses to modify the care they provide, and to maintain up-to-date local knowledge of the range of services available to people at different phases of their recovery. Judgement is important here. For example, during episodes of crisis, intensive face-to-face care may best be provided by nurses and others working in dedicated crisis resolution and home treatment (CRHT) teams or in hospital. However, although referring a service user to a crisis team may enable his or her needs to be more effectively met, the cost of doing so may be to increase the risk of cross-boundary discontinuity. Flexible continuity means making use of available local services, but also involves practitioners developing the personal capability to underpin variations in the type and intensity of the face-to-face interventions they provide to reflect changing needs. A practical example could be developing skills in evidence-based psychosocial interventions to support people with severe mental health problems and their carers. Achieving flexible care in this way means working across traditional role boundaries, provided that new areas of work that are assumed remain within the sphere of an individual's competence.

Skills to improve longitudinal continuity

Achieving longitudinal continuity of care can be a challenge in conditions of high staff turnover and scarce resources, and in contexts where services are increasingly provided by specialist teams. Longitudinal continuity is promoted by the policy of allocating single care coordinators to individual service users. Consistent care coordination, underpinned by positive interpersonal relationships between users and professionals, can promote continuity when the care of service users crosses multiple organizational and professional boundaries. CMHT care coordinators can do much to improve longitudinal continuity by actively maintaining face-to-face relations during periods of hospital admission, or when care is shared with workers based in new specialist community teams.

Skills to improve relational or personal continuity

Care coordination, which emerges as key across many of the components contributing to continuity, involves much more than the technical organization of an individual's plan of care. Effective care coordination additionally makes demands on nurses' skills in building and maintaining relationships. Strong relational continuity is likely to be of particular benefit when service users receive care from multiple teams or workers, or during phases of transition. The idea of personal continuity can also be usefully extended to relationships between members of health and social care teams. Good personal relations between nurses and other members of the mental health team, or between nurses and primary care colleagues, are likely to benefit care continuity.

✖ Practice Example

Here you are invited to consider the nursing actions that might be taken to improve continuity of care to a (fictitious) individual with severe mental health problems whose service use spans multiple agency, occupational, and organizational boundaries.

John is in his mid-forties and is a user of the local CMHT. He receives care from a community mental health nurse (CMHN), Patricia. Part of John's recovery is to make use of day services provided by a local voluntary sector organization, with the cost of this being borne by the local authority. This part of John's care plan was arranged by a colleague of Patricia's, a CMHT-based social worker. John also receives care and treatment from a CMHT-based psychiatrist and from his GP, who prescribes John's atypical antipsychotic medication and helps monitor John's diet-controlled diabetes.

»

» During periods of crisis John describes the experience of hearing voices, becomes very frightened, and misperceives the actions of those around him as threatening. Over the years he has had multiple admissions to hospital as his health has deteriorated in this way.

Good practice in improving continuity of care in everyday community mental health services is shown in Box 20.1.

Box 20.1 Continuity of care in everyday community mental health services

Promoting continuity of information

- Maintain accurate and up-to-date records using paper and/or electronic systems as per local practice, and consistent with professional standards surrounding storage and sharing of patient information.
- Care coordinator to ensure that John's care plan, once negotiated, is distributed to John and all members of his care team.

Promoting cross-boundary and team continuity

- Care coordinator to be appointed in consultation with John and with members of his care team.
- Identity and contact details of care coordinator to be clearly made known to John, his family, and other workers (including psychiatrist, social worker, GP, day services staff).
- Consistent with local policies, care coordinator to negotiate strategies for joining up ongoing care across health–social care and mental health–primary care interfaces (e.g. by maintaining regular contact with GP, by accompanying John to primary care appointments when diabetes care is reviewed, by convening care plan reviews in consultation with all care team members).

Promoting flexible continuity

- Care coordinator to take responsibility to negotiate contingency plans with John and his care team aimed at meeting needs during periods of developing and actual crisis.

Promoting longitudinal continuity

- Once identified, care coordinator to maintain regular contact with John.

Promoting relational or personal continuity

- Care coordinator to draw on personal therapeutic skills to form and maintain helpful interpersonal relationship with John and his informal carers.

For further discussion see Freeman et al. (2002).

Good practice in improving continuity of care during episodes of crisis is shown in Box 20.2.

Box 20.2 Continuity of care during episodes of crisis

Promoting continuity of information

- Consistent with professional standards and local policies surrounding storage and sharing of patient information, members of John's care team to share knowledge indicating possible evolving crisis in order to inform revision of care plan.
- In cases where new teams or workers become involved (e.g. CRHT team), care coordinator to ensure that information on John and his needs be shared across organizational boundaries (e.g. share records, participate in joint assessment).

Promoting cross-boundary and team continuity

- Care coordinator to take lead responsibility in negotiating reassessments of John's needs and in gathering relevant information.

Promoting flexible continuity

- Care coordinator to take responsibility to oversee implementation of contingency plan, and to draw on local knowledge to make use of dedicated crisis services as necessary.

Promoting longitudinal continuity

- Care coordinator to maintain ongoing contact with John and his informal carers throughout whole episode of crisis.

Promoting relational or personal continuity

- Care coordinator to maintain personal therapeutic relationship with John during episode of crisis, irrespective of other teams or workers involved or location(s) in which care is provided.

For further discussion see Freeman et al. (2002).

Health promotion

There are clear connections between the organization of care and the experience of health and well-being. Care that is fragmented is unlikely to result in needs being met. By extension, actions to improve continuity are likely to enhance health gain. Effectively joining up the contributions made by different practitioners and agencies, through strong care coordination underpinned by good interpersonal relationships between workers and users, is an important component in promoting positive health. As the discussion earlier suggests, this is particularly important during periods of transition.

Conclusion

Mental health care is a shared responsibility. NHS, local authority, and non-statutory sector organizations have important parts to play. Nurses, although the most numerous of the groups providing specialist mental health services, always work alongside representatives of other health and social care professional groups. In modern services, care is frequently fragmented across multiple teams and settings. Examples include teams based in hospitals, and teams (of various varieties) based in the community.

These factors combine to challenge the joined up delivery of mental health services, as do problems of scarce resources. Nurses, who often fulfil the vital role of care coordinator, have major contributions to make in promoting continuity of care. By drawing on personal therapeutic skills and by ensuring that care is managed effectively across the interfaces, particularly at times of transition, nurses can do much to improve the service user experience and thus promote health gain.

w Website

You may find it helpful to work through our short online quiz and scenario intended to help you to develop and apply the skills in this chapter. Please go to:

  www.oxfordtextbooks.co.uk/orc/callaghan

➤ Further reading

Freeman, G., Weaver, T., Low, J., de Jonge, E., and Crawford, M. (2002). *Promoting Continuity of Care for People with Severe Mental Illness whose Needs Span Primary, Secondary and Social Care: A Multi-method Investigation of Relevant Mechanisms and Contexts*. London: National Coordinating Centre for NHS Service Delivery and Organisation R&D.

This publication deals comprehensively with the concept of continuity of care.

Onyett, S. (2003). *Teamworking in Mental Health.* Basingstoke: Palgrave.
A valuable text dealing exclusively with the interprofessional environment in which mental health services are delivered.

✦ References

Abbott, A. (1988). *The System of Professions: An Essay on the Division of Expert Labor.* Chicago: University of Chicago Press.

Barker, P. (2001). The Tidal Model: developing an empowering, person-centred approach to recovery within psychiatric and mental health nursing. *Journal of Psychiatric and Mental Health Nursing* 3(3), 233–40.

Department of Health (1998). *Partnership in Action: New Opportunities for Joint Working Between Health and Social Services. A Discussion Document.* London: DH.

Department of Health (1999). *Effective Care Co-ordination in Mental Health Services: Modernising the Care Programme Approach*. London: DH.

Department of Health (2000). *The NHS Plan: A Plan for Investment, A Plan for Reform*. London: DH.

Department of Health (2001). *The Mental Health Policy Implementation Guide*. London: DH.

Department of Health (2006). *Reviewing the Care Programme Approach*. London: DH.

Freeman, G., Shepperd, S., Robinson, I., et al. (2001). *Continuity of Care: Report of a Scoping Exercise for the National Coordinating Centre for NHS Service Delivery and Organisation R&D*. London: National Coordinating Centre for NHS Service Delivery and Organisation R&D.

Freeman, G., Weaver, T., Low, J., de Jonge, E., and Crawford, M. (2002). *Promoting Continuity of Care for People with Severe Mental Illness Whose Needs Span Primary, Secondary and Social Care: A Multi-Method Investigation of Relevant Mechanisms and Contexts*. London: National Coordinating Centre for NHS Service Delivery and Organisation R&D.

Galvin, S.W. and McCarthy, S. (1994). Multi-disciplinary community teams: clinging to the wreckage. *Journal of Mental Health* 3(2), 157–66.

Gask, L., Sibbald, B., and Creed, B. (1997). Evaluating models of working at the interface between mental health services and primary care. *British Journal of Psychiatry* 170, 6–11.

Glasby, J. and Lester, H. (2004). Cases for change in mental health: partnership working in mental health services. *Journal of Interprofessional Care* 18(1), 7–16.

Glasby, J. and Lester, H. (2005). On the inside: a narrative review of mental health inpatient services. *British Journal of Social Work* 35, 863–79.

Gulliver, P., Peck, E., and Towell, D. (2000a). Evaluation of the implementation of the mental health review in Somerset: methodology. *Managing Community Care* 8(3), 13–19.

Gulliver, P., Peck, E., Ramsay, R., and Towell, D. (2000b). Evaluation of the implementation of the mental health review in Somerset: results from the baseline data collection. *Managing Community Care* 8(4), 16–23.

Hancock, M. and Villeneau, L. (1997). *Effective Partnerships: Developing Key Indicators for Joint Working in Mental Health*. London: Sainsbury Centre for Mental Health.

Hannigan, B. and Allen, D. (2006). Complexity and change in the United Kingdom's system of mental health care. *Social Theory and Health* 4(3), 244–63.

Hudson, B. (2002). Interprofessionality in health and social care: the Achilles' heel of partnership? *Journal of Interprofessional Care* 16(1), 7–17.

Hudson, B., Hardy, B., Henwood, M., and Wistow, G. (1999). In pursuit of inter-agency collaboration in the public sector: what is the contribution of theory and research? *Public Management* 1(2), 235–60.

Norman, I. J. and Peck, E. (1999). Working together in adult community mental health services: an interprofessional dialogue. *Journal of Mental Health* 8(3), 217–30.

Nursing and Midwifery Council (2004). *Standards of Proficiency for Pre-registration Nursing Education*. London: NMC.

Nursing and Midwifery Council (2007). *Essential Skills Clusters (ESCs) for Pre-registration Nursing Programmes*. London: NMC.

Nursing and Midwifery Council (2008). *The NMC Code of Standards of Conduct, Performance and Ethics for Nurses and Midwives*. London: NMC.

Peck, E. and Norman, I. J. (1999). Working together in adult community mental health services: exploring interprofessional role relations. *Journal of Mental Health* 8(3), 231–42.

Peck, E., Gulliver, P., and Towell, D. (2002). Governance of partnership between health and social services: the experience in Somerset. *Health and Social Care in the Community* 10(5), 331–8.

Peck, E., Towell, D., and Gulliver, P. (2001). The meanings of 'culture' in health and social care: a case study of the combined trust in Somerset. *Journal of Interprofessional Care* 15(4), 319–27.

Preston, C., Cheater, F., Baker, R., and Hearnshaw, H. (1999). Left in limbo: patients' views on care across the primary/secondary interface. *Quality in Health Care* 8, 16–21.

Ritchie, J. H., Dick, D., and Lingham, R. (1994). *The Report of the Inquiry into the Care and Treatment of Christopher Clunis*. London: HMSO.

(21) Personal and professional development

Sara Owen   Clare Fox

▼ Introduction

This chapter focuses on **personal and professional development**. In essence this means keeping up to date with changes in practice and participating in **lifelong learning**, and personal and professional development for oneself and colleagues through supervision, appraisal, and reflective practice (Department of Health [DH] 2004a). Mental health nursing students at the point of registration are required to demonstrate a commitment to **continuing professional development** and personal supervision activities, in order to enhance the knowledge, skills, values, and attitudes needed for safe and effective nursing practice (DH 2006a). After registration, it is a professional expectation that mental health nurses continue to develop their skills, knowledge, and attitudes throughout their entire careers to meet the needs of service users effectively. This expectation is clearly articulated in the Nursing and Midwifery Council Code: (NMC 2008, p. 4)

> 'you must keep your knowledge and skills up-to-date throughout your working life and you must take part in appropriate learning and practice activities that maintain and develop your competence and performance.'

So why is lifelong learning and continuing professional development so important? First, the rapidly changing nature of health and social care requires mental health nurses not only to adapt to change but also to identify the need for change and to initiate change. Second, the 'shelf-life' of knowledge and skills acquired at the point of registration becomes less and less each year, with the consequent need to continue learning throughout your professional life. These two reasons underpin the gradual trend of pre-registration nurse education becoming less about the acquisition of a defined body of knowledge and skills and more about developing capabilities in problem solving, accessing information, and continuing to learn (DH 2001).

In this chapter we will explain the concepts of lifelong learning and continuing professional development, present an ongoing cycle of learning, and demonstrate how to get the most out of **clinical supervision**, **reflective practice**, and appraisal. Throughout the chapter we continually emphasize the importance of mental health nurses taking an active role in their own personal and professional development. In the same way that service users should be viewed as active partners in their care, not passive recipients, nurses should be active participants in their own development (DH 2004a).

Learning outcomes

By the end of this chapter you should be better able to:

1 Appreciate the value of lifelong learning and continuing professional development

2 Understand the key principles underpinning clinical supervision, reflective practice, and appraisal

3 Take responsibility for your own personal and professional development, seeking and accessing development opportunities to meet your needs.

Lifelong learning and continuing professional development

Lifelong learning is the concept that '*it is never too soon or too late for learning*' (Wikipedia 2008), a philosophy that has taken root in a whole host of different organizations. Lifelong learning is attitudinal, leading to a belief that one can and should be open to new ideas, decisions, skills, and behaviours. Lifelong learning sees citizens provided with learning opportunities at all ages and in numerous contexts: at work, at home, and through leisure activities, not just through formal channels such as school and higher education. One of the reasons why lifelong learning has become so important is the acceleration of scientific and technological progress. Despite the increased duration of primary, secondary, and university education, the knowledge and skills acquired there are usually not sufficient for a professional career spanning three or four decades.

Lifelong/professional learning in the National Health Service (NHS) has been increasingly influenced by general government policy on lifelong learning. Much of this is set out in the White Paper *Learning to Succeed* (Department of Education and Employment 1999). As a major employer, the NHS and related sectors have a significant part to play in supporting and realizing this agenda. Learning and development is the key to delivering the government's vision of patient-centred care in the NHS (DH 2001). Lifelong learning is about growth and opportunity, about making sure that staff, teams, and organizations can acquire new knowledge and skills, both to realize their potential and to help shape and change things for the better. Lifelong learning is inextricably linked with the wider agenda for building, rewarding, and supporting the NHS workforce for the future so that they can:

- support changes and improvements in patient care
- take advantage of wider career opportunities
- realize their potential.

Continuing professional development is part of the process of lifelong learning for all health care professionals. It has been defined as a systematic and planned approach to the maintenance, enhancement, and development of knowledge, skills, and expertise that continues throughout a professional's career and is to the mutual benefit of the individual, the employer, and the professional body (DH 2006b). It is seen as an essential feature of maintaining competent professional practice, primarily to support quality services and protection of the public (DH 2000). There is, however, considerable variation in the interpretation and use of the term continuing professional development, ranging from formal professional qualifications to informal individualized activities (Lawton and Wimpenny 2003). To clarify this confusion, the key principles of continuing professional development are summarized in Box 21.1.

Ongoing cycle of learning

Recent changes have provided a useful new framework for professional development, the *Knowledge and Skills Framework* (**KSF**) (DH 2004b). The KSF is a competency

Box 21.1 Principles of continuing professional development

- Delivered in partnership with stakeholders, with objectives aligned to the individual's working environment and to the job they actually do.
- An integral part of the NHS Quality Framework and employers' strategies and plans must be closely linked to clinical governance plans.
- Patient-centred.
- Meets local needs as well as the personal and professional development needs of the individual.
- Increasingly focused on the development needs of clinical teams, across traditional professional boundaries and service boundaries.
- Increasingly work based. The acid test must be 'competence in doing'.
- Involves service users and carers wherever practicable in designing and evaluating the outcomes and in the delivery of learning programmes.
- Makes use of the full range of development approaches and methods, rather than relying solely or largely on formal courses.
- Is modular and attracts academic credits where possible.
- Draws on clinical audit and clinical effectiveness findings to facilitate the development of a research-aware workforce.
- Makes optimal use of new technology and distance learning.

Adapted from DH (2001, pp 40–1)

framework and a human resources tool; it defines and describes the knowledge and skills that NHS staff need to apply in their work in order to deliver quality services. It was developed as part of the NHS Agenda for Change Initiative (DH 2004c). It applies specifically to career progression and remuneration for NHS staff, and maps against pay bands in order to establish pay levels and salary increments. One of the purposes of the KSF is to support the effective learning and development of individuals and teams, with all members of staff being supported to learn throughout their careers and develop in a variety of ways, and being given the resources to do so. Although the KSF is not mental health specific, it has been highlighted as a useful framework for the continuing professional development of mental health nurses (DH 2006b).

The KSF is designed to form the basis of a development review process. This is a cycle of review, planning, development, and evaluation for all staff in the NHS that links organizational and individual development needs. The development review is a partnership process undertaken between an individual member of staff and a 'reviewer', and the annual review process is based on an ongoing cycle of learning. It has four stages:

1   A joint review between the individual and their reviewer, their line manager (or another person in that capacity), of the individual's work against the demands of their post.

2   The production of a Personal Development Plan, which identifies the individual's learning and development needs in the coming months. This is jointly agreed between the individual and their reviewer.

3   Learning and development activities by the individual supported by their reviewer.

4   An evaluation of the learning and development that has taken place and how it has been applied by the individual in their work.

Once completed, the cycle then begins again. The important thing to remember is that the current approach to continuing professional development recognizes that much learning actually takes place within the workplace and while you are doing your day-to-day job. The emphasis is on learning and development as a whole, rather than on everyone attending a set number of study days or courses.

The development review process is based on good appraisal practice. It has been designed so that organizations can combine the development review with their appraisal process in order that the two work seamlessly together to support individual development. The KSF will benefit individuals by:

- enabling them to be clear about the knowledge and skills they need to apply in their posts.

- enabling them to access appropriate learning and development.

- showing how their work relates to the work of others in their immediate team and beyond.

- identifying the knowledge and skills they need to learn and develop throughout their careers.

- providing a structure and process for the NHS to invest in an individual's learning and development throughout their working life.

Preparing for your appraisal or development review

The main purpose of the appraisal or development review is to look at the way that you are developing in relation to the duties and responsibilities of your job, and how you apply your knowledge and skills in the workplace, and to identify future development needs. It is meant to be a positive and beneficial experience for both you and your manager. This review process will form the basis of your Personal Development Plan for the coming year, so it is important that you come to the meeting prepared to discuss your progress with sufficient evidence to support what you say. The information contained in Box 21.2 suggests how you can prepare for your appraisal, the types of evidence that you can use to demonstrate how you have progressed, and how to conduct yourself during the actual appraisal meeting. It may also be helpful to read accounts written by others about the process of being appraised, such as Metcalf (2001) and Wedderburn-Tate (2005).

Box 21.2   The appraisal or development review process

Preparation

- Set aside protected time to prepare and gather evidence together for the meeting.

- Agree the time, location, and venue of the meeting with your appraiser.

- Stop and think back over the previous year: how do you think you have performed? What problems have you encountered, and how have you dealt with them? Where, if at all, have you fallen short of what was expected of you, and what were the reasons?

- Be honest with yourself—an honest self-appraisal of your strengths and weaknesses will put you in a good position to benefit from the meeting.

- Plan ahead: what do you want to achieve in the next year? What new knowledge and skills do you need to acquire? Will you need specific training?

- Think back on the goals you set yourself last year—which were achieved and which were not and why?

- Have you grasped opportunities and achieved things you did not plan?

Box 21.2 *Continued*

Types of evidence

- Verbal feedback from you or your mentor.
- Written work.
- Electronic work.
- Records of work such as minutes of meetings showing your contribution.
- Your professional portfolio containing items such as reflections on learning or practice, notes from clinical supervision session.
- Examples of conferences or study days that you have attended with evidence showing what you have learned and how that learning has benefited your practice.

Approach during the meeting

- Make sure you say what you want to say.
- Listen to and take note of your appraiser's comments.
- Raise and discuss issues.
- Be realistic about your progress and future plans.
- Demonstrate a positive attitude and take responsibility for your successes and possible shortfalls.
- Back up everything you say with reasons and fact.
- At all times keep your cool.
- Use the appraisal process to your advantage, say what you want to achieve and suggest possible development opportunities that you would like.

The appraisal or development review will then form the basis of your Personal Development Plan for the coming year. This plan will identify your individual learning and development needs and interests, together with an agreed plan for how these are to be taken forward. Here are some examples of learning and development opportunities that you may want to consider:

- Project work within your workplace
- Shadowing a colleague in a different work area or specialty
- Being mentored
- Reading books and journals
- Structured reflection on your own practice
- Clinical supervision

- Writing articles
- Using electronic resources to identify the evidence base for practice
- Joining a learning set
- Chairing meetings
- Doing some work-based or classroom teaching
- Attending conferences
- Attending study days or courses
- Developing your therapeutic skills.

Clinical supervision and reflective practice are two approaches to learning and development that are commonly used by mental health nurses. We will now look at these in more depth.

Clinical supervision

Clinical supervision has a long history within the caring professions. It was first developed in the UK in the social work profession in the 1920s, and subsequently adopted within nursing (primarily in mental health nursing) and then within midwifery. It was later included as an essential component of the 1993 strategy for nursing, *A Vision for the Future* (DH 1993). The UK Central Council for Nursing, Midwifery and Health Visiting (UKCC) position statement on clinical supervision (UKCC 1996) provided the impetus for implementation and its importance was further emphasized in *Making a Difference: Strengthening the Nursing, Midwifery and Health Visiting Contribution to Health and Healthcare* (DH 1999). Most recently , *From Values to Action* (DH 2006b) strongly suggests that all mental health nurses should engage in regular clinical supervision from a suitably trained supervisor.

There are a number of definitions of clinical supervision within the literature; two examples are highlighted in Box 21.3. There are also numerous different models of supervision that Butterworth and Faugier (1992) suggest can be divided into three types: those that focus on the supervisory relationship; those that describe the functions of the role; and developmental models that focus on the process of the supervisory relationship. Interestingly the NMC, whilst supporting the principle of clinical supervision, does not advocate a particular model of supervision. Instead it believes that the clinical supervision model selected is best left to local services in accordance with local needs. It is therefore likely that you will come across a range of different models during your career. Further information about models of clinical supervision can be found in Butterworth and Faugier (1992), Sloan and Watson (2002), and Farrington (1995).

Box 21.3 Definitions of clinical supervision

Clinical supervision is:

'A formal process of professional support and learning which enables practitioners to develop knowledge and competence, assume responsibility for their own practice and enhance consumer protection and safety of care in complex situations. It is central to the process of learning and to the scope of the expansion of practice and should be seen as a means of encouraging self-assessment and analytic and reflective skills'

Department of Health (1993, p. 36)

'A process which aims to bring practitioners and skilled supervisors together to reflect on practice, to identify solutions to problems, to increase understanding of professional issues, and, most importantly, to improve standards of care'

Department of Health (2006b, p. 64)

Box 21.4 Factors that will enhance your experience of clinical supervision

• Choose your supervisor if possible. Your decision should be based on your own developmental needs, and then matched with the skills and experience of potential supervisors.

• Establish ground rules: meeting times, places, content of the sessions, issues of confidentiality, and commitment.

• Prepare for each session in advance. Have an agenda and bring examples of pertinent practice issues with you.

• Take responsibility for making effective use of the time.

• Be willing to learn, to develop practice skills, and be open to receiving support and challenge.

• Arrange to meet with your supervisor at least every four weeks for one hour.

• Arrange the day, time, and venue in advance.

• The sessions should be conducted in work time in a venue that is private and where you will not be disturbed.

• Keep written records of the sessions. These should focus on your experiences and development, and should not contain specific patient information.

Despite the current absence of a strong evidence base for the effectiveness of clinical supervision, particularly in terms of improved patient care, there is a general view amongst mental health nurses that clinical supervision supports you in your practice (Mullarkey et al. 2001). For example, it is a useful means of helping staff to avoid burnout and job-related stress, for improving clinical performance, and for support and professional development (Clegg 2001, Mullarkey et al. 2001). There has, however, been some interesting work that has identified the important factors that impact upon the success of clinical supervision (Butterworth et al. 1997, Edwards et al. 2005). These factors have been translated into a list of activities that you could consider to enhance your own experience of clinical supervision (Box 21.4).

Reflective practice

Reflective practice is an approach in which you look at events in your practice and analyse them. It involves thinking about your work in a structured way, sometimes with the help of a reflective journal, log, or diary. Reflective practice requires a conscious effort on your part. It is not something you do automatically and it is not a grand name for the normal process of thinking about your work. Rather, it is a particular way of thinking about situations, analysing them, and learning from them. You can then try out what you have learned by building it into your practice (Manthey 2001).

Reflective practice has three components: your experiences, the reflective processes that enable you to learn from those experiences, and the action that results from the new perspectives taken. These components need to be viewed as a process through which you actively learn rather than a series of separate events. For example, when we want to learn from something that has happened to us, we need to recall our observations of the event and then reflect on those observations in some way. We do this through reflective processes that ask us to describe the experience and analyse it so that, at the end, we form some ideas or theories about it. This will then inform any action that we take as a result of the experience. Reflective learning is not simply about thinking about something that has already happened as a retrospective activity. It can also be seen as a predictive activity, a strategy for planning our learning for the future on the basis of what we already know and on what we can anticipate (Jasper 2003).

Reflection can be divided into two types: reflection-in-action and reflection-on-action. These were identified by Donald Schon (1983) as the principal ways that professionals use to conceptualize and articulate their knowledge. These two types are complex, but their essences have been summarized very clearly by Jasper (2003). For example, reflection-in-action is the way that people think and theorize about practice while they are doing it. This is often seen as an automatic activity that occurs subconsciously in practice at an everyday level. It is perceived by some people to be an intuitive process and, therefore, not reflective activity that we use deliberately. Reflection-on-action involves us in consciously exploring experience and thinking about practice after it has occurred to discover the knowledge used in the situation. It occurs through analysis, interpretation, and the recombination of information about the experience so that new perspectives are found about what has happened. This usually happens retrospectively and away from the scene of practice. Reflection-on-action can therefore be seen as an active process of transforming experience into knowledge, and involves much more than simply thinking about and describing practice.

Numerous models and frameworks have been developed for nurses to use to help them reflect on their practice. Perhaps the best known and most commonly used are Gibbs's (1988) reflective cycle and Johns's (2004) model of guided reflection. You will come across others; most are sufficiently flexible to enable you to develop them to suit your own needs. Most of the frameworks and models reflect the following fundamental stages of the reflective process:

1 Selecting a critical incident or experience to reflect on.

2 Observing and describing the experience.

3 Analysing the experience.

4 Interpreting the experience.

5 Exploring alternatives.

6 Framing action.

These frameworks also provide key questions to guide you through the process of reflecting on your practice. Whilst the format and focus of these questions vary, a typical set of questions can be seen in Box 21.5. Many nurses find keeping a journal a useful way of recording their reflections, and it is a very effective way of monitoring learning and providing evidence of your growing competence to your mentor or appraiser.

There are times when you feel that you do not have time for reflection. However, you should consider that any time you

Box 21.5 Questions to guide reflection on practice

- What happened and what were you trying to do in the situation?

- Why did you do that and how did you feel about it?

- How do you feel about it now?

- What were the service user's feelings at that time?

- How do you know that?

- Can you think of a better way of dealing with the situation?

- Having thought about the situation, what did you learn from it?

- What are your feelings about the situation now?

Manthey (2001)

spend on reflection can pay for itself many times over in the long run. The personal and professional development that can take place as a result of reflection includes:

- Reducing the theory-practice gap (Burton 2000, Carney 2000, Getliffe 1996).

- Encouraging the ability to think critically (Cotton 2001, Durgahee 1998, Foster and Greenwood 1998).

- Enhancing personal development by leading to self-awareness (Cotton 2001).

- Helping make more sense of difficult and complex practice (Driscoll and Teh 2001).

- Developing clinical knowledge and skills (Graham 2000).

- Slowing down activity, thereby providing time to process material of learning and link it to previous ideas (Moon 2002).

- Enabling greater ownership of the learning taking place (Moon 2002).

- Reminding qualified practitioners that there is no endpoint to learning about their everyday practice (Driscoll and Teh 2001).

▲ Conclusion

Mental health services have experienced a period of profound change. There is no doubt that such change will continue as services strive towards models of care that both meet the needs of service users and keep the trust and support of the public.

Mental health nursing is changing almost as rapidly as the context in which it is practised, and has developed radically in terms of its roles and responsibilities and how it is organized. The recent report *Modernising Nursing Careers* (DH 2006c) argues that the careers of all nurses must respond to the profound changes taking place in the structure of health care delivery and the need for nurses to exercise leadership to bring about change. Currently, nursing careers take different forms; some will choose to climb an upward ladder of increasing responsibility and higher financial reward, whereas other nurses choose a more lateral career journey within and between care groups and settings. Increasingly, nursing will move towards a model that supports movement between career pathways, practice, management, research, and education, and that values and rewards different career types (DH 2006c).

In order both to keep up to date with and to influence such changes, mental health nurses must take responsibility for their own continuing personal and professional development. In this chapter we have highlighted various frameworks that you will be able to use to support your practice and to plan your future educational and training needs. Reflective practice, for example, is an excellent way of highlighting the strengths and weaknesses of your practice and encouraging you to think about what you need to do to improve. This process, in turn, can provide a focus for clinical supervision where you can begin to think about your professional development and further educational opportunities. These opportunities can take many forms, ranging from work-based learning through to more formal courses. Finally, this work can feed into your annual appraisal and development review process where your continuing learning and development needs can be formally identified in your Personal Development Plan. This continuous cycle of reflection, identification of development needs, learning, and application to practice is the essence of lifelong learning—a philosophy that needs to underpin the career pathways of all mental health nurses.

w Website

You may find it helpful to work through our two short scenarios intended to help you to develop and apply the skills in this chapter. Please go to:

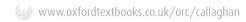 www.oxfordtextbooks.co.uk/orc/callaghan

➤ Further reading

Bond, M. and Holland, S. (2001). *Skills of Clinical Supervision for Nurses: A Practical Guide for Supervisees, Clinical Supervisors and Managers.* Buckingham: Open University Press.
This book provides practical guidance for supervisees, emphasizing self-empowerment and developing the reflective skills necessary to make the full use of clinical supervision.

Cutcliffe, J., Butterworth, T., and Proctor, B. (2001). *Fundamental Themes in Clinical Supervision.* London: Routledge.
This looks at how clinical supervision has developed and explores a range of issues such as education and training in clinical supervision, and current research activity.

Johns, C. (2004). *Becoming a Reflective Practitioner.* London: Blackwell.
This is a practical guide to using reflection in everyday clinical practice.

Rolfe, G., Freshwater, D., and Jasper, M. (2001). *Critical Reflection for Nursing and the Helping Professions: A User's Guide.* London: Palgrave Macmillan.
A good introduction to the literature on reflective practice.

✦ References

Burton, A. J. (2000). Reflection: nursing's practice and education panacea? *Journal of Advanced Education* 31(5), 1009–17.

Butterworth, T. and Faugier, J. (1992). *Clinical Supervision and Mentorship in Nursing.* London: Chapman and Hall.

Butterworth, T., Carson, J., White, E., Jeacock, J., Clements, A., and Bishop, V. (1997). *It is Good to Talk: An Evaluation Study in England and Wales.* Manchester: School of Nursing, Midwifery and Health Visiting, University of Manchester.

Carney, M. (2000). The development of a model to manage change: reflection on a critical incident in a focus group setting. An innovative approach. *Journal of Nursing Management* 8, 265–72.

Clegg, A. (2001). Occupational stress in nursing: a review of the literature. *Journal of Nursing Management* 9, 101–6.

Cotton, A. H. (2001). Private thoughts in public spheres: issues in reflection and reflective practices in nursing. *Journal of Advanced Nursing* 36(4), 512–19.

Department of Education and Employment (1999). *Learning to Succeed.* Cm. 4392. London: The Stationery Office.

Department of Health (1993). *A Vision for the Future: Report of the Chief Nursing Officer.* London: DH.

Department of Health (1999). *Making a Difference: Strengthening the Nursing, Midwifery and Health Visiting Contribution to Health and Healthcare.* London: DH.

Department of Health (2000). *Continuing Professional Development: Quality in the New NHS.* London: DH.

Department of Health (2001). *Working Together, Learning Together: A Framework for Lifelong Learning in the NHS.* London: DH.

Department of Health (2004a). *The Ten Essential Shared Capabilities: A Framework for the Whole of the Mental Health Workforce.* London: DH.

Department of Health (2004b). *The NHS Knowledge and Skills Framework and the Development Review Process.* London: DH.

Department of Health (2004c). *Agenda for Change— Final Agreement.* London: DH.

Department of Health (2006a). *Best Practice Competencies and Capabilities for Pre-registration Mental Health Nurses in England: The Chief Nursing Officer's Review of Mental Health Nursing.* London: DH.

Department of Health (2006b). *From Values to Action: The Chief Nursing Officer's Review of Mental Health Nursing.* London: DH.

Department of Health (2006c). *Modernising Nursing Careers: Setting the Direction.* London: DH.

Driscoll, J. and Teh, B. (2001). The potential of reflective practice to develop individual orthopaedic nurse practitioners and their practice. *Journal of Orthopaedic Nursing* 5, 95–103.

Durgahee, T. (1998). Facilitating reflection: from the sage on the stage to a guide on the side. *Nurse Education Today* 18, 158–64.

Edwards, D., Cooper, L., Burnard, P., et al. (2005). Factors influencing the effectiveness of clinical supervision. *Journal of Psychiatric and Mental Health Nursing* 12, 405–14.

Farrington, A. (1995). Models of clinical supervision. *British Journal of Nursing* 4(15), 876–8.

Foster, J. and Greenwood, J. (1998). Reflection: a challenging innovation for nurses. *Contemporary Nurse* 7, 165–72.

Getliffe, K. A. (1996). An examination of the use of reflection in the assessment of practice for undergraduate nursing students. *International Journal of Nursing Studies* 33(4), 361–74.

Gibbs, G. (1988). *Learning by Doing: A Guide to Teaching and Learning Methods.* Oxford: Further Education Unit, Oxford Polytechnic.

Graham, I. W. (2000). Reflective practice and its role in mental health nurses' practice development: a year-long study. *Journal of Psychiatric and Mental Health Nursing* 7, 109–17.

Jasper, M. (2003). *Beginning Reflective Practice.* Cheltenham: Nelson Thornes.

Johns, C. (2004). *Becoming a Reflective Practitioner,* 2nd edn. Oxford: Blackwell Science.

Lawton, S. and Wimpenny, P. (2003). Continuing professional development: a review. *Nursing Standard* 17(24), 41–4.

Manthey, M. (2001). Reflective practice. *Creative Nursing* 7(2), 3–5.

Metcalf, C. (2001). The importance of performance appraisal and staff development: a graduating nurse's perspective. *International Journal of Nursing Practice* 7(1), 54–6.

Moon, J. (2002). *PDP Working Paper 4: Reflection in Higher Education Learning.* York: Learning and Teaching Support Network Generic Centre.

Mullarkey, K., Keeley, P., and Playle, J. F. (2001). Multiprofessional clinical supervision: challenges for mental health nurses. *Journal of Psychiatric and Mental Health Nursing* 8, 205–11.

Nursing and Midwifery Council (2008). *The Code: Standards of Conduct, Performance and Ethics for Nurses and Midwives.* London: NMC.

Schon, D. (1983). *The Reflective Practitioner: How Professionals Think in Action.* London: Temple Smith.

Sloan, G. and Watson, H. (2002). Clinical supervision models for nursing: structure, research and limitations. *Nursing Standard* 17(4), 41–6.

UK Central Council for Nursing, Midwifery and Health Visiting (1996). *Position Paper on Clinical Supervision for Nursing and Health Visiting.* London: UKCC.

Wedderburn-Tate, C. (2005). Appraisal time. *Nursing Standard* 19(15), 69.

Wikipedia (2008). *Lifelong learning.* en.wikipedia.org/wiki/Lifelong_education [accessed 9 Apr 2008].

22 Leadership and management

Neil Brimblecombe

▼ Introduction

From the day that a mental health nurse qualifies, they will require skills in both leadership and management. This chapter discusses the range of managerial and leadership activities that mental health nurses may engage with and some of the specific skills that are required to make those roles effective. The aim of the chapter is to enable readers to be able to identify the difference and similarity between leadership and management skills, to identify activities that will require those skills to be applied, and to consider which skills they themselves possess or may need to develop in the future.

Learning outcomes

By the end of this chapter you should be better able to:

1 Discuss the difference between leadership and management

2 Describe how leadership and management roles are central to mental health nursing practice

3 Define the key skills/competencies required to lead successfully.

What are leadership and management?

These two terms are often used interchangeably and, indeed, very often they go together. 'Management' typically refers to an administrative function linked with formal authority coming from a particular job role. Leadership can encompass this, but can also refer more broadly to setting a direction of travel or providing a 'vision'. To see leadership simply as a reflection of the way that managerial functions

are carried out (e.g. Martin and Henderson 2001) provides a narrow view that does not take into account that leadership does not always need to be linked to a management role in health care settings. All registered mental health nurses will need both management and leadership skills, although how frequently and the manner in which they are applied will vary markedly according to the nature of the role that the nurse is employed in.

When do mental health nurses lead?

All nurses need to utilize leadership skills. These may or may not be formally recognized in their job descriptions. Figure 22.1 provides examples of roles requiring leadership skills that may be informal (i.e. not necessarily linked with a management position) and those more formal roles where it is recognized within an organization that leadership activities are inherent in that role.

A mental health nurse may provide leadership for a team occasionally on particular issues (see Practice Example 1), whereas a team leader is expected to provide leadership most of the time (as well as managing the team).

Values and leadership

'Management is doing things right; leadership is doing the right things.'

Peter F. Drucker

Effective leadership (and indeed management) is a good thing only if the changes that are being created are in line with the values of mental health nursing. Therefore, all mental

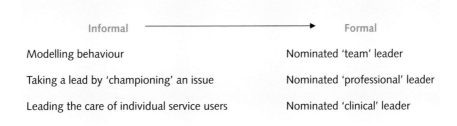

Figure 22.1 Formal and informal leadership.

✖ Practice Example 1

'Informal' leadership roles

Afraz is still a third-year student nurse, but has shown leadership skills during his placement on a low secure unit. He has instigated a project on introducing the recovery approach to the unit. He did this by initially raising the possible benefits to service users of adopting this approach in a discussion at a team meeting. Since then, with the support of his manager, he has been gathering information and working closely with an advocate in looking at how the current service could develop to become more recovery focused. Particular skills that Afraz has used have been role modelling—demonstrating enthusiasm for the project, and using empathy—to understand why some staff were anxious about change. He responded effectively to their concerns by finding another low secure unit where the recovery approach was already successfully embedded in practice and, with the help of his ward manager, arranged for staff to visit there.

health nurses need continually to be challenging themselves as to 'why' change is happening, with the central question being 'within the limits of resources, is this change really in the best interests of service users and carers?' Whilst this may seem a banal and unnecessary reminder, the reality is that in the midst of complex organizational demands the needs of service users and carers sometimes seem less immediately important than organizational imperatives. Some questions that may help are:

- Is there any evidence available to suggest that these changes/actions will be beneficial to service users or carers?

- Have we engaged with service users and carers to ascertain their views?

- Does this development make sense in terms of the philosophy of mental health nursing/the organization/the NHS? For example, is it congruent with the principles of the recovery approach (Department of Health [DH] 2006a).

The importance of leadership skills

The importance of the leadership role for all nurses is recognized in statutory regulations and national good practice guidance. The *Best Practice Competencies and Capabilities for Pre-registration Mental Health Nurses in England* (DH 2006b, p. 21) points out the need for all mental health nurses to have a working knowledge of '*how effective leadership contributes to effective care delivery*'. The Nursing and Midwifery Council's *Standards of Proficiency for Pre-registration Nursing Education* refer to the nurse being able to '*Enhance the professional development and safe practice of others through peer support, leadership, supervision and teaching*'. Specifically, the standards state that nurses should be able to '*Demonstrate effective leadership in the establishment and maintenance of safe nursing practice*' (NMC 2004, p. 5). It is noteworthy that what is referred to here is *leadership* rather than *management*.

Practice Example 2 illustrates the leadership role of a newly qualified nurse in an acute admission ward setting.

✖ Practice Example 2

Leadership in clinical roles

Jane is a recently qualified mental health nurse working on an acute admission ward. She is a key worker for John, who has had numerous admissions with psychotic symptoms and is typically verbally abusive and aggressive towards staff. He is under the care of the assertive outreach team, and has a long history of drug abuse.

Jane's **leadership** role includes leading the delivery of the multidisciplinary care plan day to day and **leading** the raising of issues that need to be discussed and addressed by the MDT. She also **leads** by modelling a positive attitude to John on the ward when others sometimes have negative attitudes towards him owing to his abusiveness. She **leads** and **manages** by providing supervision and support to the care assistants on the ward, helping translate the care plan into actions for them.

Jane also has to **manage** her own occasionally negative feelings towards John through using clinical supervision and **manages** the organizational aspects of his care, such as setting up meetings, and ensuring that he has medication arranged when he goes on leave and receives appropriate input when she is not on duty.

Skills for successful leadership

Transactional vs. transformational skills

Transactional leadership refers to leadership through management, where authority is used to give instructions directly to staff. Typically, this approach is linked with formal management relationships. However, it is striking that, in mental health care, certain roles are still at times assumed to have authority to provide instruction, even in the absence of a formal management relationship. For example, assumptions of authority are still sometimes found in relationships between senior medical staff and other professions (Brimblecombe 2005).

Transformational leadership is an approach that seeks to support change, not by direct authority, but by supporting staff to take forward and own change themselves. This requires engaging with them so that they willingly transform themselves and the ways in which they work. Undoubtedly, inspiring others is a key aspect of this approach. George Eliot (1876, p. 387) wrote: '*The strongest principle of growth lies in human choice*'. Successful transformational leadership lets staff see themselves and their roles differently. Generally, this approach to leadership is advocated as the best model. Certainly having the enthusiastic engagement of staff is better than forcing them into action, simply because outcomes are more likely to be lasting. However, historically there is a health service tradition of trying to manage change through instruction rather than engagement; indeed, Tate contends that, to date, nurses have typically been '*more managed than led*' (Tate 1999, p. 60). Although transformational approaches are generally the best approach to leadership, there will still be times when a more transactional approach is needed, as is illustrated in Practice Example 3.

✖ Practice Example 3

Transactional vs. transformational leadership

A new manager started work in an adolescent unit. She immediately had major concerns regarding inadequate risk assessment processes and a lack of clear boundaries for the service users. She felt that immediate change was essential and shared her concerns with the staff group, seeking their engagement in moving to safer practice. However, when they did not seem to take on the urgency of the situation, she decided to issue clear instructions about safer assessment processes and what was not acceptable behaviour by service users, together with a clear explanation of why this action was being taken.   »

» Once the new processes had been put in place, she set up a series of staff meetings to look formally at the impact of change. She also tried to work with the staff on their feelings about enforced change and to set up forums in which future developments could be discussed.

The team leader started by trying to take a transformational approach to leadership, but owing to her belief regarding the urgency of the situation, she then used managerial authority and demonstrated a transactional approach. However, once the immediate risks were being managed, she returned to trying to engage with the staff in a transformational manner.

Developing leadership skills—what is needed

Whilst some would suggest that leaders are born not made, any admired leader has a number of skills and attributes that can be developed to varying degrees through training and practice. Some of these will include:

- Communication skills (see Chapters 6–8)—an ability to convey ideas and concepts clearly, whether in informal conversation or in public speaking.

- Resilience—inevitably leaders in the health service will experience adverse events, funding will be withdrawn, some staff will be apathetic, day-to-day demands may get in the way of plans, reorganizations may change who makes decisions. To overcome this and still provide effective leadership requires an ability to 'bounce back' from adversity. This does not imply a lack of feeling, but anyone planning to lead should know that this will not always be easy.

- Empathy—an ability to understand others' viewpoints is important, as only by doing so will the leader be able to recognize and respond to others' objections to change or their difficulties in implementation. In the health service it is often easier for someone to lead who is from a similar clinical background to staff, as at least they know they have had some of the same experiences. If they do not share a similar background, they will need to show that they understand those experiences.

- Clarity of vision—a leader needs to be able to articulate exactly what their vision is and what the benefits will be. Benjamin Disraeli said: '*I must follow the people. Am I not their leader?*'. The most effective leadership visions are those that are experienced as their own by those who follow.

- Trustworthiness—no one will want to have a leader who will abandon those whom they lead. Leadership is a reciprocal relationship. Consistently, a willingness both to support colleagues and to share their difficulties helps to convey that the leader is someone who can be trusted.

In addition to these skills, successful leaders will normally need to have a sophisticated understanding of the political and organizational context in which they are working and adjust their style to respond to this (Burdett Trust for Nursing 2006). Those who have a single approach to leadership may be successful in some circumstances, but may cease to be so when the context in which they are working changes; for example, see the 'ruthless leader' on the next page.

The exercises in Box 22.1 will help to develop the skills described above. They can be applied in all student placements or after qualifying in your work environment.

Box 22.1 Activities to develop leadership skills

Communication

Carry out a presentation to the multidisciplinary team. Ensure that helpful feedback is gathered. Do not accept sweeping comments such as 'It was fine'. Find out which bits really were fine and which could have been more effective.

Resilience

Identify at least one point during your placement where you felt deflated and in some way inadequate. Reflect on this in supervision, with particular recognition that such events happen in practice and how they can be made positive learning experiences. If the events that led to these feelings were out of your control, identify strategies that led you to recognize the challenge to self-esteem, but then helped you to move on.

Empathy

Identify at least one situation where you had a very different view from a colleague. Spend time in supervision thinking about how they might have come to hold such a view. The aim is not to think about whether they

Box 22.1 *Continued*

were right or wrong, but rather to understand why they held that view.

Clarity

Identify an instance in your placement where someone gave a striking example of clarity of vision, for example during a clinical or management discussion. It does not matter whether you agreed with their vision; you should look at how they managed to convey such a clear view.

Trustworthiness

Identify a colleague you encountered during your placement who you felt you could absolutely trust. Consider what it was about them that helped you feel this about them. Was it their interest in others? Was it a concrete example of trustworthiness? Or was it simply the way they were with others? Think about what you would need to do to convey trustworthiness to others.

The 'ruthless leader'

It is undoubtedly true that some leaders are effective in producing change whilst ignoring many of the principles above, with the exception of clarity of vision. Some seem able to ignore the feelings of staff and ruthlessly push through change regardless—a truly transactional approach. Such leadership may occasionally be useful where change is urgently needed. In the words of a Russian proverb: '*The same hammer that shatters the glass forges the steel*'. However, it is unlikely that this style of leadership will support a healthy organization in the long term. Ruthless leaders tend not to stay around long in organizations, soon moving on to the next 'problem to be sorted'.

From Values to Action and leadership

From Values to Action: The Chief Nursing Officer's Review of Mental Health Nursing (DH 2006a) recognized the importance of strong management and leadership in mental health nursing. In particular, it identified the importance of ward managers having leadership skills, as well as management skills, in order to lead and develop the complex and responsive multidisciplinary care required by service users in inpatient care settings. Modern inpatient environments are very complex organizationally and clinically, with challenges arising from working with many different community-based teams, a range of different professions, and widely varying need in terms of the people admitted to their services. Leadership is essential in such settings, in terms of setting agendas for the team to take forward, in providing a positive role model of clinical interaction, and through the subtleties of leading a team where not all will be line managed by the ward manager. Additionally the role encompasses many management functions, organizing staffing (including recruitment and performance management when staff are not performing well), ensuring the physical environment is safe and appropriate, and managing the complex interactions between ward and community-based services—a truly demanding role needing the highest level of leadership and management skills!

From Values to Action also highlighted the importance of professional leadership more generally within mental health nursing, and that it was vitally important for individual nurses to be able to seek support from a nominated professional lead in relation to professional issues, such as those arising from ethical and interdisciplinary issues. Nurses can feel professionally isolated working in the increasing range of services that are not managed by health care personnel. It is important that leadership on professional issues is available to all mental health nurses. This does not mean that there will be someone who will tell them what to do, but rather will lead thinking about, and advise on, professional issues, such as ethical conundrums and interprofessional challenges.

When do mental health nurses manage?

Most of this chapter has related to leadership, particularly stressing the idea that leadership does not always have to be through management roles. However, this is not to deny the importance of management skills in mental health nursing. Nurses will certainly also need management skills in every role. This will vary in scope from managing teams, physical and financial resources to managing one's own time and emotions, and the care of individual service users. Figure 22.2 illustrates the range of management roles for mental health nurses.

Skills for management

As with leadership skills, managerial skills can be developed. Johnstone (2006) argues that many clinicians actually lack fundamental management skills with consequent ill effect on any services that they may manage. Although a detailed discussion of managerial skills is beyond the remit of this chapter, a

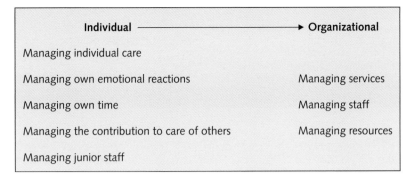

Figure 22.2 Individual and organizational management.

few of the managerial activities carried out are listed below, together with examples of when these might be carried out by a typical ward manager:

- Finance—ensuring good use of staff to minimize use of expensive agency staff.
- Planning—being involved with planning groups regarding the future structure of services (e.g. links with crisis/home treatment services).
- Communication—passing on information about Trust-wide and national developments to staff and considering the implications for the ward with them.
- Analysis—looking at patterns of need amongst service users and using this information to plan future training for staff.
- Performance management—providing annual appraisals to staff and dealing with issues of poor performance.
- Setting standards—establishing standards with the ward team (e.g. about responding to visitors and phone calls).

- Recruitment—ensuring suitable staff are employed in sufficient numbers and with appropriate skills and attitudes.

Practice Example 4 illustrates the range of managerial activities that a nurse who does not formally manage anyone might be involved with.

Pulling together good management and good leadership

Shirey (2006) provides a useful list of five practices that she sees as being essential to both good management and leadership:

1 Balancing the tension between production and efficiency

2 Creating and sustaining trust throughout the organization

✖ Practice Example 4

Management in clinical roles
Sheila is a community mental health nurse working in an older people's team. Although she does not line manage anyone, she nevertheless has a range of management functions that are core to her role. These include:

- Managing the placement of students, negotiating about how to spend time, and providing advice, guidance, and instruction.

- Managing her own time, prioritizing between the diverse needs of the 25 service users for whom she is the community key worker, and balancing this against demands of allowing sufficient time for new assessments, professional and team meetings, continuous professional development, and the need to complete high-quality records.

- Managing the budgets for individual service users in negotiation with the service user and multidisciplinary team.

3 Actively managing the process of change

4 Involving workers in decision making pertaining to work design and work flow

5 Using knowledge management to establish the organization as a learning organization.

These practices pull together management skills with leadership skills; only by the two being used together will the leader manager be truly successful.

 ## Conclusion

This chapter has emphasized that all mental health nurses are, and need to be, both managers and leaders. Different roles and different career pathways will require nurses to utilize these skills to a greater or lesser extent at different times. Skills for both roles can be defined and developed. Good management and leadership are vital in supporting the provision of excellent care to service users.

 ## Website

You may find it helpful to work through our short online quiz and scenario intended to help you to develop and apply the skills in this chapter. Please go to:

www.oxfordtextbooks.co.uk/orc/callaghan

References

Brimblecombe, N. (2005). **The changing relationship between mental health nurses and psychiatrists in the United Kingdom.** *Journal of Advanced Nursing* 49(4), 344–53.

Burdett Trust for Nursing (2006). *Who Cares, Wins. Leadership and the Business of Caring.* London: BTFN.

Department of Health (2006a). *From Values to Action: The Chief Nursing Officer's Review of Mental Health Nursing.* London: DH.

Department of Health (2006b). *Best Practice Competencies and Capabilities for Pre-registration Mental Health Nurses in England: The Chief Nursing Officer's Review of Mental Health Nursing.* London: DH.

Eliot, G. (1876). *Daniel Deronda.* Book VI, Chapter XLII. http://www.bookrags.com/ebooks/7469/387.html [accessed 30 July 2008].

Johnstone, A. (2006). Managing effective teams. In: *Oxford Handbook of Mental Health Nursing* (ed. P. Callaghan and H. Waldock), p. 306. Oxford: Oxford University Press.

Martin, V. and Henderson, E. (2001). *Managing in Health and Social Care.* London: Routledge.

Nursing and Midwifery Council (2004). *Standards of Proficiency for Pre-registration Nursing Education.* London: NMC.

Shirey, M. R. (2006). Authentic leaders creating healthy work environments for nursing practice. *American Journal of Critical Care* 15(3), 256–67.

Tate, C. W. (1999). *Leadership in Nursing.* London: Churchill Livingstone.

Index

The index entries appear in word-by-word alphabetical order.